Scar
Scleredema
Scleroderma

ATROPHY

Aplasia cutis congenita
Corticosteroid (topical)
Lichen sclerosus et atrophicus
Lupus erythematosus
Morphea
Necrobiosis lipoidica diabeticorum
Postinflammatory
Scar
Striae
Trauma

NODULE/CYST

Calcinosis cutis
Congenital vascular malformation
Epidermoid cyst
Granuloma annulare
Infection
Lipoma
Pilar cyst
Panniculitis
Sarcoidosis
Tumor
Vasculitis

HAIR LOSS

Alopecia areata/totalis/univer
Atopic dermatitis
Cutis aplasia
Dermatophyte
Drugs
Hair shaft abnormalities
Infection
Lichen planopilaris
Linear morphea
Lupus erythematosus
Nevus sebaceous
Telogen effluvium
Trauma
Trichotillomania

HAIR GROWTH

Anorexia nervosa
Dermatomyositis
Drug
Familial
Hypertrichosis lanuginosa

NAIL ABNORMALITIES

Candidiasis
Dermatophyte
Epidermolysis bullosa
Ingrown nail
Lichen planus

Median nail dystrophy

MOUTH LESIONS

Aphthous stomatitis
Autoimmune blister diseases
Candidiasis
Congenital vascular malformation
Drug
Epidermolysis bullosa
Erythema multiforme
Geographic tongue
Hand-foot-and-mouth disease
Herpangina
Herpes simplex
Lichen planus
Lupus erythematosus
Neurofibroma
Thyroglossal duct cyst
Toxic epidermal necrolysis
Trauma
Wart

SKIN MANIFESTATIONS OF AIDS

MACULES

Drug
Exanthem
Pellagra

PAPULES

Acquired ichthyosis
Aspergillosis
Bacillary angiomatosis
Basal cell carcinoma
Cryptococcosis
Dermatophyte
Drug
Eczema
Eosinophilic folliculitis
Granuloma annulare
Insect bite
Kaposi's sarcoma
Lichen planus
Melanoma
Molluscum contagiosum
Nummular eczema
Papular mucinosis
Pityriasis rubra pilaris
Polymorphous light eruption
Psoriasis

Reiter's disease
Scabies
Seborrheic dermatitis
Syphilis
Warts
Xerosis

PUSTULES

Atypical mycobacteria
Bacterial infection
Candidiasis
Dermatophyte
Herpes simplex/zoster
Histoplasmosis
Folliculitis
Impetigo
Scabies

BLISTERS

Herpes simplex/zoster
Porphyria cutanea tarda

ULCERS

Atypical mycobacteria
Herpes simplex/zoster

Kaposi's sarcoma
Leishmaniasis
Sporotrichosis

HAIR

Straight hair
Telogen effluvium

NAILS

Candida paronychia
Onychomycosis
Pityriasis rubra pilaris
Psoriasis
Reiter's disease
Yellow nails

MOUTH

Aphthous stomatitis
Candidiasis
Enanthem (HIV-associated)
Herpes simplex/zoster
Histoplasmosis
Kaposi's sarcoma
Oral hairy leukoplakia
Xerostomia

Adult and Pediatric Dermatology:

A Color Guide to Diagnosis and Treatment

Lowell A. Goldsmith, M.D.
James H. Sterner Professor of Dermatology
Dean, School of Medicine and Dentistry
University of Rochester
Rochester, New York

Gerald S. Lazarus, M.D., F.A.C.P.
Professor of Dermatology
Dean, School of Medicine
University of California, Davis
Davis, California

Michael D. Tharp, M.D.
The Clark W. Finnerud, MD, Professor and Chairman
Department of Dermatology
Rush-Presbyterian-St. Luke's Medical Center
Chicago, Illinois

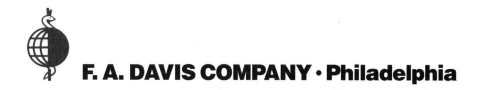
F. A. DAVIS COMPANY · Philadelphia

F. A. Davis Company
1915 Arch Street
Philadelphia, PA 19103

Printed in the United States of America

Last digit indicates print number: 10 9 8 7 6 5 4 3 2

Medical Editor: Robert W. Reinhardt
Medical Developmental Editor: Bernice M. Wissler
Production Editor: Roberta Massey
Cover Designer: Steven Ross Morrone

As new scientific information becomes available through basic and clinical research, recommended treatments and drug therapies undergo changes. The authors and publisher have done everything possible to make this book accurate, up to date, and in accord with accepted standards at the time of publication. The authors, editors, and publisher are not responsible for errors or omissions or for consequences from application of the book, and make no warranty, expressed or implied, in regard to the contents of the book. Any practice described in this book should be applied by the reader in accordance with professional standards of care used in regard to the unique circumstances that may apply in each situation. The reader is advised always to check product information (package inserts) for changes and new information regarding dose and contraindications before administering any drug. Caution is especially urged when using new or infrequently ordered drugs.

Library of Congress Cataloging-in-Publication Data

Goldsmith, Lowell A., 1938–
   Adult and pediatric dermatology : a color guide to diagnosis and
treatment / Lowell A. Goldsmith, Gerald S. Lazarus, Michael D. Tharp.
      p.   cm.
   Includes bibliographical references and index.
   ISBN 0-8036-0146-8 (alk. paper)
   1. Dermatology—Atlases. 2. Pediatric dermatology—Atlases.
I. Lazarus, Gerald S., 1939–   . II. Tharp, Michael D. 1949–   .
III. Title.
   [DNLM: 1. Skin Diseases—diagnosis. 2. Skin Diseases—pathology.
3. Skin Diseases—therapy.   WR 141 G624a 1997]
RL81.G55   1997
616.5—dc20
DNLM/DLC
for Library of Congress   96-26032
                                                                            CIP

For Carol Goldsmith, who quietly endured this book, a second time, while on sabbatical in England. For Marion, Joe, and Audrey Lazarus, who made the second edition possible, and the late Sandra Lazarus, who made the first edition a reality, and for Robin, Kristin, Kelly, and Kathryn Tharp, for their support and encouragement.

Preface

Fifteen years have passed since we published a book entitled *Diagnosis of Skin Disease*. Those years have been marked with the flourishing of molecular dermatology and the introduction of several new classes of effective therapeutic agents. Related to the cataclysmic changes in the financing of health care, many primary care practitioners, both M.D.s and nurses, have sought to learn the fundamentals of dermatologic diagnosis and therapy. It is remarkable, and in some ways not surprising, that the classification system for skin diseases of the past 200 years continues into the opening days of this new third millennium despite profound scientific and social changes. We believe this completely revised version of our earlier book will be useful for students learning dermatologic diagnosis for the first time, for those practicing primary care, and for residents during their study of dermatology. For the accomplished dermatologist, we have included sufficient doses of the arcane so that there is a glittering gem to find among what may be familiar discussions.

This book is a natural outgrowth of our previous book. Its name reflects the addition of new material, including a therapy section for each disease, and recognizes that this book contains useful material of interest in caring for both adults and infants.

The two authors of the earlier text are now joined by Michael D. Tharp, M.D., who was a trainee who worked on our initial volume. While training dermatology residents, students, and other personnel, all three authors have observed that establishing the presumptive diagnosis is necessary before using the comprehensive texts in dermatology and the computer-based information services. The arrangement of our book allows the reader to get to first base—although other sources may be necessary to get to home plate, no one scores without touching first base.

We approach with humility the task of trying to characterize a disease in a few sentences and one or two photographs. As a model, we use nature field guides, realizing that distinguishing species is not the same as designating diseases within one organ system of one species. Our age faces the challenge of information organization and presentation, and we have crafted this new book to help the reader penetrate the rubric of dermatology.

LOWELL A. GOLDSMITH, M.D.
GERALD S. LAZARUS, M.D., F.A.C.P.
MICHAEL D. THARP, M.D.

Acknowledgments

A number of our friends and colleagues have provided us with illustrative material. To them we offer thanks: Mr. Ron Mitchell of the Audiovisual Department of the Durham Veterans Administration Hospital; Dr. Peyton Weary and Dr. Louis E. Harman, Jr., Department of Dermatology, University of Virginia Medical School; Dr. E. V. Zegarelli, Dean Emeritus, School of Dental and Oral Surgery, Columbia University; Dr. Leonard Harber and Dr. Marc Grossman, Department of Dermatology, Columbia University of Physicians and Surgeons; Dr. Rudolf Baer, Department of Dermatology, New York University School of Medicine; Dr. Robert Howell, School of Dentistry, University of North Carolina, Dr. Rodney P. R. Dawber, Slade Hospital, Oxford; Dr. Terence J. Ryan, United Oxford Hospitals; Professor Malcolm Greaves, St. Johns Hospital for Diseases of the Skin, London; Dr. Peter Samman (deceased), Westminster, London; Drs. Byron Croker and Bernard Fetter, Department of Pathology, Duke University Medical School; Dr. Charles Grupper, Rothschild Hospital, Paris; Drs. Thomas Fitzpatrick and Howard Baden, Department of Dermatology, Harvard Medical School; Dr. Michael Fisher, Division of Dermatology, Albert Einstein College of Medicine; Dr. Ervin Epstein, Jr., Department of Dermatology, University of California, San Francisco; Drs. John Haserick, Pinehurst, NC, Gloria Graham, Wilson, NC, Harrison Turner, Greenborough, NC; Dr. Stanley Foster, Communicable Disease Center, Atlanta, Georgia; Dr. Aaron Lerner, Department of Dermatology, Yale University School of Medicine; Dr. Howard Rosenman, Dr. Frances Pascher (deceased), and Dr. Clayton E. Wheeler, Jr., Department of Dermatology, University of North Carolina.

Appreciation is also extended to Mr. Bob Blake (retired) of the Audiovisual Department, Duke University Medical Center, for designing the artwork; Ms. Judith Thorpe, for producing the original distribution diagrams; Dr. Doug Kress (University of Pittsburgh), for his creativity in developing the treatment tables; Drs. Janet Hickman and Alexander Chiaramonti, for taking special photographs for this book. We are extremely grateful to our former colleagues at Duke, including the late Dr. J. L. Callaway, who played a pivotal role in the development of *Diagnosis of Skin Disease*. His extensive collection of kodachromes is the basis of our clinical photographs. Through the years, he provided encouragement and advice. The authors of this book owe a great debt to Dr. Callaway for his helpfulness, creativity, and humanity. Drs. Robert Gilgor, Brian Jegasothy, and Sheldon Pinnell provided us with constant stimulation and willingly shared their clinical expertise.

Contents

How To Use This Book

This book aids correct dermatologic diagnosis by utilizing clinical observation. It can be used by the neophyte health care provider or the accomplished dermatologist. It also presents the basics of dermatologic therapy.

Diagnosis

- Read the chapter on the examination of the skin and become familiar with the dermatologic terms described in the Guide to Clinical Diagnosis.
- Examine the patient.
- Decide on the category of lesions and presentation using the Guide to Clinical Diagnosis—e.g., blisters or diffuse red papules.
- Turn to the appropriate chapter and select the best category for your patient. Each category is marked at the top of the page.
- Review the listed diseases in a category or subcategory. The typical distribution is diagrammed and a characteristic clinical photograph is presented. If the choices appear inappropriate, go to the front of the chapter, where additional diseases that may present with similar morphologies are listed.
- Accomplished dermatology diagnosticians will find the diagnostic index at the back of the book an excellent refresher for complete differential diagnosis.

Therapy

- Read the chapter on therapy before attempting to treat patients.
- Note the entry on therapy for the specific disease. If you are uncertain about the diagnosis of a disease, go to a comprehensive textbook of dermatology or obtain consultation from a knowledgeable dermatologist.

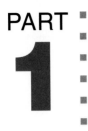

PART

Introduction

Chapter 1

Guide to Clinical Diagnosis

ABSCESSES are circumscribed collections of pus that involve the deeper layers of the skin.

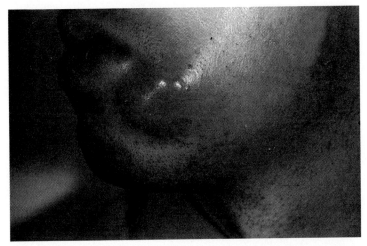

ATROPHY is loss of substance in the skin. Superficial atrophy is characterized by loss of skin markings, fine wrinkling, variation in pigmentation, and transparency of the skin so that vessels are easily seen. Dermal and subcutaneous atrophy produces a depression that is covered by normal-appearing skin.

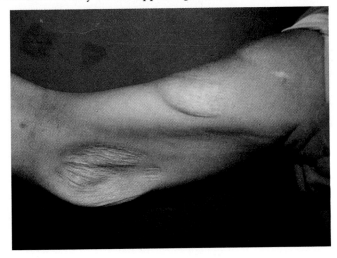

BLISTERS are sharply marginated, elevated lesions that contain clear fluid. Small blisters (<1 cm) are called **VESICLES**. Blisters >1 cm are known as **BULLAE**.

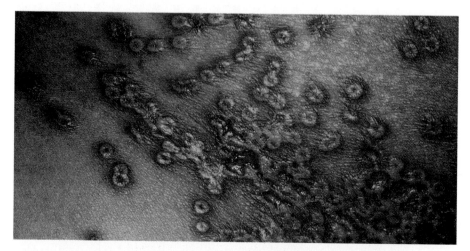

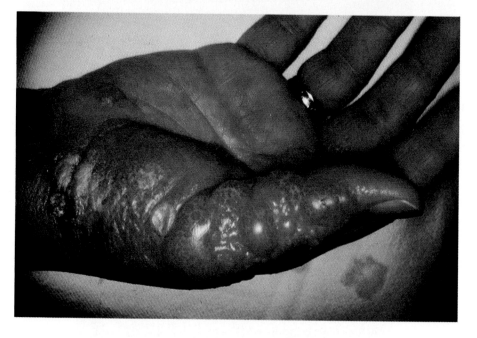

CRUSTS are yellow-brown to black circumscribed collections of serum and inflammatory cells on the surface of the skin. They may be due to inflammation or infection.

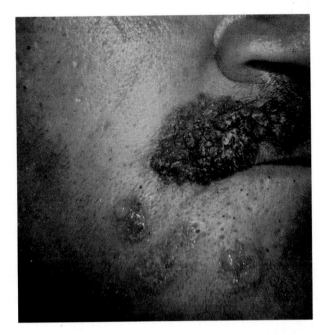

CYSTS are very sharply circumscribed, often movable, compressible, space-occupying lesions in the skin. As with nodules, the skin can often be moved over the lesion.

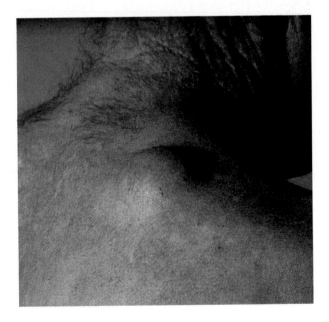

EROSIONS are moist, red, shiny, circumscribed lesions that lack the upper layer of the skin. These lesions are almost always secondary to the rupture of a blister. Linear erosions caused by scratching are known as **EXCORIATIONS**.

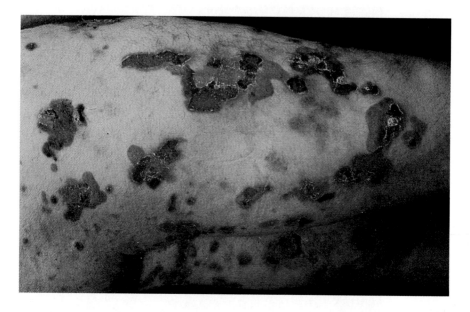

LICHENIFICATION is thickening of the skin accompanied by accentuation of the skin markings. It is usually secondary to chronic rubbing of the skin, most often related to itching.

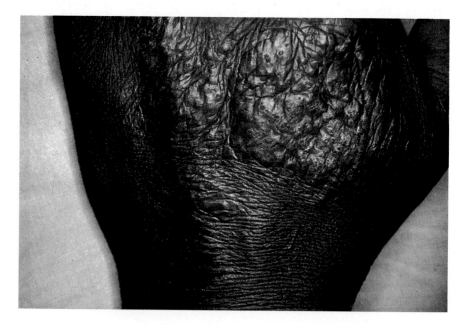

MACULES are flat lesions that are observed because of a change in color. They are usually circumscribed, but diffuse disorders of pigmentation are discussed in Chapter 3.

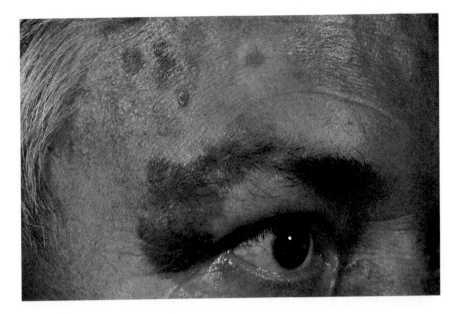

NODULES are elevated lesions that are located deep in the cutis. The most important characteristic of these lesions is that the skin can be moved over the lesion.

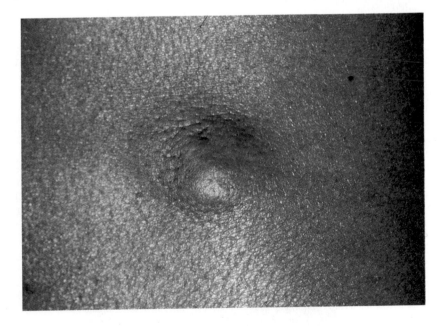

PAPULES are lesions that are raised above the skin. **PLAQUES** are papules >1 cm in diameter. The surface of these lesions may be smooth or irregular and scaly.

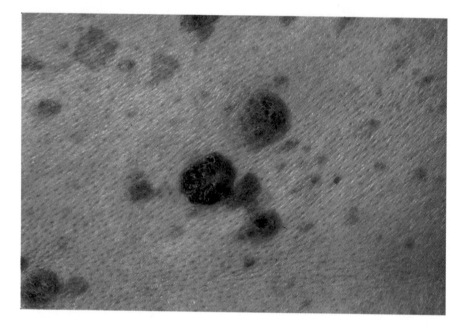

PUSTULES are focal accumulations of inflammatory cells and serum in the skin. Nicking a pustule releases yellow-white purulent material.

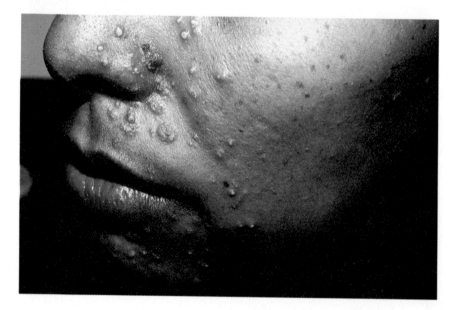

SCALES are white to tan flakes on the skin. They are different from crusts.

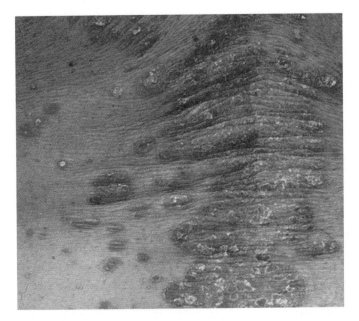

SCLEROTIC LESIONS are flat to slightly elevated and are discovered because palpation of the skin reveals hardness and thickening. This is sometimes referred to as **INDURATION**.

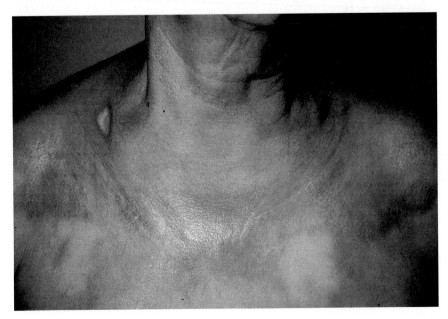

SINUSES are connections between the surface of the skin and an underlying structure.

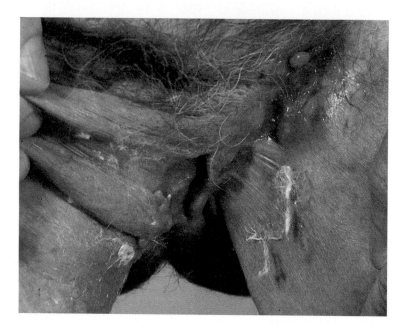

ULCERS are depressed lesions in which the epidermis and at least part of the dermis have been lost. These lesions frequently heal with scarring.

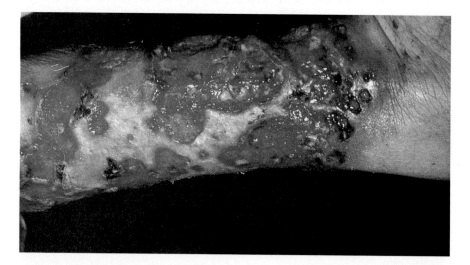

Chapter 2

■ ■ ■ ■ ■ ■ ■ ■ ■ ■ ■ ■ ■ ■ ■ ■ ■ ■

Examination of the Skin

EXAMINING THE SKIN

The Patient
The patient must undress completely for an adequate skin examination. Looking at an isolated lesion without examining the patient completely may lead to misdiagnosis or nondiagnosis of potentially serious lesions. Explaining the reason for complete disrobing even when the chief complaint is a single papule increases patient compliance. When performing a skin examination, the entire integument should be examined. Gloves are worn for examination of the genitals, intraoral palpation, and palpation of potentially infectious lesions that are moist, hemorrhagic, or crusted. Wearing gloves for the complete examination may stigmatize the patient and is not necessary unless there is a concern about infection.

Lighting
Good lighting, either artificial or natural, is essential for a good skin examination. Fixed or standing lighting frees both hands for examination or manipulation of lesions.

Oblique illumination (side lighting) of a slightly elevated papule confirms its raised character by the shadow it casts. This should be done in a dimly lit or dark room.

Intense light (e.g., the head of an ophthalmologic penlight) is used to transilluminate cystic lesions and reveal the homogeneity of the structure. Focused, intense light should not be used for the complete examination because it can wash out important details.

Wood's Light
The Wood's lamp ("black light") produces long-wave ultraviolet rays (360-nm peak

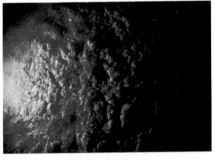
Side lighting

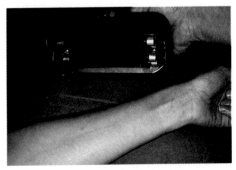
Wood's lamp

UVA range) with relatively low energy. No special precautions are required for its routine use. Melanin absorbs strongly at 360 nm, so that minor losses of melanin are accentuated. Hypopigmented areas are paler than normal skin, and depigmented areas are stark or milk white under Wood's light. The Wood's lamp is especially useful in the diagnosis of vitiligo or the hypopigmentation of tinea versicolor in their early stages. Certain conditions have characteristic fluorescent patterns (Table 2–1). The lamp is also useful for checking urine specimens for uroporphyrins (pink fluorescence), characteristic of porphyria cutanea tarda. Multiple exogenous substances, including lint, dyes, and lipstick, can fluoresce on the skin.

Magnifying Glasses

Magnifying lenses (5× to 10×) should be strong enough to allow the physician to observe lesions easily. Lenses are especially useful for detecting altered skin markings and contours in tumors, and especially melanoma. Lenses are also used to observe nail fold telangiectasia in connective tissue diseases or to detect the subtle surface changes (Wickham's striae) in lichen planus. When mineral oil or immersion oil is placed on the skin, the stratum corneum becomes more transparent, revealing deeper structures in more detail. This technique allows easier visualization of telangiectases, Wickham's striae, and similar findings. Episcopes or dermatoscopes allow the examination of skin lesions under magnification with excellent illumination and permit resolution of fine detail and size. They are especially useful

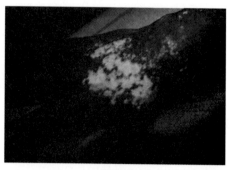

Vitiligo

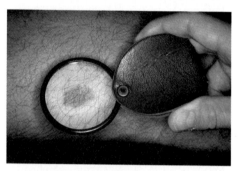

Magnifying lens

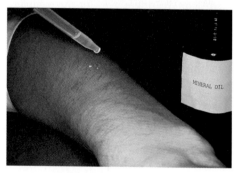

Application of mineral oil

TABLE 2–1. **Fluorescent Characteristics of Certain Conditions**

Characteristics	Conditions
Yellow-green fluorescence of hair	*Microsporum canis*
Yellow-green fluorescence of skin	*Pseudomonas* infection
	Atabrine ingestion (nails also fluoresce)
Coral fluorescence of toes, axillae, groin	Erythrasma infection

for viewing complex pigmented lesions and melanomas.

Compression

Observing the changes in a skin lesion with compression (diascopy) is often useful in the diagnosis of skin diseases. Compression may be performed with a magnifying glass, microscope slide, or clear plastic plate. These instruments are all considered *diascopes*. Blue to red lesions that blanch when compressed are vascular lesions, and their gradual refilling is observed by seeing the red color return. Purpuric lesions do not blanch completely with pressure; raised, purpuric, nonblanchable lesions indicate vasculitis. Compression of brown to yellow-brown papules may reveal the apple-jelly nodules of granulomatosis.

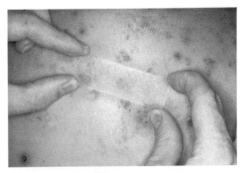

Diascopy

Palpation of Skin Lesions

Palpation reveals the lesion's depth, extension, texture, firmness, and fixation to underlying structures of skin. Light pressure can reveal a thrill in a vascular lesion, implying an arteriovenous malformation. Lateral compression of dermatofibromas causes them to become depressed and to indent the overlying skin *(Fitzpatrick's sign)*. Firm stroking of apparently normal skin can induce histamine release, redness, and edema; this phenomenon, known as *dermographism*, is accentuated in urticaria. Stroking of individual papules leading to local erythema and edema (and, rarely, vesiculation) is diagnostic of urticaria pigmentosa. This phenomenon is named *Darier's sign*. Stroking the skin of atopic patients produces a white line without a red phase (white dermographism). In nevus anemicus, firm rubbing makes the surrounding normal skin bright red but does not induce erythema in the hypopigmented skin.

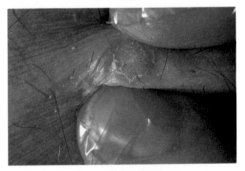

Fitzpatrick's sign

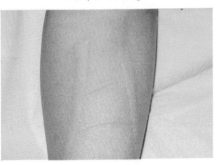

Dermographism

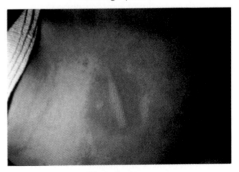

Darier's sign

In blistering diseases, rubbing apparently normal skin may induce new blisters; this occurs in patients with pemphigus vulgaris and toxic epidermal necrolysis *(Nikolsky's sign)*. Extension of an intact blister by applying pressure to the lesions *(Asboe-Hansen sign)* indicates an intraepidermal blister.

SPECIAL DIAGNOSTIC PROCEDURES

Organism Identification

Organism identification is essential for the rational treatment of skin infections and infestations. Procedures important for dermatology are outlined in this section; standard infectious-disease and microbiology texts should be consulted for further details. Superficial crusts, exudate, and medications should be swabbed with alcohol to remove saprophytes and secondary contaminating bacteria.

Gram's Stain for Bacteria and *Candida*

1. Air dry the slide.
2. Cover with 1% crystal violet for 15 seconds. Wash with water.
3. Cover with Gram's iodine for 15 seconds. Wash with water.
4. Decolorize for 15 seconds with acetone-alcohol. Wash with water.
5. Cover with 2.5% safranin for 15 seconds. Wash with water and air dry.
6. Examine with 10×, 40×, and oil immersion lenses.

Potassium Hydroxide (KOH) Preparation for Fungus

1. Cleanse skin of any ointment with an alcohol swab.
2. With the edge of a microscope slide or a scalpel, scrape the skin vigorously onto a second microscope slide. The best areas for scraping are:
   a. Inner surface of a blister roof, or the blister base
   b. Moist, macerated areas, such as between toes
   c. Rim of lesion
   d. Under nail or under paronychial fold
   e. Base of a plucked hair
3. Place a drop of 10% KOH on the scale-covered slide and apply a coverslip.

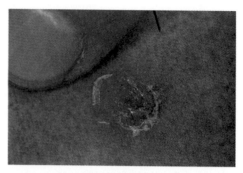

Nikolsky's sign

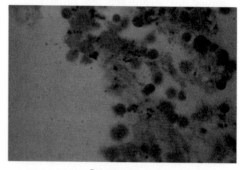

Gram's stain

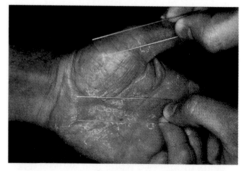

Scraping

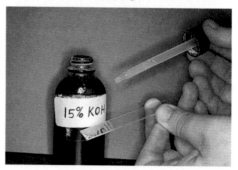

Use of potassium hydroxide

4. Warm gently. Avoid actual boiling, because it causes the KOH to crystallize.
5. Examine with a microscope with 10× and 40× objective at low illumination. This is achieved by setting a low level of light and racking the condenser down.

Small amounts of scrapings on a slide frequently yield the best results because the cover slip rests on the slide, producing the best optical properties. Potassium hydroxide hydrolyses the epidermal proteins but not the fungal elements. The cell envelopes of the stratum corneum remain and should not be confused with fungi.

India Ink Stain for *Cryptococcus*
A smear of an exudate is mixed with 1 small drop of commercial India ink and a coverslip is applied. If the preparation is too dark, water may be added to dilute the ink. The large, translucent capsules of the *Cryptococcus*, with a small central nucleus that may contain a nucleolus, are seen. The buds have a narrow base; blastomycosis and other fungi have a broad base.

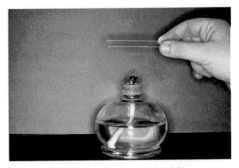
Heating potassium hydroxide

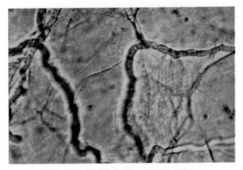
Dermatophyte, KOH preparation

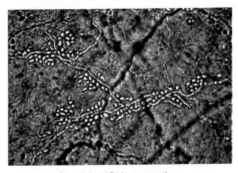
Candida, KOH preparation

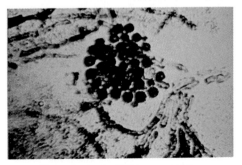
Tinea versicolor, KOH preparation

Acid-Fast Stain

In suspected lepromatous leprosy and orificial tuberculosis, direct stains may be positive. In other forms of cutaneous leprosy and cutaneous tuberculosis, the chance of a positive smear is so small that a direct smear is not indicated. *Nocardia* in mycetomas will also stain with the acid-fast stain.

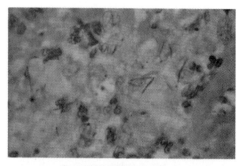

Leprosy, acid-fast stain

Tzanck Smear for Giant Cells

A Tzanck smear is very important in the diagnosis of patients with vesicles. The demonstration of multinucleated giant cells indicates that the causative agent is either herpes simplex or varicella-zoster virus. The procedure is as follows:

1. Select a fresh, umbilicated vesicle.
2. Unroof the vesicle with a scalpel blade.
3. Gently scrape the base of the vesicle with the scalpel and smear scrapings onto a microscope slide.
4. Fix with 95% alcohol.
5. Stain with Wright's or Giemsa stain, using the technique that is used for routine white cell differential counts.
6. Examine under the microscope, using the 10× or 40× objective. A positive preparation demonstrates very large multinucleated giant cells with deep blue cytoplasm or enlarged cells with a high nuclear-cytoplasmic ratio. Examination with the oil immersion objective often is required in equivocal cases.

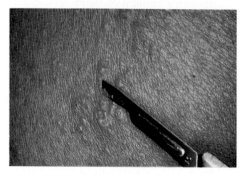

Scraping blister

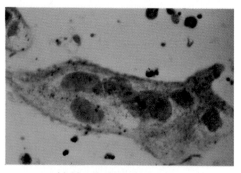

Multinucleated giant cell

Dark-Field Microscopic Examination for Syphilis

With a special condenser (dark field) and a funnel stage for the lens, any microscope can be converted to a dark-field microscope. The condenser causes an oblique beam of light to refract off objects too small to be seen by conventional optics. The narrow organism causing syphilis, *Treponema pallidum*, is such an organism. Dark-field examination for organisms can be positive even before the most sensitive serologic tests for syphilis confirm the diagnosis. Dark-field examinations are difficult to do, and examinations of specimens from the oral cavity are especially difficult to interpret, because normal spirochetes in the oral flora resemble *T. pallidum*.

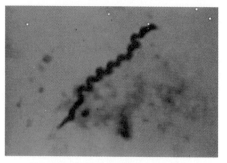

T. pallidum in a dark-field preparation

The procedure is as follows:

1. Put on gloves.
2. Clean the surface of the lesion with dry gauze and rub vigorously.
3. Compress the lesion between the gloved fingers.
4. Touch a coverslip to the drop of serum arising on the surface of the lesion.
5. Drop the coverslip on a drop of saline on the slide and examine immediately. *Do not allow the specimen to dry out.* Remember to put oil between the condenser and slide as well as between the coverslip and objective.

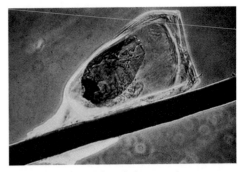

Nit on hair

Examination for Lice
Nits (eggs of lice) on pubic, axillary, scalp, or other hairs may be examined directly with the microscope. Organisms or empty, highly refractile egg cases are easily observed with 10× objective.

Examination for Scabies
Scabetic mites may be removed from burrows with a scalpel after applying 10% potassium hydroxide or mineral oil to the suspected burrow. The oil optically clears the stratum corneum, enhancing visualization of the mite. Application of a tetracycline solution (500 mg tetracycline in 20 mL glycerin and 80 mL absolute ethanol), followed 1 minute later by shining a Wood's lamp on the skin, accentuates the burrow. Burrows fluoresce a brilliant green, allowing easy removal of a suspected organism. A small drop of ink placed on the opening of the burrow and then rapidly removed with a tissue may also reveal tracks.

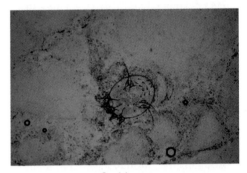

Scabies

Culture Techniques
Sabouraud's medium is useful for the isolation of most fungi. It is available commercially, stored cool, and then incubated with specimens at room temperature. Sabouraud's medium with cycloheximide (actidone) and chloramphenicol suppresses bacterial and saprophytic fungi. It is very important not to use this medium if *Cryptococcus* is suspected, because cycloheximide suppresses the growth of *Cryptococcus*.

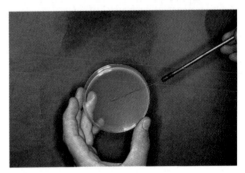

Fungal culture

Mycobacteria from skin lesions may be cultured using special media. Certain atypical mycobacteria that cause skin disease grow best at 32°C, and this should be noted when submitting specimens if the presence of mycobacteria is suspected.

Patch and Skin Testing

Patch testing is essential in the evaluation of contact dermatitis. *Fisher's Contact Dermatitis*, edited by Reitschel and Fowler, is an excellent and complete reference on the subject. In brief, the suspected antigen is applied under an occlusive dressing (a Finn chamber, Band-Aid, or A1-Test strip) and is left undisturbed for 2 to 4 days. Then the test site is inspected for erythema, vesiculation, or induration. The test sites should be observed 1 hour, 24 hours, and 48 hours after removing the patch. Kits with dozens of antigens are available. Direct patch testing with suspected material (shoe lining, clothing, etc.) is often positive and useful. Kits of reagents for patch tests are available from several sources, including the American Academy of Dermatology. The 20 most common antigens are now available on two self-adhesive patches (T.R.U.E. test, Glaxo-Wellcome, Nashville, TN). Scratch testing, which detects the presence of specific IgE antibodies, is not commonly used in dermatology.

Intradermal skin tests with *Candida* (0.1 mL of a 1:100 dilution of *Candida albicans* glycerosaline extract, Bayer Pharmaceuticals, Spokane, WA) and streptokinase-streptodornase (Varidase, Lederle Pharmaceuticals, Wayne, NJ, 100 and 25 units, respectively) and sensitization to dinitrochlorobenzene are often used if a patient is suspected of having abnormalities of cellular immunity. Sensitizing with dinitrochlorobenzene is performed with a 2-mg dose (dissolved in 0.1 mL acetone) applied to 9 cm² of skin. A challenge dose of 100 µg in 0.1 mL is given after 2 weeks.

Biopsies

Skin Punch Biopsy

Skin punch biopsy, when properly performed, involves minimal scarring. The physician should always ask the patient

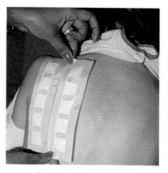

Applying patch tests

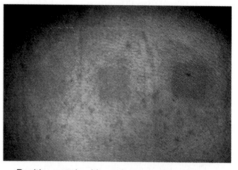

Positive patch with erythema and papules

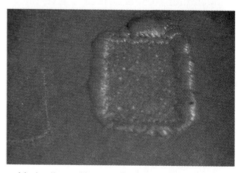

Markedly positive patch test with blistering

about ingestion of anticoagulants or aspirin and about allergy to lidocaine (Xylocaine) before doing a biopsy. The procedure is performed as follows:

1. Wear sterile gloves.
2. Clean skin with alcohol.
3. Infiltrate with 1% to 2% lidocaine with or without 1:1000 epinephrine.
4. Rotate punch of 2- to 6-mm diameter (usually 4-mm) into lesion.
5. Lift specimen with pick-up and cut base of lesion, which should contain fat.
6. Routinely fix in 10% formalin. Fixation in ethanol is necessary for the preservation of urates and the glycosaminoglycans found in scleredema and pretibial myxedema.
7. Achieve hemostasis by pressure alone or by pressure and by applying 25% or 30% aluminum chloride trichloroacetic with a cotton swab to a wound that has been blotted dry. Biopsies made using a 2- to 3-mm punch can be allowed to heal by secondary intention. The lesion produced by a 4- to 6-mm punch should be closed with a suture. Biopsies on cosmetically important sites often heal better with a suture.

Excision Biopsy

Excision biopsy is performed using standard surgical techniques, and the wound is always closed with sutures. Excision biopsy should be used for best cosmetic results, total removal of malignant lesions with adequate margins, and deep nodular lesions including panniculitis; for obtaining adequate tissue for histology and culture; or for study of the rim of a lesion.

Special Microscopic Examinations of Biopsy Tissue

Polarization Microscopy

In foreign-body reactions or granulomas, tissue should be examined by polarizing microscopy to identify deposition of silica or other foreign materials. Polarization detects doubly refractile cholesterols, urates, and various other crystals.

Polarization of the hair is diagnostic for trichothiodystrophy and shows alternating bands of birefringence (see p. 498).

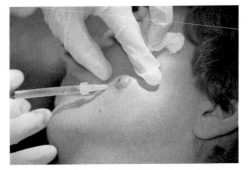
Injecting Xylocaine

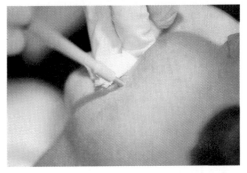
Screwing punch into skin

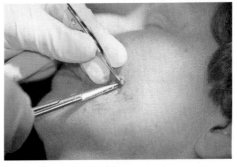
Removing the biopsy specimen

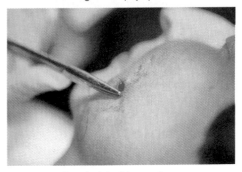
Suturing the biopsy site

Special Staining Microscopy

Evaluating tissue with certain stains should be specified if specific diseases are suspected (Table 2–2).

Immunofluorescence Microscopy and Immunochemistry

Deposits of immunoglobulins and complement in skin have diagnostic significance in several serious skin diseases. These direct immunofluorescent studies (Table 2–3) are performed by staining a biopsy from a patient with fluoresceinated antihuman immunoglobulin or anticomplement reagents and then examining the tissue under a fluorescent microscope. Indirect immunofluorescence tests a patient's serum for the presence of circulating autoantibodies. The basement membrane zone can be enhanced by preincubation overnight in 1 mol/L sodium chloride, a technique that allows more precise localization of the immune reactants.

Immunohistochemical techniques are used for identification of intracellular filaments (keratins, vimentin, desmins), T- and B-cell markers, S-100 protein, and organisms. Details of these tests are available in histopathology texts listed in the Bibliography.

TABLE 2–2. **Special Stains Used in Diagnosis**

Stain	Tissue Element	Disease or Organism
Acid-fast	Mycobacteria	*Nocardia;* actinomycoses, leprosy, tuberculosis, atypical mycobacteria
Alcian blue	Glycosaminoglycans	Scleredema, pretibial myxedema, sclerosmyxedema
Avidin-fluorescein	Mast cells	Mastocytosis
Congo red	Amyloid	Amyloid, lichen amyloid, macular amyloid
DOPA	Melanin	Nevi, amelanotic melanoma
Giemsa	Mast cell granules, multiple organisms	Mastocytosis, leishmaniasis, histoplasmosis, etc.
Periodic acid-Schiff	Polysaccharides, basement membranes	Deep fungus, lupus erythematosus
Silver	Fungi	Deep fungus
Verhoeff's	Elastic fiber	Pseudoxanthoma elasticum, perforating disorders
von Kossa's	Calcium	Calcinosis cutis, calcifying epithelioma

TABLE 2–3. **Immunofluorescent Studies Used in Diagnosis**

Disease	Immunofluorescent Findings	
	Skin (Direct Technique)	*Serum (Indirect Technique)*
Acquired epidermolysis bullosa	Linear IgG along the dermal-epidermal junction.	Positive in 40% of patients
Bullous pemphigoid	Linear deposition of IgG and complement at basement membrane between epidermis and dermis.	Positive in 70% of patients
Dermatitis herpetiformis	Clumps of IgA and complement in the upper dermis immediately below the dermal/epidermal basement membrane.	No detectable circulating antibodies
Lupus erythematosus	Clumps of immunoglobulin (especially IgG) and complement in upper dermis immediately below the dermal/epidermal basement membrane.	Antinuclear antibodies, especially in systemic lupus erythematosus
Linear IgA bullous dermatosis	Linear deposits of immunoglobulin along the dermal/epidermal basement membrane.	Positive in 30%–70% of patients
Pemphigus	IgG is present intercellularly in the epidermis. It is almost impossible to make the diagnosis of pemphigus in an untreated patient without this finding.	Positive in 90% of patients

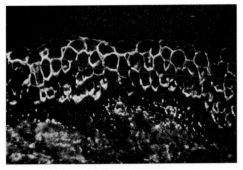

Pemphigus vulgaris

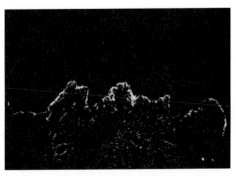

Bullous pemphigoid

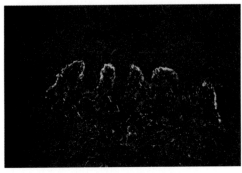

Dermatitis herpetiformis

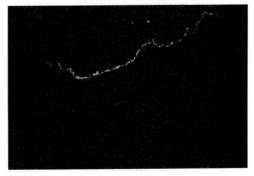

Lupus erythematosus

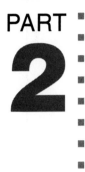

PART

2

Diseases

Chapter 3

■ ■

Macules

Macules are flat, circumscribed lesions that are apparent because of a color change. This chapter also deals with diffuse changes in color.

At times it is difficult to determine whether a lesion is a flat macule or a raised papule. Side lighting the lesion in a dark room with a flashlight aids in proper identification; papular lesions cast a shadow (see p. 11). Brown macules are caused by melanin, hemosiderin, or drug pigment. Blue macules result from melanin, hemosiderin, or drug pigment deposited deep in the dermis. Hypopigmented macules are caused by lack of melanin or decreased blood supply in the skin. Red macules are due to blood. Red macules that blanch completely when compressed are vascular in origin and are discussed in this chapter. If red macules cannot be blanched, then blood has extravasated from vessels, and this is known as *purpura*. Purpura is discussed on page 58.

MAJOR CATEGORIES

Blue Macules
Congenital
Acquired

Brown Macules
Generalized hyperpigmentation
Non–sun-exposed areas
Palms and soles
Sun-exposed areas

Purple Macules and Purpura

Red Macules
Transient
Exanthems
Reticulated
Scattered
Configurate

White Macules
Congenital
Acquired

DIAGNOSTIC OBSERVATIONS
Color: blue, brown, purple, red, white.
Can lesions be blanched with pressure?
Is the lesion circumscribed or diffuse?
Are lesions single or multiple?
Are lesions confined to sun-exposed areas?
Determine whether lesions are acquired or congenital, appear abruptly, or are transient (last <24 hours).
Is the lesion atrophic?

BLUE MACULES

DIAGNOSTIC OBSERVATIONS
Location, age of onset, other medical conditions. Blue macules are a result of deposition of melanin, hemosiderin, exogenous or drug pigment in the dermis.

MAJOR CATEGORIES

Congenital

Mongolian spot (congenital dermal melanocytosis)
Nevus of Ota or Ito

Acquired

Blue nevus
Drug-induced blue macule
Erythema dyschromicum perstans
Maculae caeruleae
Malignant melanoma
Ochronosis
Tattoo

Congenital Blue Macules

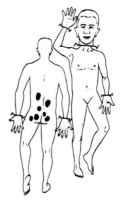

Mongolian Spot
(Congenital Dermal Melanocytosis)

■ **Morphology**
Poorly defined, blue to blue-black flat lesions.

■ **Distribution**
Trunk and buttocks but may occur anywhere.

■ **Patient Profile**
Disease present at birth. Common in Asians and blacks. Asymptomatic. Fades with age.

■ **Diagnosis**
Biopsy reveals dermal melanocytes.

■ **Treatment**
None necessary.

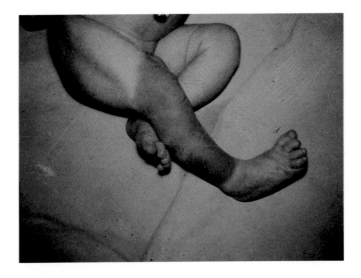

Nevus of Ota or Ito

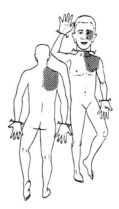

▪ **Morphology**
Flat blue-gray to brown lesions.

▪ **Distribution**
Nevus of Ota: Trigeminal nerve distribution including scleral and buccal mucosa.
Nevus of Ito: Shoulder.

▪ **Patient Profile**
Disease present at birth or may occur in young adulthood. Common in Asians. Glaucoma or melanoma may occur.

▪ **Diagnosis**
Distribution pattern is diagnostic. Biopsy reveals dermal melanocytosis.

▪ **Treatment**
Cosmetic cover-up or laser.

Acquired Blue Macules

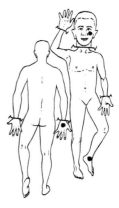

Blue Nevus

▪ Morphology
Sharply circumscribed, flat to raised uniform blue lesion. Several millimeters to several centimeters in size.

▪ Distribution
Face, lower arm, hand, and forehead near scalp but may be anywhere.

▪ Patient Profile
Adolescent, adult. Asymptomatic.

▪ Diagnosis
Biopsy reveals dermal melanocytes.

▪ Treatment
Excision for cosmesis or concern about melanoma.

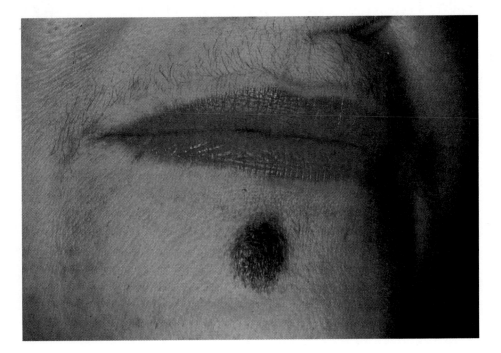

Drug-Induced Blue Macule

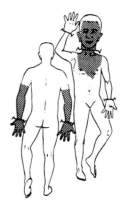

▪ Morphology
Gray-blue metallic pigmentation diffusely distributed over body or in large plaques.

▪ Distribution
Most common on sun-exposed areas but entire body and mucous membranes may be involved. Trauma often has a role in localization in patients receiving minocycline and antimalarial.

▪ Patient Profile
Patient takes phenothiazines, chloroquine, hydroxychloroquine, quinacrine (Atabrine), gold, minocycline, amiodarone, or silver-containing medications, or has occupational exposure to silver nitrate.

▪ Diagnosis
Biopsy reveals increased melanin and deposition of drug.

▪ Treatment
Very slow fading with time. Surgical removal of focal lesions. Cosmetic covering of lesions.

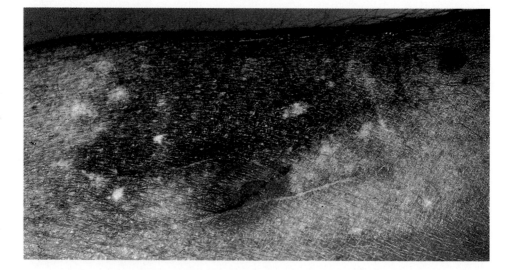

Erythema Dyschromicum Perstans

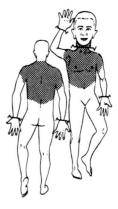

■ Morphology
Macules are initially red and develop a distinct ashy, blue-gray color. Lesions range from a few millimeters to many centimeters. Occasionally a slightly raised border is noted.

■ Distribution
Trunk and proximal extremities.

■ Patient Profile
Hyperpigmented young adults from Central and South America.

■ Diagnosis
Biopsy reveals deposition of melanin in epidermal cells and dermal melanophages.

■ Treatment
Fades slowly. Cosmetic cover.

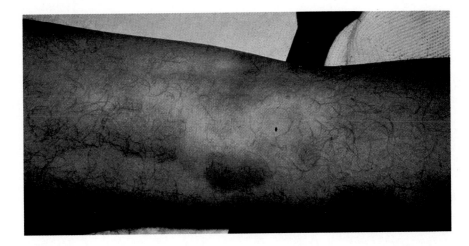

Maculae Caeruleae

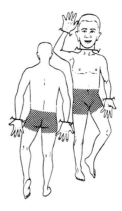

▪ Morphology
Discrete 0.5- to 1-cm blue-gray macules.
Crusts and excoriations are common.

▪ Distribution
Lower abdomen and upper thigh.

▪ Patient Profile
Patient has pubic lice. Similar lesions occur from the silver present in acupuncture
needles.

▪ Diagnosis
Lesions are secondary to louse bites. Diagnosis depends on demonstration of lice.

▪ Treatment
Overnight application of 5% permethrin
(Elimite) to kill the lice.

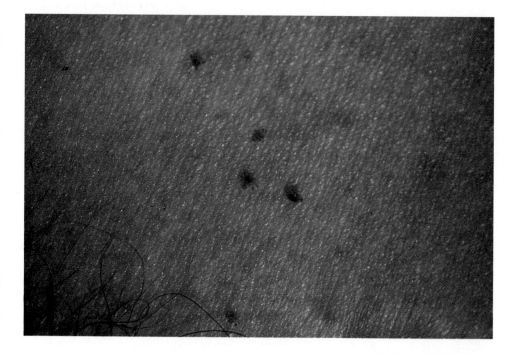

Malignant Melanoma

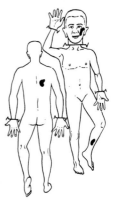

■ Morphology
Blue, black, or brown variegated, flat lesions that often have areas of white and red pigmentation. The borders of the lesions are irregular, and there may be notches. Skin markings are altered. Careful examination with a hand lens and side lighting often reveals irregularity of surface. Lesions may ulcerate and form nodules.

■ Distribution
Light-exposed areas but lesions can occur anywhere. In males, lesions commonly appear on the upper back and shoulder; in females, on the legs.

■ Patient Profile
Usually middle-aged adults of both sexes. Patient may have atypical moles and a family history of melanoma. Disease uncommon in blacks; when it does occur in this group, lesions develop on palms, soles, and under nails. Prognosis is directly related to thickness of the lesions, determined microscopically. Patients with lesions <0.76 mm thick have over 99% 5-year survival. Lesions <1 mm thick should be removed, with a 1-cm margin.

■ Diagnosis
Look for the ABCD changes associated with malignant melanoma: asymmetry, border irregularity, color variation (red, blue, white), and diameter >4 to 6 mm. A flat, blue lesion with variation in color and alteration of skin markings requires that the lesion be biopsied. Careful examination for adenopathy is important for staging. An episcope is useful for detailed examination of lesion. Histologic examination demonstrates melanoma.

■ Treatment
Excision appropriate to size and depth of the lesion.

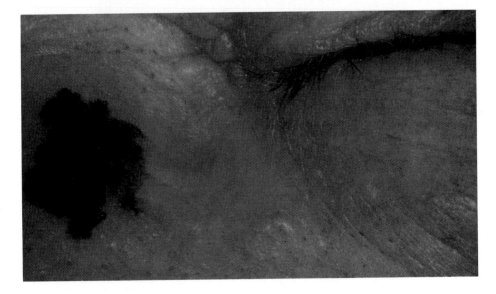

Ochronosis

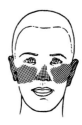

▪ **Morphology**
Poorly circumscribed, blue-black macules.

▪ **Distribution**
Eyes, ears, cheeks, nasal cartilage.

▪ **Patient Profile**
Adults with autosomal recessive genetic disease. Evidence of black urine and arthritis with calcification of the intervertebral disks. Condition develops after use of hydroquinone in high concentrations as a skin bleaching agent.

▪ **Diagnosis**
Homogentisic acid in urine. Homogeneous material in dermis.

▪ **Treatment**
None available.

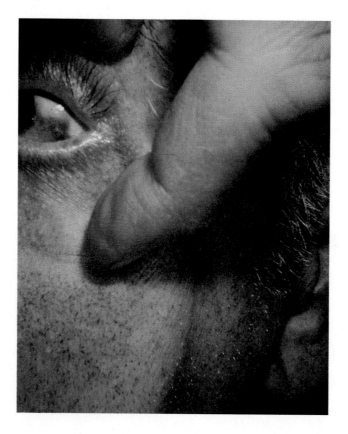

Tattoo

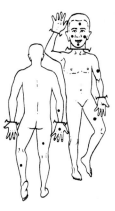

▪ Morphology
Sharply circumscribed, flat, blue pigment with irregular shape.

▪ Distribution
Anywhere, especially areas of trauma.

▪ Patient Profile
Tattoo applied by artist, self-induced, or caused by pencil leads, cinders, amalgams, or abrasions in coal miners.

▪ Diagnosis
Biopsy reveals deposition of abnormal pigment.

▪ Treatment
Surgical removal or laser.

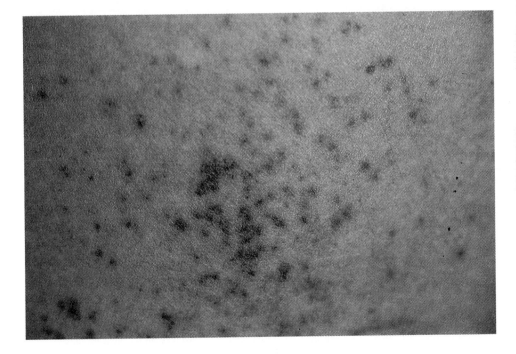

BROWN MACULES

<table>
<tr><td>

DIAGNOSTIC OBSERVATIONS
Brown color is generalized, distributed primarily in sun-exposed areas, scattered randomly on body.

</td></tr>
</table>

MAJOR CATEGORIES

Generalized
Common causes (Table 3-1)
Rare causes:
  Acromegaly
  Central nervous system disease: Schilder's disease, catatonic schizophrenia
  Chronic disease: infection, lymphoma, neoplasia
  Felty's syndrome

TABLE 3–1. **Common Causes of Generalized Pigmentation**

Disease	Constitutional Symptoms and Signs	Other Signs and Findings
Addison's disease (Nelson's syndrome)	Weakness, orthostatic hypotension	Hair loss, oral hyperpigmentation
Biliary cirrhosis	Pruritus	Xanthoma, especially on palm
Cushing's syndrome, exogenous ACTH (MSH) or ACTH-secreting tumors	Weakness, hypertension, truncal obesity, diabetes	Striae, acne, hirsutism, purpura
Drug-induced hyperpigmentation	History of atabrine, azidothymidine, amiodarone, busulfan; chloroquine, cytotoxin; 5-fluorouracil; bleomycin; dibromomannitol; psoralens, topically or systemically; topical nitrogen mustard	
Hemochromatosis	Diabetes, hepatomegaly, anorexia, weight loss, heart disease	Hair loss, koilonychia, ichthyosis-like changes
Hyperthyroidism	Weight loss, tremor, restlessness	Increased sweating, vitiligo
Malignant melanoma with generalized melanomatosis	Hepatomegaly, melanuria (grossly)	Tumor metastases, primary melanoma by history
POEMS (adult onset)	Polyneuropathy, dysglobulinemia with paraproteins, neuropathy, diffuse hyperpigmentation, hypertrichosis, papilledema, lymphadenopathy	
Porphyria cutanea tarda (and variegate porphyria)	Diabetes, elevated ethanol intake, hepatomegaly	Milia, bullae, hypertrichosis
Scleroderma	Atonic esophagus and gut, decreased diffusing capacity in lung	Raynaud's phenomenon, calcinosis cutis, telangiectasia
Whipple's disease	Malabsorption, cachexia, arthritis, lymphadenopathy	
Wilson's disease	Liver failure	Kayser-Fleischer ring

Gaucher's disease, Niemann-Pick disease
Pheochromocytoma
POEMS syndrome
Pregnancy
Preasthmatic attack melanoderma
Sprue with malabsorption
Vitamin B_{12} deficiency
Wilson's disease

Localized (in Sun-Exposed or Non–Sun-Exposed Areas)
Acanthosis nigricans
Becker's nevus
Café au lait spots: Albright's syndrome, neurofibromatosis
Erythrasma
Fungal infection
Lentigo syndromes
Mastocytosis (telangiectasia macularis eruptiva perstans, urticaria pigmentosa)
Nevi
Postinflammatory hyperpigmentation: der-matitis, dyskeratosis congenita, fixed drug eruption, incontinentia pigmenti, lichen planus, macular amyloid, pinta
Progressive pigmentary purpura
Stasis dermatitis
Tinea versicolor

On Palms and Soles
Acral lentiginous melanoma
Cronkhite-Canada syndrome
Secondary syphilis
Talon noir
Tinea nigra palmaris

In Sun-Exposed Areas
Actinic lentigo
Berlock dermatitis
Drug-induced hyperpigmentation
Freckle (ephelis)
Lentigo maligna
Melasma
Pellagra
Xeroderma pigmentosum

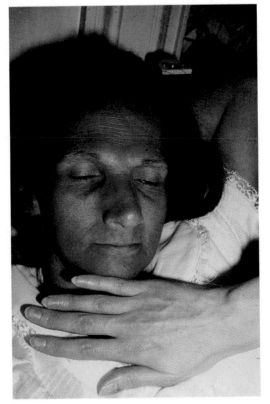

Addison's disease

Localized Brown Macules

Acanthosis Nigricans

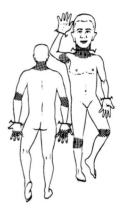

▪ Morphology
Brown to black plaques with accentuation of skin marking producing a velvety appearance. Skin tags often present.

▪ Distribution
Symmetric; axillae, neck, knuckles, and elbows. Oral or palmar lesions suggest associated adenocarcinoma.

▪ Patient Profile
In younger patients, lesions are often associated with obesity, endocrinopathy, and insulin resistance; in older patients, with adenocarcinoma. Syndromes or diseases associated with acanthosis nigricans include Lawrence-Seip, Rud's, Crouzon's, Bloom, Wilson's, Prader-Willi, ataxia-telangiectasia, and polycystic ovary disease.

▪ Diagnosis
Biopsy demonstrates acanthosis of the epidermis.

▪ Treatment
Treatment of underlying disease. Topical 12% lactic acid or retinoic acid.

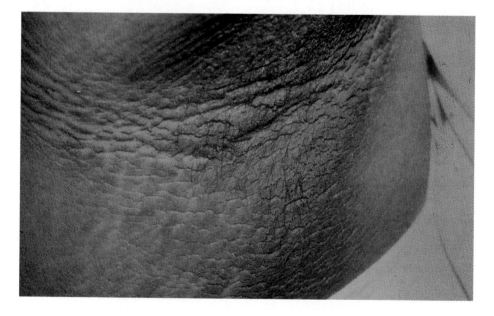

Becker's Nevus

■ **Morphology**
Irregularly pigmented brown to black flat lesions. Satellite macules may develop beyond the lesion and form a geographic configuration. Coarse, dark hairs may appear in the lesion.

■ **Distribution**
Anywhere, but most common on shoulders and trunk.

■ **Patient Profile**
Disease starts in childhood. More common in males than in females. Usually noted during adolescence; accentuated by sun exposure. No malignant potential.

■ **Diagnosis**
Biopsy with increased pigment but no melanocytic hyperplasia or nevus cells.

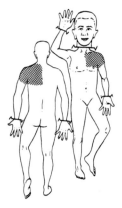

Often underlying smooth muscle hamartoma.

■ **Treatment**
Surgical excision; laser.

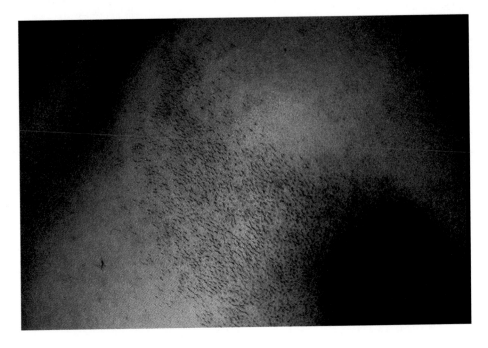

Café au Lait Spot

▪ Morphology
Uniformly pigmented, tan, nonscaly, oval to irregularly shaped macules. Lesions are usually >0.5 cm.

▪ Distribution
Most commonly on trunk but can occur anywhere. Lesions are not usually found on mucosal surfaces.

▪ Patient Profile
Ten percent of normal individuals have one to three café au lait spots; more than 5 lesions suggest neurofibromatosis.

▪ Diagnosis
Biopsy of a café au lait spot in neurofibromatosis usually demonstrates giant melanosomes in melanocytes. This feature is usually missing in common café au lait spots and in Albright's syndrome. Café au lait spots may be associated with pulmonary stenosis and mental retardation.

▪ Differential Diagnosis
See Table 3-2.

▪ Treatment
None necessary.

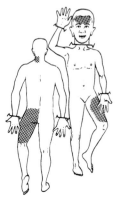

Albright's syndrome

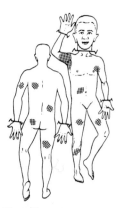

Neurofibromatosis

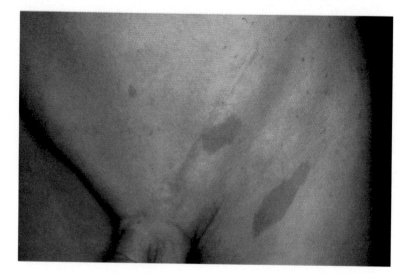

TABLE 3–2. **Differential Diagnosis of Albright's Syndrome and Neurofibromatosis**

Characteristics	Albright's Syndrome	Neurofibromatosis
Color	Tan	Tan
Size	2–20 cm	2–12 cm
Shape	Irregular, jagged, or geometric	Smooth, oval, regular
Number	Multiple or single	5 or more café au lait spots suggest neurofibromatosis
Distribution	Often unilateral	Bilateral
Associated skin lesions	None	Pedunculated or plexiform neurofibroma and axillary freckling are highly suggestive
Associated systemic lesions	Premature puberty, bony dysplasia	Premature puberty, pheochromocytoma, optic and cranial nerve tumors, mental retardation
Family history	No	Positive family history, autosomal dominant

Erythrasma

▪ **Morphology**
Reddish-brown, poorly marginated, scaling lesions.

▪ **Distribution**
Symmetric. Axillae, groin, and toe webs are commonly involved.

▪ **Patient Profile**
Most common in adult men.

▪ **Diagnosis**
With a long-wavelength ultraviolet lamp (Wood's lamp), the lesions demonstrate coral red fluorescence. If the patient has bathed within 24 hours, fluorescence is difficult to detect. Fungal scrapings are negative.

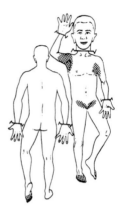

▪ **Treatment**
Topical 2% erythromycin solution bid × 7 days and prn.

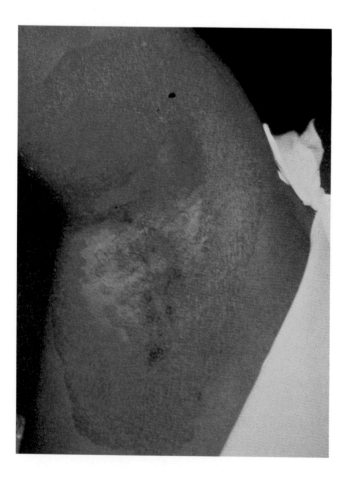

Fungal Infection
(Dermatophyte)

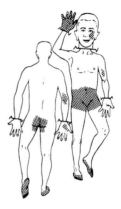

■ Morphology
Brown, circular, polycyclic, arciform, and annular lesions with some scaling. Lesions tend to spread peripherally with central clearing. Can have darker papular regions (Majocchi's granuloma).

■ Distribution
Anywhere, but most commonly on palms, soles, thighs, and trunk.

■ Patient Profile
Any age; both sexes. Slowly enlarging, slightly pruritic lesions. Fungal infections also common in HIV-positive patients.

■ Diagnosis
Potassium hydroxide preparation reveals septate hyphae for dermatophytes and yeast, hyphae in tinea versicolor and budding yeast, and pseudohyphae in candidia-sis. Fungal cultures grow dermatophytes or *Candida*.

■ Treatment
Limited infections: topical antifungals and dry powders for 3 to 4 weeks or until clear. Widespread or resistant infection: systemic antifungal agents.

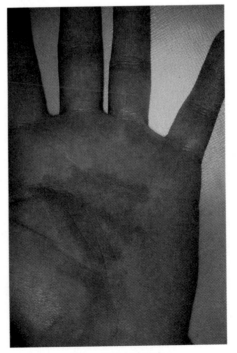

Tinea nigra palmaris

Lentigo Syndromes

▪ **Morphology**
Macular tan to black lesions, ranging from 1 mm to 1 cm in size, that do not increase in color with sun exposure.

▪ **Distribution**
Distribution aids in diagnosis of various multiple lentiginous syndromes. Common lentigos may be anywhere.

▪ **Patient Profile**
One or more lentigos are frequently present in normal individuals.

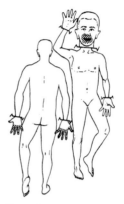

Peutz-Jeghers syndrome

▪ **Diagnosis**
When multiple lesions are found, consider:

Centrofacial lentiginosis: Horizontal band of lentigines on face associated with bony abnormalities and mental retardation. Inherited as autosomal dominant; may be associated with anhidrotic ectodermal dysplasia.

Eruptive lentiginosis: Numerous lesions erupting suddenly in adolescence may evolve into pigmented nevi.

Generalized lentiginosis: Multiple lesions appear singly, in crops, or in a dermatomal distribution. May begin in infancy. No genetic factor is demonstrable.

LAMB or NAME syndrome: Multiple lentigines, especially on the face; mucosal and cardiac myxomas; blue nevi often associated with endocrine disorders. Autosomal dominant and X-linked forms. A mnemonic for **n**evi, **a**trial myxomas, **m**yxoid neurofibromas, **e**philides. Also

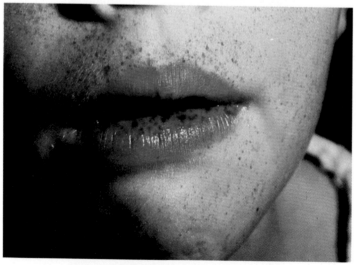

Peutz-Jeghers syndrome

associated with other pigmented, testicular, and pituitary growth-hormone–secreting tumors.

Laugier-Huziker syndrome: This condition occurs in adults. Discrete macular hyperpigmentation of the lips and buccal mucosa. Palms and soles often involved.

LEOPARD syndrome: Lentigos are present at birth and increase in number until puberty. Inherited as autosomal dominant. The name is an acronym: lentigo, ECG abnormalities, ocular hypertelorism, pulmonic stenosis, abnormalities of the genitalia, retardation of growth, deafness.

Moynahan syndrome: Multiple symmetric lentigines, congenital mitral stenosis, genital hypoplasia, and mental deficiency constitute this rare syndrome.

Peutz-Jeghers syndrome: Lentigos are often present at birth and increase in number during childhood. Lesions are most marked on the face, in the mouth, and on hands. There is associated gastrointestinal (GI) polyposis and premature puberty. Polyps are usually benign, but malignant degeneration has been observed in gastric and colonic polyps.

POEMS syndrome: The name is a mnemonic for **p**olyneuropathy, **o**rganomegaly, **e**ndocrinopathy, **m**yeloma-like protein, and **s**kin lesions. The most common skin changes are hyperpigmented macules, scleroderma-like lesions, hirsutism, hyperhidrosis, and angiomas.

■ **Treatment**
Surgical excision; laser.

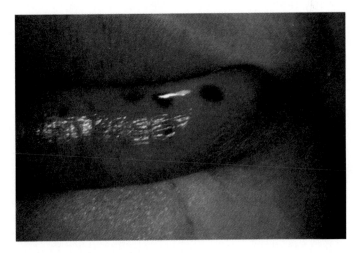

LAMB or NAME Syndrome

Mastocytosis
(Urticaria Pigmentosa, Telangiectasia
Macularis, Telangiectasia Perstans)

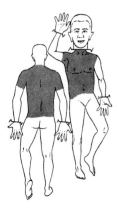

▪ Morphology
Single or multiple tan (urticaria pigmentosa) or reddish-brown (telangiectasia
macularis eruptiva perstans), nonscaly
macules that become red and raised if
stroked (Darier's sign). In young children,
blisters may occur over the lesions with
stroking.

▪ Distribution
Trunk and proximal extremities. Lesions
are uncommon on palms, soles, or mucosal surfaces.

▪ Patient Profile
Brownish macular lesions are uncommonly present at birth but develop during
the first years of life. In 75% to 80% of
affected children the lesions clear spontaneously by adolescence. The telangiectatic
lesions usually begin in adulthood and
rarely resolve.

▪ Diagnosis
The production of urticaria by stroking a
brown macular lesion is pathognomonic.
Biopsy reveals dermal infiltration by mast
cells.

▪ Treatment
Ultra-high-potency topical steroids with
occlusion overnight for 6 weeks. PUVA
therapy. Systemic antihistamines may be
needed.

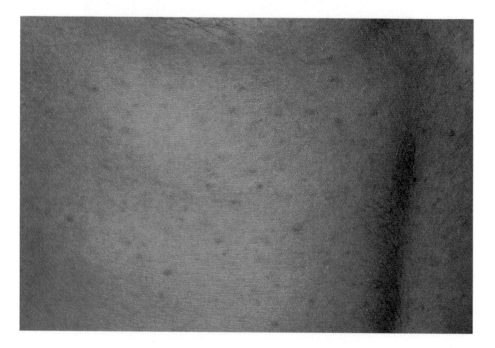

Nevi

▪ Morphology
Macular, uniform, brown to black lesions, usually several millimeters in diameter, that may be minimally to moderately raised above the surface of the skin. The lesions are usually sharply circumscribed and have a regular, round border.

▪ Distribution
Anywhere.

▪ Patient Profile
Disease begins in childhood but may become more prominent in adolescence or during pregnancy. In patients with multiple lesions, atypical mole syndrome (see p. 149) should be considered.

▪ Diagnosis
Uniformity in color and size suggests the diagnosis. Biopsy shows nests of nevus cells in the epidermis. In some families, p16 mutations may be found by DNA analysis.

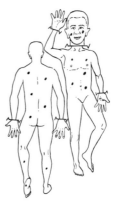

▪ Treatment
Follow-up for ABCD changes: **a**symmetry, **b**order irregularity, **c**olor variegation (red, white, blue), **d**iameter >4 to 6 mm. Patients with 12 moles >5 mm in diameter or 50 moles >2 mm in diameter probably represent those having atypical mole syndrome, and they should be followed up closely every 6 to 12 months for evidence of potential melanoma. Complete surgical excision of suspicious lesions.

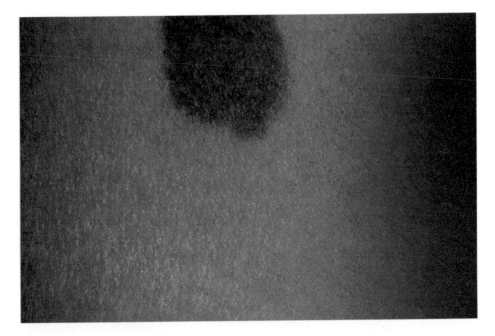

Postinflammatory Hyperpigmentation

A variety of dermatoses are associated with stimulation of melanocytes and/or disruption of the dermal-epidermal junction, resulting in deposition of melanin in the dermis. These hyperpigmented lesions are flat and follow the distribution and configuration of the original inflammatory dermatoses. Almost any dermatitis may cause hyperpigmentation.

The diseases listed below are characterized by their hyperpigmentation:

Dermatitis (see p. 243).

Dyskeratosis congenita: This dermatosis occurs in adolescent males and is characterized by reticulated brown pigment on the trunk, abnormal nails, and oral lesions, which may become carcinomas. Condition should be followed up closely for evidence of malignancy.

Fixed drug eruption: This disease is characterized by one or several sharply circumscribed erythematous plaques, which may blister and heal with marked hyperpigmentation. The lesions always recur in exactly the same spot. The offending drug should be identified and avoided.

Incontinentia pigmenti (see p. 300): The brown hyperpigmentation appears in linear and whorl-like configurations and persists for years after the appearance of acute lesions. Often blistering or papular lesions precede the hyperpigmentation. The disease is limited to females; ocular, dental, and neurologic disorders occur. Genetic counseling is provided, if necessary.

Lichen planus (p. 139): Discrete areas of hyperpigmentation, sometimes with atrophy, occur on flexor surfaces of the wrists and on the extremities.

Macular amyloid: Large, pruritic brown plaque is present on upper trunk. Frequently seen in dark-complexioned people. Biopsy reveals deposition of amyloid in dermis. Not associated with systemic amyloidosis. Treatment with topical steroids class II to III.

Pinta. Hyperpigmentation and hypopigmentation occur after papular and scaling lesions completed on the trunk, face, and buttocks; colors range from white to blue to brown. This disease has a positive serologic test for syphilis and occurs almost exclusively in Central and South America. Organisms can be demonstrated on scrapings of lesions using dark-field microscopy; serologic test for *Treponema* (STS) is positive. Treatment with penicillin.

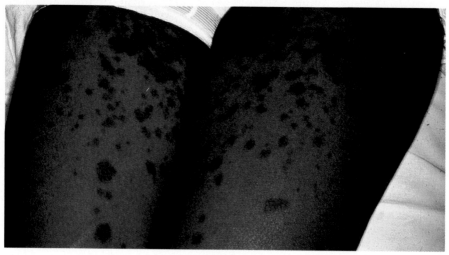

Lichen planus

Progressive Pigmentary Purpura

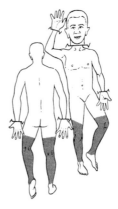

■ Morphology
Reddish-brown, punctate, petechial lesions that become rust to brown-colored macules. Lesions may be scattered and progressive (Schamberg's disease), annular (Majocchi's disease), associated with small, lichenoid papules (Gougerot and Blum dermatosis), or itchy (Lowenthal's disease).

■ Distribution
Usually confined to lower extremity; usually spares soles of feet.

■ Patient Profile
Adult form more common in men. Gradual onset of petechial lesions with chronic course. Lesions usually asymptomatic.

■ Diagnosis
Bleeding and clotting studies are normal. Skin biopsy reveals capillaritis.

■ Treatment
Pressure stockings; oral ascorbic acid. Class II to IV topical steroids.

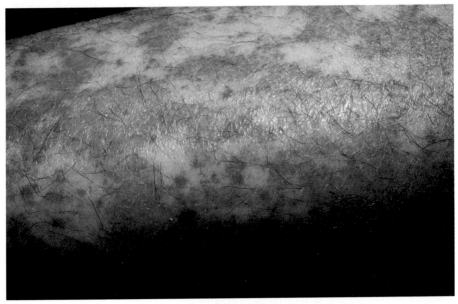

Schamberg's disease

Stasis Dermatitis

▪ **Morphology**

Brown, mottled hyperpigmentation flecked with red and purple; there may be scaling and thinning of the epidermis. There is evidence of pitting edema, varicosities, and venous insufficiency. Ulceration may be present.

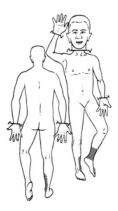

▪ **Distribution**

Lesions are most marked over the medial malleoli but can be either medial or lateral. Often bilateral.

▪ **Patient Profile**

Usually adult women. Lesions itch.

▪ **Diagnosis**

Hyperpigmentation and dermatitis over the medial malleoli in a patient with venous insufficiency and varicosities suggest this diagnosis. Stasis dermatitis in children and young adults suggests the possibility of arteriovenous (AV) fistulae, hemoglobinopathy, or hereditary anemia. Frequent associated contact dermatitis from topicals, especially neomycin. Tests for venous hypertension, such as plethysmography, may be necessary.

▪ **Treatment**

Elevation, pressure dressing, zinc oxide-gelatin (Unna) boots, and elastic support stockings with pressure at least 25 mm Hg. Class II to III topical steroids for surrounding dermatitis.

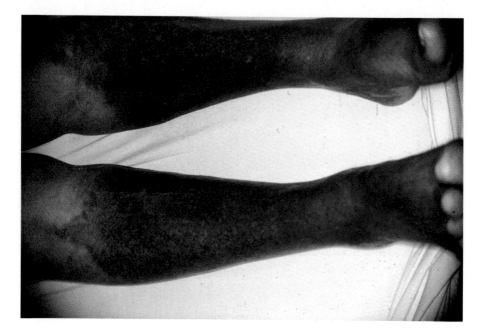

Tinea Versicolor

■ **Morphology**
Flat to slightly elevated brown papules and plaques that scale when rubbed. Areas of hypopigmentation may be seen.

■ **Distribution**
Upper trunk, shoulders, neck, proximal arms, occasionally face, and, rarely, below waist.

■ **Patient Profile**
Usually adolescents or young adults of both sexes. Lesions may be slightly pruritic.

■ **Diagnosis**
Lesion scrapings fixed with potassium hydroxide preparation reveal large spores and thick hyphae.

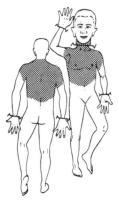

■ **Treatment**
Topical antifungals, short course of oral ketoconazole, Selsun shampoo to affected skin. Patients should be advised that normal pigmentation returns slowly.

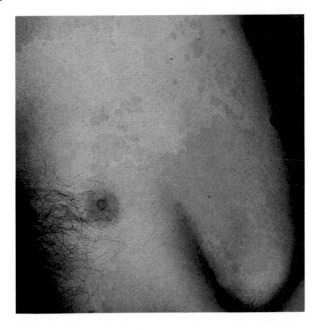

Brown Macules on Palms or Soles

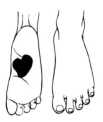

Acral lentiginous melanoma

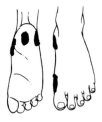

Talon noir

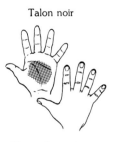

Tinea nigra palmaris

DIAGNOSTIC OBSERVATION
Brown macules on palms and soles are frequently a normal finding in hyperpigmented people, especially blacks.

Acral lentiginous melanoma: Usually pigmented brown to black stippled, jagged plaques distributed asymmetrically on palms or soles. Occurs primarily in blacks and Asians. Biopsy reveals nests of atypical melanocytes. Treated with excisional surgery.

Cronkhite-Canada syndrome: Diffuse hyperpigmentation of palms, spotty pigmentation of dorsum of hands, alopecia, nail dystrophy, GI polyposis, and malabsorption.

Junctional nevus: Brown to black macule with intact skin markings.

Secondary syphilis: May present with scaly brown macules limited to the palms bilaterally. Treatment: see STD, page 588.

Talon noir: Dotlike black lesions of sole due to trauma. Lesions can be pared off. Blood and blood breakdown products are found on biopsy. Treatment: paring with scalpel to remove lesion.

Tinea nigra palmaris: Sharply circumscribed brown to black nonscaly lesions that resemble stains and that are confined to the palms or soles suggest this diagnosis. Potassium hydroxide preparations of scrapings reveal dark, branched hyphae. Treatment: topical antifungals.

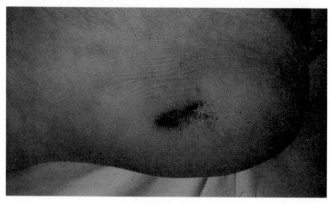

Talon noir

Brown Macules in Sun-Exposed Areas

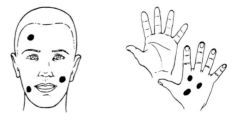

Actinic Lentigo

▪ Morphology
Sharply circumscribed, nonscaling macules with uniform brown color. May be associated with small hypopigmented, slightly atrophic lesions.

▪ Distribution
Sun-exposed areas, especially on face and dorsum of hands.

▪ Patient Profile
Disease begins in adult years and occurs in fair-skinned individuals of both sexes. Le-sions do not fade if patient avoids sun exposure.

▪ Diagnosis
Biopsy reveals increased numbers of normal melanocytes.

▪ Treatment
Cryotherapy. Retin-A. Lasers. Sunscreens to prevent new lesions.

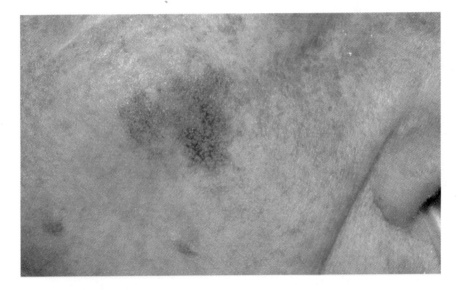

Berlock Dermatitis

▪ Morphology
Brown, streaky, geometric macules that may begin with erythema, blistering, or scaling.

▪ Distribution
Neck, anterior chest, hands, and legs.

▪ Patient Profile
Usually females who apply perfume or cologne containing oil of bergamot and are exposed to sun. Lesions also follow application of cosmetics containing lime or exposure to plants containing furocoumarins, such as rotten celery, parsley, dill, or a variety of weeds. The pigment is accentuated with Wood's light. Biopsy reveals melanocytic hyperplasia.

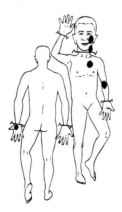

▪ Treatment
Bleaching with hydroquinone-containing creams; Retin-A. Sunscreens to prevent new lesions.

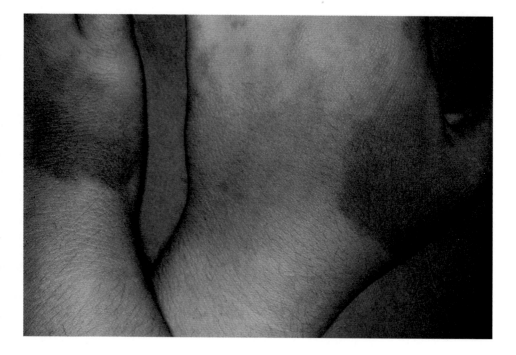

Drug-induced Hyperpigmentation

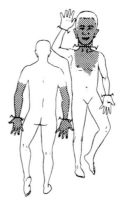

■ **Morphology**
Gray-blue to brown hyperpigmented macules.

■ **Distribution**
Dorsum of hands and other light-exposed areas. Increased pigmentation may be seen intraorally and in nail beds.

■ **Patient Profile**
Individuals have a history of chronic ingestion of chlorpromazine, chloroquine, silver (argyria), nose drops (argyria), gold (chrysiasis), amiodarone (especially nose), zidovudine (AZT), or bleomycin.

■ **Diagnosis**
Gray-blue to brown hyperpigmentation in a patient taking one of the above drugs that fades over months to years once therapy is discontinued suggests drug-induced hyperpigmentation. Brown, linear, irregular (flagellate) lesions are seen after systemic bleomycin therapy.

■ **Treatment**
Laser for dermal pigment destruction.

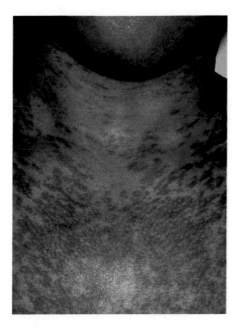

Freckle
(Ephelis)

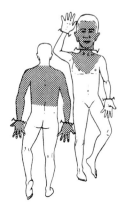

▪ Morphology
Numerous small, brown, nonscaly macules that become more prominent with sun exposure.

▪ Distribution
Lesions are most marked in sun-exposed skin.

▪ Patient Profile
Disease begins in childhood and affects both sexes. Patients have fair skin, blonde or red hair, and blue eyes. Often autosomal dominant trait. Lesions become prominent with sun exposure and fade with no sun exposure.

▪ Diagnosis
Freckles fade with lack of sun exposure; lentigos persist all year.

▪ Treatment
Sunscreens for prevention.

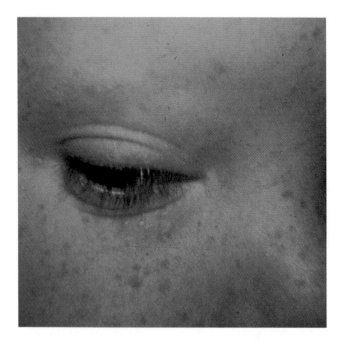

Lentigo Maligna

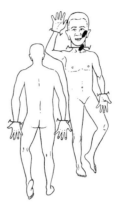

■ **Morphology**
Macules have variation in pigmentation. Lesions contain brown, blue, and black pigment that may have a reticulated or stippled pattern. Borders are frequently jagged and irregular. Fine skin markings are retained.

■ **Distribution**
Sun-exposed areas, especially face and neck.

■ **Patient Profile**
Usually older, fair-skinned individuals of both sexes. Lesions begin as flat, uniformly brown, and sharply circumscribed and develop mottling of pigmentation and irregularity of border. As the lesion enlarges, variation in color occurs.

■ **Diagnosis**
Lentigo maligna is a premalignant lesion that may go on to develop lentigo maligna melanoma. It is differentiated from lentigo by its variation in pigment. Biopsy reveals increased numbers of dysplastic melanocytes. The melanocytes are vacuolated, hyperchromatic, and limited to the epidermis. The upper dermis may contain melanocytes and inflammatory cells.

■ **Treatment**
Surgical excision.

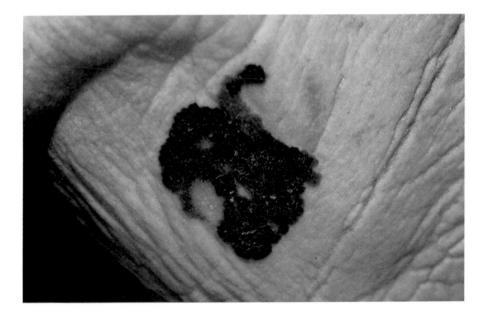

Melasma

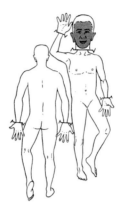

▪ Morphology
Blotchy, symmetric, nonscaly, hyperpigmented macules.

▪ Distribution
Forehead, cheeks, chin, and upper lips. Lesions are not usually seen on dorsum of hands or anterior chest.

▪ Patient Profile
Very common in postpubescent females but may rarely be seen in males. Hyperpigmentation usually occurs during pregnancy (mask of pregnancy) or while taking oral contraceptives. This lesion usually is not associated with endocrinopathy.

▪ Diagnosis
Patchy hyperpigmentation in pregnant females or in females taking oral contraceptives suggests this diagnosis.

▪ Treatment
Hydroquinone and retinoic acid topically. Sunscreens with UVA and UVB protection. Chemical peels.

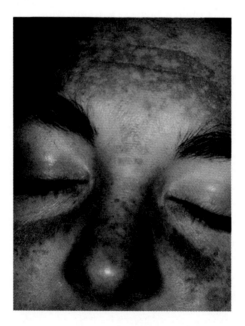

Xeroderma Pigmentosum

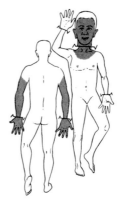

▪ Morphology
Multiple, frecklelike macular lesions in sun-exposed areas. Actinic keratoses (see p. 236), atrophy of skin, basal cell carcinomas (see p. 144), squamous cell carcinomas (see p. 263), and melanomas (see p. 146) are also found.

▪ Distribution
Sun-exposed areas of skin and lower lip and eye.

▪ Patient Profile
Lesions begin in early childhood. May be associated with mental retardation, neurologic disease, photophobia, excessive lacrimation, and prolonged erythema after sunburn.

▪ Diagnosis
Fibroblasts and lymphocytes in this disease demonstrate DNA repair defects after ultraviolet irradiation. Rothmund-Thomson syndrome does not have a DNA repair defect.

▪ Treatment
Sun-protective clothes, high-SPF sunscreens, and opaque sunscreens. Oral retinoids may retard appearance but do not prevent lesions.

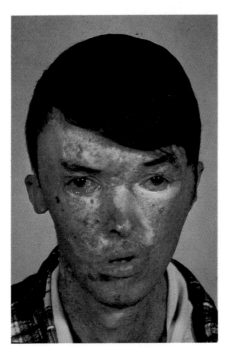

PURPLE MACULES AND PURPURA

DIAGNOSTIC OBSERVATIONS

Purpura results from blood leaking from vessels into the skin and mucous membranes. The hallmark of purpura is inability of pressure to blanch the red-purple lesion. Small lesions, <3 mm, are called *petechiae*. Larger lesions are called *ecchymoses*. Purpura goes through a series of characteristic color changes: Lesions begin as bright red or blue, then become purple, yellow, brown, and then fade. To diagnose purpura, a microscope slide is placed on the lesion and pressed firmly (diascopy). If a significant amount of red-purple remains, there is purpura.

Purpuric lesions may be flat or raised. Careful palpation of purpuric lesions helps to determine whether they are raised: Raised or palpable purpura indicates vasculitis. Palpable purpura may occur as a shower of numerous lesions or as sparse, scattered lesions. Almost all causes of palpable purpura are very serious. The physician should evaluate all patients with purpura for underlying disease.

Caput succedaneum: edema and purpura of the scalp in newborns due to trauma of labor

Dysproteinemia

Ecchymoses: trauma, senile purpura, venous stasis, clotting abnormalities, Cushing's syndrome, corticosteroid usage, chronic renal disease, primary amyloidosis, psychogenic purpura

Platelet abnormalities

Progressive pigmentary purpura

Scurvy

Severe physical exertion

Viral infections: Wiskott-Aldrich syndrome, histiocytosis X

Dysproteinemia

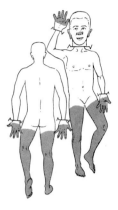

■ **Morphology**
Crops of petechiae and occasionally ecchymoses.

■ **Distribution**
Acral, lower extremities; sometimes ears and tip of nose.

■ **Patient Profile**
Profile depends on type of dysproteinemia.

Cryoglobulinemia: Associated with Raynaud's phenomenon, cold urticaria, dizziness, and epistaxis.

Hyperglobulinemic purpura: May be associated with arthritis, xerostomia, anemia, and hepatosplenomegaly.

Macroglobulinemia: Associated with dilated vessels and hemorrhage in the optic fundi, mental confusion, anemia, weight loss, hepatosplenomegaly, and lymphadenopathy.

■ **Diagnosis**
The finding of abnormal proteins by serum electrophoresis, immunoelectrophoresis, rheumatoid factor determinations, or presence of cryoglobulins establishes this diagnosis. Bone marrow biopsy is helpful with diagnosis of primary paraproteinemia with plasmacytosis. Skin biopsy reveals thrombi in dermal vessels that may be associated with leukocytoclastic vasculitis.

■ **Treatment**
Treatment for underlying disease may include plasmapheresis or antimetabolites. Avoidance of cold if cryoglobulins or macroglobulins are present.

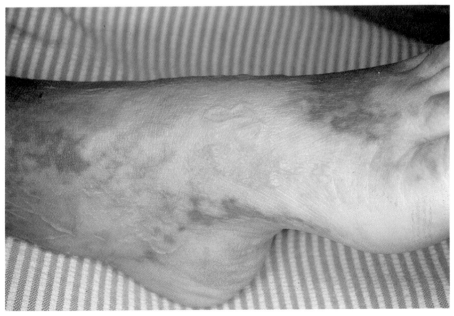

Cryoglobulinemia

Ecchymoses

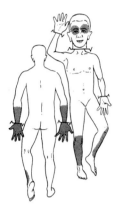

▪ Morphology
Red to blue macular plaques that are often geometric in shape and that become purple, yellow, brown, and gradually fade.

▪ Distribution
Anywhere.

▪ Patient Profile
Profile depends on cause. Includes all the causes of petechiae plus:

Trauma: It is the most common cause of ecchymoses.

Senile purpura: Condition is very common and occurs in older patients in areas of sun exposure.

Venous stasis: Condition is frequently associated with varicose veins. Petechiae and ecchymoses occur over the medial malleoli.

Clotting abnormalities: In young patients with numerous lesions, hemophilia, Ehlers-Danlos syndrome, and circulating anticoagulants associated with collagen vascular disease should be considered.

Cushing's syndrome and chronic use of topical or systemic corticosteroids: Both produce ecchymoses, thinning of skin, and atrophy.

Chronic renal disease: Ecchymoses may be linear because of scratching.

Primary amyloidosis: Patients with this condition have traumatic "pinch purpura," especially around the eyes.

Psychogenic purpura: Patients may traumatize their skin intentionally for secondary gain.

▪ Diagnosis
Skin biopsy is not helpful except in amyloidosis. A search should be made for the etiologies suggested above in patients with extensive purpura.

▪ Treatment
Decreasing trauma. Minimizing corticosteroid usage.

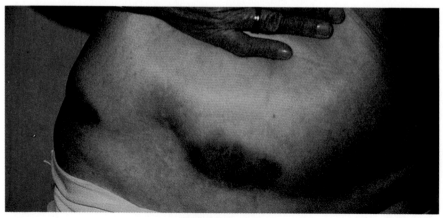

Psychogenic purpura

Platelet Abnormalities

■ Morphology
Red, flat, nonblanchable petechiae. Petechiae may be associated with larger ecchymoses and oral blisters. Lesions may be in
straight lines in areas of trauma.

■ Distribution
Dependent, traumatized, or acral areas.
Petechiae may be found in mucous mem-
branes.

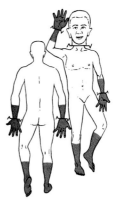

■ Patient Profile
Depends on underlying causes. Ingestion
of drugs, severe viral infections, β-hemolytic streptococcal infections, leukemia,
lupus erythematosus, idiopathic thrombocytopenic purpura, and paroxysmal noc-
turnal hemoglobinuria are prominent
causes of decreased platelet levels. Qualita-
tive platelet defects in thrombasthenia may
also cause petechiae. Severe physical stress
may induce petechiae without an underlying defect; for example, severe vomiting
may produce periorbital petechiae.

■ Diagnosis
All patients with petechiae should be
evaluated for platelet number and function. Von Willebrand's disease presents
with a similar clinical picture but is characterized by a deficiency of factor VIII and
vascular fragility.

■ Treatment
Treatment of underlying disease. Platelet
transfusions.

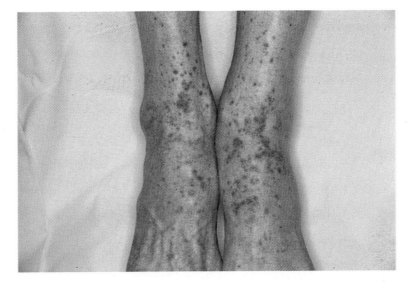

Progressive Pigmentary Purpura

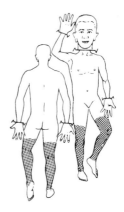

▪ Morphology
Reddish-brown, punctate, petechial lesions that become rust-colored to brown macules. May be pruritic. Lesions may be scattered and progressive (Schamberg's disease), annular (Majocchi's disease), associated with small lichenoid papules (Gougerot and Blum dermatosis), or itchy (Lowenthal's disease).

▪ Distribution
Symmetric. Usually confined to lower extremities; spares soles of feet.

▪ Patient Profile
Gradual onset with chronic course. Lesions usually asymptomatic.

▪ Diagnosis
Bleeding and clotting studies are normal, and skin biopsy reveals capillaritis.

▪ Treatment
Leg elevation, support stockings, medium-strength corticosteroid (class II to IV). Avoidance of aspirin and NSAIDs.

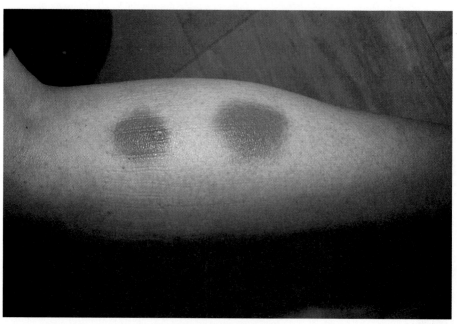

Schamberg's disease

Scurvy

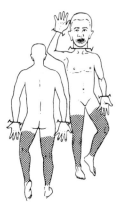

■ Morphology
Perifollicular petechiae are associated with keratotic plugs in hair follicles and tightly curled hairs.

■ Distribution
Symmetric; primarily lower extremities. Gums may be swollen and hemorrhagic. Petechiae occur on bulbar conjunctiva.

■ Patient Profile
Patients have inadequate intake of vitamin C. Children may have bone tenderness, epistaxis, and hematuria. Adults often have myalgia and fatigue.

■ Diagnosis
Low ascorbic acid in serum. Prompt correction with vitamin C is diagnostic.

■ Treatment
Ascorbic acid (1 g/day); restoration of proper nutrition.

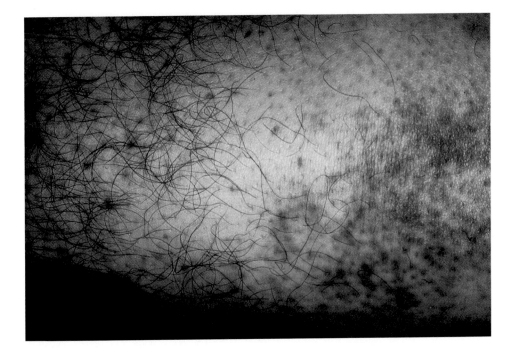

Viral Infection and Immune Disorders

Viral exanthems may become petechial. Measles; atypical measles; rubella; hepatitis; dengue; cytomegalovirus; echoviruses 4, 7, and 9; coxsackievirus A9, and respiratory syncytial virus infection have been reported to be petechial.

Wiskott-Aldrich syndrome: These diagnoses are suggested by the presence of petechiae in eczematous or seborrheic dermatitis-like lesions.

Histiocytosis X: Petechiae in young children may also be associated with histiocytosis X.

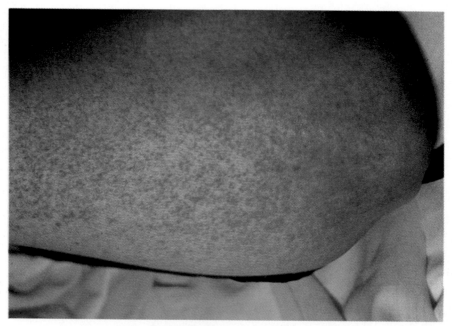

Purpura following a viral exanthem

RED MACULES

DIAGNOSTIC OBSERVATIONS
The lesions in this section are red, circumscribed, flat lesions. Red-blue color remaining after compression of a lesion indicates that blood is outside the blood vessels; this is known as purpura. Purpuric macules are discussed in the section on purpura (see p. 58). The number of lesions, a netlike reticulated or telangiectatic appearance of lesions, presence of fine scaling, and duration of lesions should be observed.

MAJOR CATEGORIES
Exanthems
Reticulated
Scattered
Telangiectasia
Transient

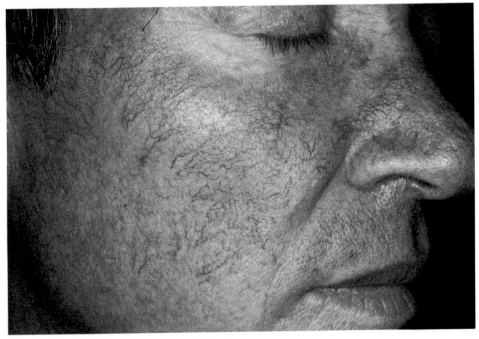

Telangiectases

Red Exanthems

DIAGNOSTIC OBSERVATIONS

These diseases present with the sudden appearance of multiple lesions. The physician should determine whether the patient has associated lymphadenopathy, prodrome, enanthem, or associated symptoms. Drug-induced eruptions must be considered in the differential diagnosis of all exanthematous eruptions regardless of the age of the patient.

MAJOR CATEGORIES

Exanthems with Adenopathy (Table 3–3)

Exanthems without Adenopathy (Tables 3–4 and 3–5)

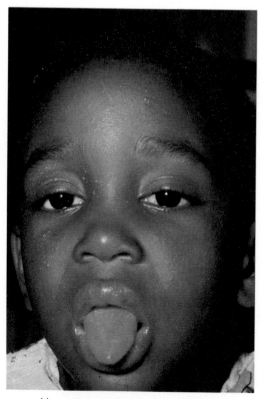

Mucocutaneous lymph node syndrome

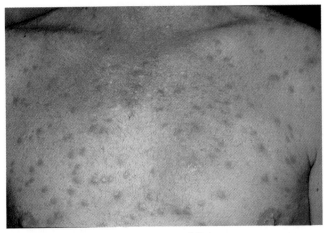

Secondary syphilis

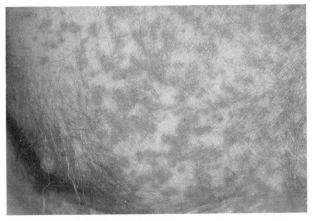

Drug eruption

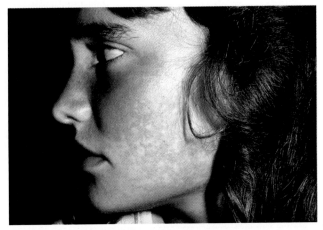

Erythema infectiosum

TABLE 3–3. Exanthems Associated with Significant Systemic Adenopathy

Disease	Time of Year	Age Range	Incubation Period	Prodrome	Enanthem
Brucellosis	Any time	Any age	5–30 days	Headache, malaise, and fever.	
Collagen vascular disease, systemic lupus erythematosus, rheumatoid arthritis	Any time	Usually children or young adults			May have oral lesions
Cytomegalovirus	Any time	Infants; patients on chemotherapy or after cardiac surgery and immunosuppression	Variable		Variable
Echovirus 16, Boston exanthem	Any time, epidemic	Children		Fever may precede eruption for several days. Eruption appears and fever abates.	No
Gianotti-Crosti syndrome	Any time	Young children		Fever, malaise, upper respiratory infection.	No
HIV infection, primary	Any time	Adults, most commonly	3–6 wks	Fever, lethargy, headache.	Erosions
Infectious mononucleosis	Any time	Young adults	7–21 days	Fever, malaise, myalgia.	Pharyngitis, petechiae at junctions of hard and soft palates
Mucocutaneous lymph node syndrome, Kawasaki's disease	Not established	Children		Hectic fever.	Redness of lips, strawberry tongue
Rubella, German measles	Spring	Childhood	12–25 days	Mild fever, headache, sore throat.	Petechiae on soft palate—Forchheimer's sign
Syphilis, congenital	Any time	Congenital	Days to wks	Fever, adenopathy, rhinorrhea.	White mucous patches on oral and genital mucosa
Syphilis, secondary	Any time	Any age	3 wks to 3 mos	History of chancre (see p. 464). In females, history of chancre may be difficult to obtain.	Mucous patches, oral and genital lesions
Toxoplasmosis	Any time	Congenital or acquired			

+/− Variable feature; + often present; ++ prominent clinical feature; +++ may be a major complaint.

Eruption	Petechiae	Fever	Other Clinical Features	Diagnosis
Macules and papules.		++	Hepatosplenomegaly.	Specific agglutinins.
Hivelike lesions, may have ringlike or arci-form configuration.	+/−	Variable	Signs of systemic lupus erythematosus or Still's disease.	Appropriate serologic tests.
Nondescript macular and papular exanthem.	+	+	Hepatosplenomegaly, thrombocytopenia, hepatitis, lymphocy-tosis, neurologic damage in newborns.	Viral cultures, serologic tests.
Vesicles rare.		+++		Viral culture.
Red papules on face, extremities, buttocks; become plaques and occasionally scales.		+/−	Hepatosplenomegaly.	Persistent skin lesions in a child with hepato-splenomegaly suggest this diagnosis.
Eruption, macules and papules.	Uncom-mon	+	Leukopenia, depressed CD4+ counts.	Isolation of HIV, p24 antigen in blood; sera-conversion by ELISA and Western blot.
Edema of upper lids, ery-thematous macules and papules. Skin rash common in patients who take ampicillin or allopurinol.	Uncom-mon	Yes	Hepatosplenomegaly, Guillain-Barré syn-drome, encepha-lopathy.	Atypical mononuclear cells or serologic test for mononucleosis.
Reddening and indura-tion of palms and soles, followed by desquama-tion, truncal maculo-papular rash.		Yes	Pyuria, leukocytosis, increased sedimenta-tion rate, injection of bulbar conjunctivae, myocardial infarction, thrombocytosis, coro-nary artery aneurysms.	Common in Japan, but worldwide. Staph exo-toxin responsible for many features.
Begins on face and rap-idly spreads down to trunk in hours, clears in same progression; to-tal course 2–3 days.		Mild	Encephalitis, monoar-ticular arthritis in adult females. Congenital rubella syndrome if mother infected during first trimester.	Antibody titers.
Sharply circumscribed, erythematous macules and papules on entire body, especially palms and soles. May blister in babies.	Uncom-mon	+	Hepatosplenomegaly, hepatitis, neuritis, meningitis, periostitis.	Serologic test for syphilis, dark-field examination.
Sharply circumscribed, ham-colored papules with slight scale, lesions over entire body but especially palms and soles.	Uncom-mon	+	Hepatosplenomegaly, hepatitis, neuritis, meningitis.	Serologic test for syphilis, dark-field examination.
Macules, papules spare feet, palms, and soles.	++	++	Hepatitis, pneumonitis, meningoencephalitis, chorioretinitis.	Mouse inoculation, sero-logic tests.

TABLE 3–4.Common Exanthems Not Associated with Systemic Lymphadenopathy

Disease	Time of Year	Age Range	Incubation Period	Prodrome	Enanthem
Collagen vascular disease, systemic lupus erythematosus, rheumatoid arthritis, rheumatic fever	Any time	Usually children or young adults	—	—	May have oral lesions
Drug-induced eruption	Any time	Any age	Days to mos	—	Unusual
Enterovirus, echovirus, or coxsackievirus	Late summer and fall	Children, but any age	1–2 wks	Fever, malaise, nausea and vomiting, diarrhea, meningismus	Occasionally, depends on specific virus
Erythema infectiosum, parvovirus B19	Sporadic	5–15 yrs	5–10 days	Uncommon, but sore throat and upper respiratory infection do occur	Uncommon
Infectious hepatitis	Any time	Any age	6 wks to 6 mos	Fever, fatigue, malaise, poly-articular arthritis	Uncommon
Measles	Winter, early spring	Childhood	10–14 days	Cough, coryza, conjunctivitis, fever	Suffusion of buccal mucosa, followed by white Koplik's spots
Rocky Mountain spotted fever	Spring, summer, and fall	Any age	3–12 days	History of tick bite, high fever, headache, malaise, arthralgia, photophobia	No
Roseola infantum (echovirus 16 may be very similar)	Any time	6–24 mos	5–15 days	Anorexia, restlessness, occasional vomiting, diarrhea	No
Scarlet fever	Winter	Childhood	2–4 days	Fever, headache, sore throat, nausea and vomiting	Injected, purulent sore throat with petechiae, strawberry tongue

+/− Variable feature; + often present; ++ prominent clinical feature; +++ may be a major complaint.

Eruption	Petechiae	Fever	Other Clinical Features	Diagnosis
Hivelike lesions, may have ringlike or arciform configuration.	+/−	Variable	Signs of systemic lupus erythematosus or Still's disease.	Appropriate serologic tests.
Symmetric macules or papules. May migrate. May be very pruritic.	No	Uncommon but occurs		All patients with exanthems should be carefully questioned about drugs.
Erythematous macules and papules begin on face and neck, spread to rest of body.	Especially coxsackieviruses A-5 and B-3	Yes	Headache, meningismus, diarrhea, myalgias.	Serologic tests. Patients with petechiae may mimic meningococcemia.
Eruption begins on cheek with slapped-face appearance. Spares bridge of nose and perioral area. Lacelike reticulated lesions on trunk, extensor arms, and thighs. May remit and exacerbate over 2-wk period.	No	Variable	Aplastic crisis in those with hemolytic anemias. Fetal death. Acute arthralgia in adults.	Clinical. ELISA and B19 DNA determination by polymerase chain reaction.
Measleslike rash or hivelike rash.	+/−	++	Development of icterus, hepatic tenderness and enlargement.	Abnormal liver function tests and serology for hepatitis B.
Red macules begin on back of neck, then spread over face and upper trunk in 48 h. Lesions become papular and may be confluent over face. Fades over 3- to 5-day period.	Only when very severe	+	Encephalopathy, pneumonitis, thrombocytopenia, otitis media in infants and children.	Giant cells in secretions or biopsies, antibody titer.
Eruption 2–6 days after prodrome. Begins at wrist and ankles and goes to palms and soles, then centrally on face; becomes petechial.	+++	+++	Vasculitis, photophobia, hepatosplenomegaly, meningoencephalitis.	Weil-Felix reaction is positive for OX19 and OX2; complement fixation antibody and skin biopsy.
Fever defervesces, then 2–4-mm red macules appear on neck and posterior trunk; spares face and extremities.	No	Disappears before onset of rash	Occasional postoccipital lymph node.	Rash follows defervescence of high fever. Herpesvirus 6.
Erythematous papules: back of neck, axilla, groin, spreads to trunk. Face may be spared. Circumoral pallor. Fades in 3–7 days with scaling in sheets, especially on hands and feet.	Petechiae in flexural creases	+++	Rheumatic fever, erythema nodosum, erythema multiforme, vasculitis.	Throat culture for β-hemolytic streptococcus.

TABLE 3–5. **Uncommon Exanthems Not Associated with Systemic Lymphadenopathy**

Disease	Time of Year	Age Range	Incubation Period	Prodrome	Enanthem
Acrodynia	Any time	3 mos to 8 yrs	Swelling, cyanosis, coldness of palms and soles	No.	No
Infectious hepatitis	Any time	Any age	Variable	Malaise, fever, and loss of appetite.	Rare
Rat-bite fever (*Spirillum minus*)	Any time	Any age	1–4 wks after rat bite	History of rat bite. Healed wound becomes red and purulent, adenopathy develops.	No
Typhoid fever	Summer and fall	Any age	3–21 days	Diarrhea, fever, headache, leukopenia, splenomegaly.	No
Typhus		Any age	1–2 wks	Lice bites, high fever, headache, malaise.	No

+ Often present; ++ prominent clinical feature; +++ may be a major complaint.

Eruption	Petechiae	Fever	Other Clinical Features	Diagnosis
Palms and soles, red and scaly.	No			Urine mercury level elevated.
Red papules on trunk and proximal extremities, spares face.	Occasional	Occasional	Hepatitis, arthralgias	Liver function tests, hepatitis-associated antigen.
Sparse macular or papular rash.	No	++		Dark-field examination of pus reveals spirochete.
Rose spots, 10–100 erythematous papules periumbilically or on back.	Occasional	+	Septicemia, diarrhea, fistulae, meningoencephalitis, osteomyelitis	Stool cultures, blood cultures, serology.
Exanthem appears after 6 days. Begins on trunk and moves peripherally. Becomes petechial but not papular.	+++	+++	Central nervous system disease, uremia, bradycardia	Weil-Felix reaction, OX-2 negative, OX-19 positive.

Reticulated Red Macules

Erythema ab igne
Erythema infectiosum
Larva migrans
Livedo reticularis

DIAGNOSTIC OBSERVATIONS
Reticulated red macules are arranged in a broad, vascular, lacelike pattern.

Erythema Ab Igne

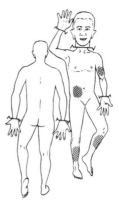

■ **Morphology**
Reddish-brown, reticulated, nonscaly, non-blanchable plaques. Telangiectases, keratoses, and squamous cell carcinomas may arise in these lesions.

■ **Distribution**
Symmetric; develops on shin but can occur on any heat-exposed area.

■ **Patient Profile**
Adult females who expose their legs to a heating fire or element. May also occur in blacksmiths and steelworkers.

■ **Diagnosis**
Biopsy reveals endothelial swelling, perivascular infiltrate, and melanin throughout the epidermis and dermis.

■ **Treatment**
Avoidance of infrared radiation to the skin by using firescreens and avoiding heating pads.

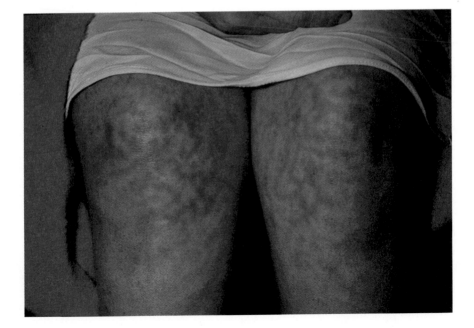

Erythema Infectiosum

▪ Morphology
Red lesions coalesce into large, red, swollen polycyclic or reticulated plaques with peripheral white rims.

▪ Distribution
Cheeks have a "slapped face" appearance. Extremities.

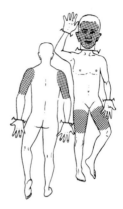

▪ Patient Profile
Children and young adults. Eruption lasts 6 to 10 days, and warmth or rubbing accentuates the lesions.

▪ Diagnosis
This viral illness caused by parvovirus B19 has a 6- to 10-day incubation period. This infectious exanthem is characterized by a reticulate pattern of erythema and is self-limited.

▪ Treatment
None necessary.

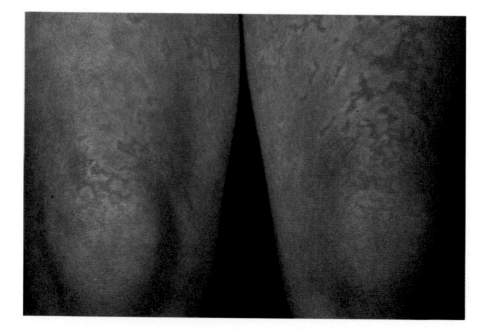

Larva Migrans

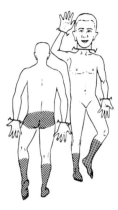

■ **Morphology**
Red, threadlike, serpentine lines, arcs, and loops that are about 3 mm in diameter. The lines extend a few millimeters to several centimeters per day and may have tiny vesicles, erosions, and crusts.

■ **Distribution**
Anywhere, but most commonly feet, legs, buttocks, and trunk.

■ **Patient Profile**
Any age, both sexes. Extremely pruritic lesions. Patient has usually been in a warm, moist, sandy area in Central America, South America, or the southeastern United States.

■ **Diagnosis**
This disease is caused by dog hookworm larvae migrating through the skin. Occasionally, a larva can be demonstrated by scraping the skin at the advancing border of the lesion or in a biopsy.

■ **Treatment**
Liquid nitrogen to advancing edge of lesion; topical or oral thiabendazole.

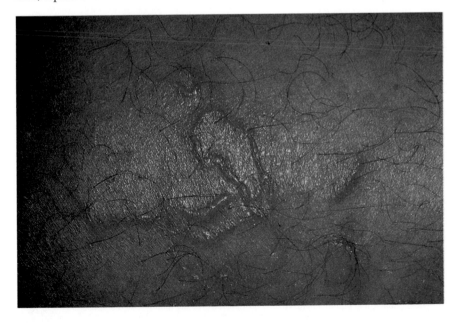

Livedo Reticularis

■ **Morphology**
Red-blue, netlike mottling that blanches on pressure and may last minutes to hours.

■ **Distribution**
Most common on lower extremities but can include the rest of the body, except for the face and neck.

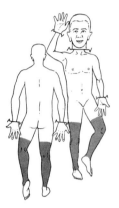

■ **Patient Profile**
Livedo may be either a primary event or secondary to an underlying disease. The patient profile depends on the cause.

Cutis marmorata: Occurs in newborn infants and is a physiological response to cold. This is more common in Cornelia de Lange's and Down syndromes.

Idiopathic livedo reticularis: Occurs predominantly in young adult females, with livedo exacerbated by cold. Lesions may be associated with tingling and burning. Cutaneous ulcerations sometimes occur with vasculitis. Some patients have circulating anticardiolipin.

The following diseases have been associated with episodes of livedo reticularis:

Arterial emboli, air emboli (decompression after diving)

Arteriosclerosis

Calciphylaxis: from calcified vessels associated with chronic renal disease (alteration in plasminogen activator inhibitor and proteins)

Collagen vascular disease: polyarteritis nodosa, rheumatoid arthritis, lupus erythematosus, dermatomyositis, rheumatic fever

Dysproteinemia and cryoglobulinemia

Pancreatitis, hyperparathyroidism

Syphilis, tuberculosis

Thrombocythemia

■ **Diagnosis**
The blanchable reticulate pattern is diagnostic of this vascular event. A thorough search for the cause should be made.

■ **Treatment**
Identification and treatment of underlying cause.

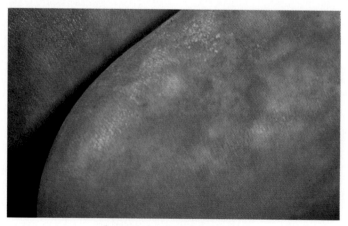

Systemic lupus erythematosus

Scattered Red Macules

DIAGNOSTIC OBSERVATIONS

These lesions are few in number and irregularly distributed. They evolve and often have anatomic distribution. Drug eruptions should always be considered when a patient has scattered red macules.

Atopic dermatitis
Burns
Cellulitis
Dermatomyositis
Drug eruptions
Erysipelas
Fixed drug eruption
Herpes zoster
Intertrigo
Leprosy
Lupus erythematosus
Seborrheic dermatitis

Atopic Dermatitis

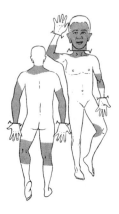

▪ Morphology
Red to red-brown, slightly scaly, poorly circumscribed lesions. There is accentuation of the skin markings, lichenification. Scratch marks and excoriations are common. Lesions may become infected and crusted. Lesions heal with hyperpigmentation and hypopigmentation. Edema of eyelids, conjunctivitis, and rhinitis are common.

▪ Distribution
Symmetric. Infants: cheeks, scalp, trunk, and lower legs. Children older than 4 years and adults: antecubital and popliteal space, thighs, and neck. At any age eruption may become generalized.

▪ Patient Profile
Lesions are extremely pruritic. Disease usually begins in infancy and early childhood, remits in late childhood, and flares up in adolescence. Lesions clear in many adult patients, but 40% persist. Many patients have asthma, rhinitis, and autosomal dominant ichthyosis.

▪ Diagnosis
Pruritic eruption in an atopic patient suggests the diagnosis of atopic dermatitis. Many patients have elevated IgE levels.

Biopsy reveals nonspecific psoriasiform dermatitis. Atopic eczema frequently becomes infected with bacteria and less commonly with herpesvirus (see p. 306).

▪ Treatment
Therapy is difficult. Systemic antihistamine to decrease pruritus; medium- to high-potency topical steroids (class II or III), oral antibiotics (antistaphylococcal), and mupirocin to nares, hydration, emollients, and avoidance of skin irritants. Refractory cases may need tars, UVB, and UVA.

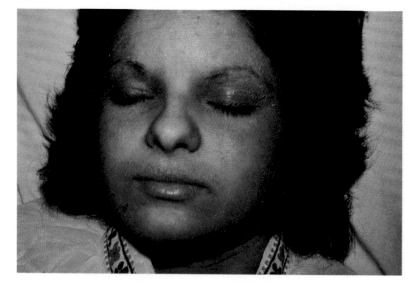

Burns

The early stage of a burn caused by the sun, heat, friction, or x-ray may appear as flat, red areas. Diagnosis is obvious, based on the progression of the lesion and patient history.

■ Treatment
Local skin care. Cleansing, moisturizers, and treatment of secondary infection if it occurs.

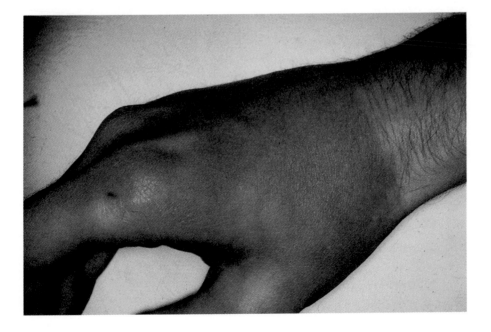

Cellulitis

▪ Morphology
Unilateral erythematous flat, tender lesion. In the case of a deeper infection, necrotizing fasciitis and purpura may be present.

▪ Distribution
Anywhere, unilateral.

▪ Patient Profile
Rapid onset of tender lesion often associated with fever. Occurs at all ages. *Streptococcus* and *Staphylococcus* are common causes. *Haemophilus influenzae* may cause cellulitis in children, although it is now rare with *H. influenzae* vaccine. In immunosuppressed patients, bacterial and fungal (*Cryptococcus*) organisms may cause cellulitis. Postoperative and diabetic patients at risk for necrotizing fasciitis.

▪ Diagnosis
Established by Gram's stain and culture from recovered fluid injected into the site. Culture and special stains of skin biopsy from the involved site may be necessary for identifying some bacterial and fungal organisms. Mixed anaerobes are common in necrotizing fasciitis. Eosinophils without organisms within lesions in Wells' syndrome.

▪ Treatment
Systemic antibiotics appropriate for the recovered organism.

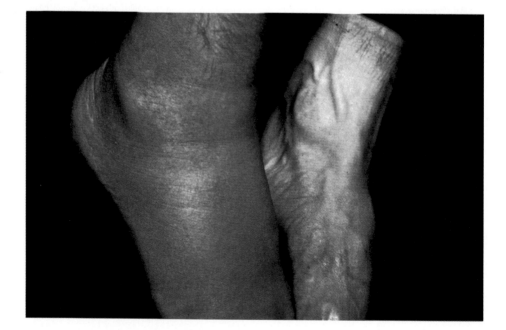

Dermatomyositis

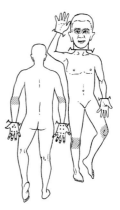

■ Morphology
Pink to bright red, poorly circumscribed oval lesions that may have fine scaling and atrophy.

■ Distribution
Symmetric. Periorbital and over extensor aspects of joints and extremities.

■ Patient Profile
Children and adults of both sexes. Lesions are nonpruritic. Proximal muscle weakness is almost always present, although the skin lesions may occur without muscle lesions.

■ Diagnosis
The combination of skin lesions and muscle weakness is very suggestive of the diagnosis of dermatomyositis. Careful muscle testing, electromyography, measurements of muscle enzymes, and muscle biopsy may be necessary to establish the diagnosis. Skin biopsy shows basal cell vacuolization, epidermal atrophy, and increased mucopolysaccharides in the dermis. Older patients with dermatomyositis must be carefully evaluated for associated malignancies, often adenocarcinomas, generally of a type common in individuals of the same sex without dermatomyositis.

■ Treatment
Systemic steroids are the initial form of treatment, to which antimetabolites may have to be added. UVA and UVB sunscreens. Immunoglobulin infusions are effective in some patients.

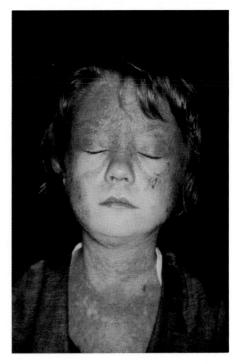

Erysipelas

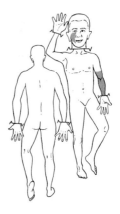

▪ Morphology
Red, warm, sharply marginated plaque that is indurated and may be painful. In more advanced lesions, purpura and vesicles may be seen.

▪ Distribution
Extremities, face.

▪ Patient Profile
Adults or children. Patient may be systemically ill with high fever and toxicity. Lesions are tender and rapidly change size within hours. Linear streaking from inflamed lymphatics may be present.

▪ Diagnosis
Erysipelas should be considered for any rapidly progressive, red, warm plaque. In older patients, the presentation is more subacute. Lesions can progress to streptococcal gangrene on the face or to cavernous sinus thrombosis. The cause of this disease is *Streptococcus hemolyticus*. Can occur in a linear pattern on the saphenous vein donor site for coronary artery bypass. In children, *Haemophilus* cellulitis may cause an erysipelas-like lesion. In immunosuppressed patients, *Cryptococcus* may cause an erysipelas-like illness. Diagnosis depends on demonstration of streptococci in aspirates of the lesion by Gram's stain and culture. Biopsy shows acute inflammation and organisms. Erysipeloid should be considered in hand lesions of people who have contact with fish or animals. In Central and South America, erysipelas-like lesions of the eyelid may be due to Chagas' disease. *Vibrio vulnificus* infection in those with liver disease or immunodeficiency produces cellulitis.

▪ Treatment
Systemic antibiotics.

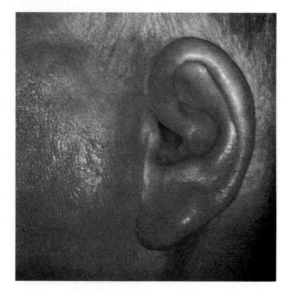

Fixed Drug Eruption

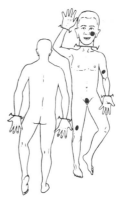

■ **Morphology**
One or more sharply marginated red plaques that may blister and that heal with marked hyperpigmentation.

■ **Distribution**
Anywhere, but commonly the extremities and genitals.

■ **Patient Profile**
Adults of both sexes. Patient ingests drug, especially ASA, NSAIDs, phenolphthalein-containing laxatives, barbiturates, tetracycline, and minocycline, and within several days develops lesions.

■ **Diagnosis**
Red lesions associated with drug ingestion and recurring in exactly the same location suggests this diagnosis. Provocative test with the suspected drug can confirm the diagnosis.

■ **Treatment**
Avoidance of the offending agents and its chemical congeners.

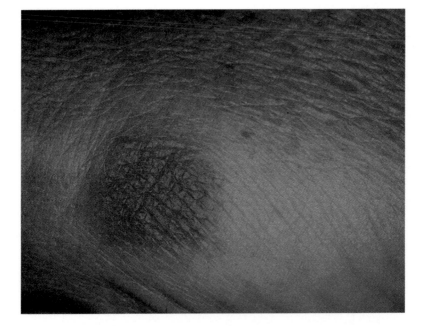

Herpes Zoster

■ Morphology
Grouped, flat, red lesions that become edematous papules and vesicles.

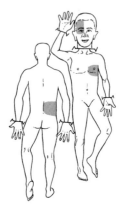

■ Distribution
Herpes zoster begins in a dermatomal distribution. Thoracic, cervical, trigeminal, and lumbrosacral involvement are most common. Ophthalmic zoster may involve the ciliary body and appears clinically as macules leading to vesicles on the tip of the nose. Vesicles or erosions in the mouth may be seen when the mandibular and maxillary branches of the trigeminal nerve are affected.

■ Patient Profile
The disease is most common in patients older than 40 years and in HIV-positive and other immunosuppressed patients. Frequently begins with pain and burning in a dermatomal distribution. After 3 to 4 days, groups of erythematous macules and papules erupt, which develop into characteristic umbilicated vesicles. Lesions and surrounding skin frequently are hypoalgesic or dysesthetic.

■ Diagnosis
Groups of macules in a dermatomal distribution are suggestive. Evolution of these lesions into umbilicated vesicles is diagnostic. Tzanck's preparation reveals multinucleated giant cells. Contact with herpes zoster through a previously infected patient can result in varicella. Biopsy shows reticular and ballooning degeneration of the epidermis, multinucleated giant cells, and intranuclear inclusions.

■ Treatment
Acyclovir (800 mg five times a day) until lesions are crusted, usually 7 to 10 days, or famciclovir (500 mg three times a day) for 7 days. Symptomatic pain relief.

Intertrigo

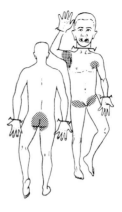

▪ Morphology
Pink to red lesions with slight scaling and erosions.

▪ Distribution
Skinfolds: under pendulous breasts, on obese abdomen, groin, buttocks, axillae; diaper area.

▪ Patient Profile
Obese patients with deep skin folds and poor hygiene. Young babies, especially those still in diapers.

▪ Diagnosis
Potassium hydroxide preparations are negative for fungus.

▪ Treatment
Local care, especially drying of the area, results in clearing of disease. Topical class IV to V corticosteroids are often helpful. Weight reduction in obese individuals.

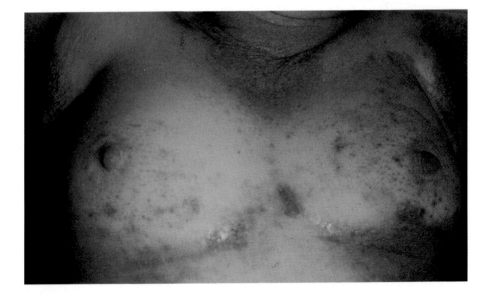

Leprosy

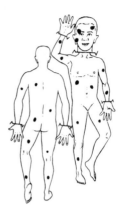

■ Morphology
Several poorly circumscribed, persistent, pinkish, flat areas.

■ Distribution
Anywhere.

■ Patient Profile
Young adults living in endemic areas for leprosy.

■ Diagnosis
Sensation may be normal in the indeterminate lesions of leprosy. Biopsy reveals a perivascular round-cell infiltrate. Organisms may be very sparse in the tissue.

■ Treatment
Antilepromatous drugs.

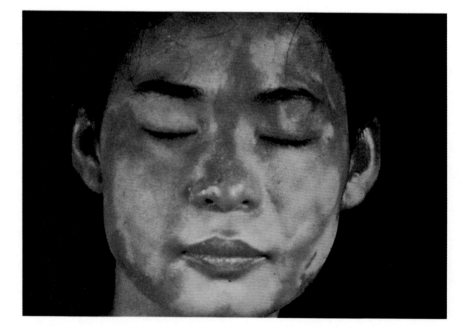

Lupus Erythematosus

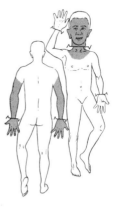

■ Morphology
Single or multiple sharply marginated red areas that have irregular fine scale. Loss of skin markings, hyperpigmentation, hypopigmentation, atrophy, and telangiectasia may be present. Nonscaling papules on the upper trunk in a reticulated pattern have been termed *reticulated erythematosus mucinosis.*

■ Distribution
Face, especially malar eminences; ears; scalp; sun-exposed areas of extremities, neck, upper chest, palms, and soles are most frequently involved.

■ Patient Profile
Most common in young adult women. Patients may have renal, rheumatologic, or neuropsychiatric disease in systemic lupus erythematosus.

■ Diagnosis
Biopsy demonstrates an atrophic epidermis, basal cell vacuolization, thickening of the basement membrane, and perivascular and periadnexal round-cell infiltrate in the dermis. Immunofluorescent examination of the skin reveals deposition of immunoglobulin and complement at the dermal-epidermal basement membrane.

■ Treatment
Complete evaluation for systemic manifestations is necessary. Antimalarials, systemic corticosteroids, and antimetabolites for patients with systemic involvement (kidney, central nervous system, lung) are often necessary. UVA and UVB sunscreens.

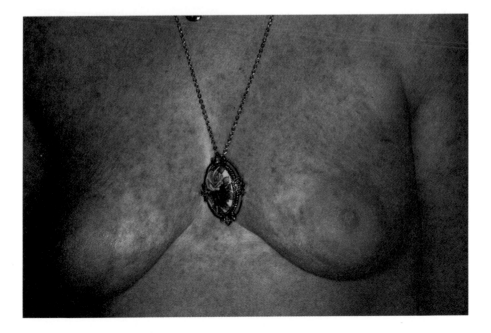

Seborrheic Dermatitis

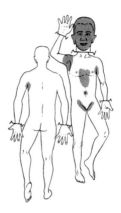

▪ Morphology
Poorly circumscribed, flat, red lesions with greasy scale. Discrete papules and sometimes pustules are seen. Secondary infection of the lesions with crusting may occur.

▪ Distribution
Symmetric. Scalp, eyebrows, eyelids, retro-auricular areas, cheeks, beard, anterior chest, axillae, and groin are most commonly involved. Seborrheic dermatitis may be generalized.

▪ Patient Profile
Both sexes. In early childhood, scalp is involved with cradle cap, as well as diaper area. In infancy, persistent, severe seborrheic dermatitis associated with diarrhea and deficiency of the fifth component of complement is called *Leiner's disease*. The presence of petechiae in severe seborrheic dermatitis in a young child should suggest the possibility of histiocytosis X. In adults, seborrheic dermatitis is very common; it is more severe in patients with Parkinson's disease. Seborrheic dermatitis flares up in HIV-positive patients with low CD4 counts.

▪ Diagnosis
Psoriatic lesions are sharply circumscribed, definitely raised, and the scale is whiter and more compact than that seen in seborrheic dermatitis. The biopsy shows a psoriasiform dermatitis and is not diagnostic.

▪ Treatment
Class II to III corticosteroids with class IV to V corticosteroids in intertriginous sites and the face. Topical ketoconazole alone or with corticosteroids can be effective. Tar- and sulfur-containing shampoos.

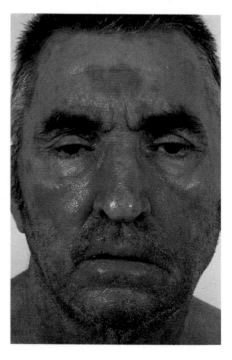

Telangiectasia

DIAGNOSTIC OBSERVATIONS

Telangiectases are flat and have a linear or netlike pattern. Telangiectases are permanently dilated blood vessels. The vessels are usually <1 mm wide and may be linear, pointlike (punctate), or starburst (stellate) in shape. When compressed, telangiectases blanch completely. They may be seen by themselves or associated with other skin signs. The associated skin signs and locations of the telangiectases are helpful in their differential diagnosis. Telangiectases are found in many normal people. They may begin in childhood and sometimes have a dermatomal distribution. Star-shaped telangiectases are usually above the waist, and gentle compression of the central punctum permits demonstration of pulsation. The appearance of many new telangiectases requires consideration of a variety of diseases or conditions, including pregnancy, liver disease, Cushing's syndrome, carcinoid syndrome, polycythemia, endogenous or exogenous estrogen, and rosacea. Congenital syndromes that may have telangiectasia with internal and especially neurologic involvement include neonatal lupus, Goltz's syndrome, and the Rothmund-Thomson syndrome.

MAJOR CATEGORIES

Telangiectatic Lesions without Other Skin Changes
Ataxia-telangiectasia
Essential telangiectasia
Hereditary hemorrhagic telangiectasia (Osler-Weber-Rendu disease)
Lupus erythematosus
Nevus flammeus
Posterior nail fold telangiectasia
Scleroderma
Telangiectasia macularis eruptiva perstans

Telangiectasia with Other Skin Changes
Actinically damaged skin
Atrophy from systemic or topical administration of corticosteroids
Dermatomyositis
Goltz's syndrome
Lupus erythematosus
Necrobiosis lipoidica diabeticorum
Poikiloderma atrophicans vasculare
Radiodermatitis
Rare childhood diseases with atrophy
Rosacea
Scleroderma
Telangiectasia and prominent hyperpigmentation

Telangiectatic Lesions without Other Skin Changes

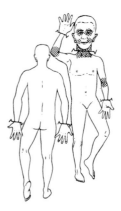

Ataxia-Telangiectasia

▪ Morphology
Fine telangiectases associated occasionally with sclerodermatous change on nose.

▪ Distribution
Symmetric; bulbar conjunctiva, pinna, face, neck, and antecubital fossa.

▪ Patient Profile
Autosomal recessive trait. Nystagmus and cerebellar ataxia usually begin at ages 2 to 3. Sinus and lung infections common. IgA and IgE are decreased; T-cell function is depressed.

▪ Diagnosis
Diagnosis made from clinical and laboratory findings. Rothmund-Thomson syndrome, Fabry's disease, and Bloom syndrome are extremely rare diseases that appear in childhood; telangiectases on the face comprise part of their clinical picture.

▪ Treatment
Telangiectases can be treated with a laser.

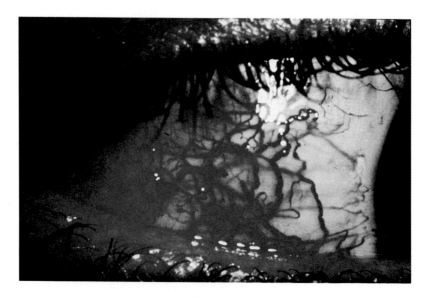

Essential Telangiectasia

■ **Morphology**
Numerous diffuse, fine telangiectases.

■ **Distribution**
Symmetric. Telangiectases often begin on thighs and spread to trunk.

■ **Patient profile**
Females, adolescence to age 50. May be familial.

■ **Diagnosis**
Diagnosis is made on the basis of clinical presentation and absence of other diseases.

■ **Treatment**
Laser.

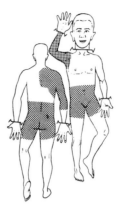

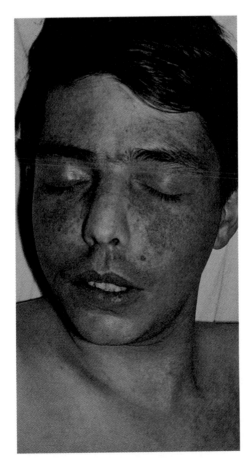

Hereditary Hemorrhagic Telangiectasia
(Osler-Weber-Rendu Disease)

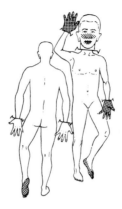

▪ Morphology
Punctate, linear, or polyangular lesions with an eccentric punctum.

▪ Distribution
Mucous membranes, especially nose and mouth. Central part of face, fingers, palms, and soles.

▪ Patient Profile
Autosomal dominant inheritance. Nosebleeds begin in childhood. Telangiectases appear in 20s and 30s. Gastrointestinal bleeding and pulmonary AV fistulae occur, as do cerebral abscesses.

▪ Diagnosis
Differential diagnosis includes the CREST syndrome of scleroderma.

▪ Treatment
Laser for cosmetic effects.

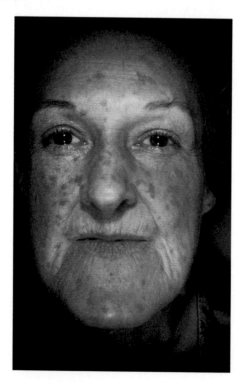

Lupus Erythematosus

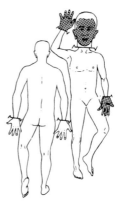

■ Morphology
Large telangiectatic macules. Erythematous, scaly plaques, hyperpigmentation and hypopigmentation, and atrophy are present.

■ Distribution
Especially palms, soles, and face but can occur anywhere.

■ Patient Profile
Patient usually has systemic lupus erythematosus with serositis, rheumatologic complaints, renal disease, and fever.

■ Diagnosis
Serologic tests for systemic lupus erythematosus (see p. 252) confirm the diagnosis.

■ Treatment
Systemic evaluation mandatory. Therapies include antimalarials, systemic steroids, and antimetabolites for patients with more systemic involvement. UVA and UVB sunscreens; sun-protective clothing. Isotretinoin and thalidomide have been used for more resistant cutaneous lupus.

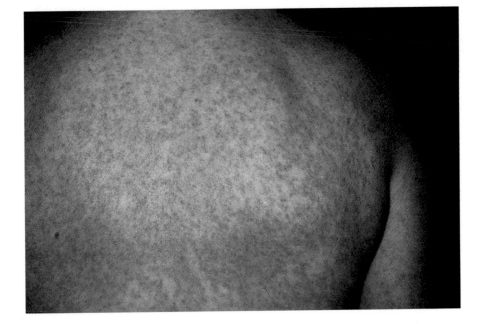

Nevus Flammeus
(Port-Wine Stain)

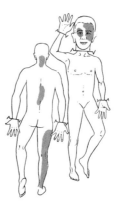

▪ Morphology
Flat, pink to blue, well-circumscribed lesions without distinct individual vessels.

▪ Distribution
Eyelids, nape of neck, mid-forehead. Lesions may occur in the distribution of the I and II branches of the trigeminal nerve (Sturge-Weber syndrome), extremities, or back.

▪ Patient Profile
Lesions are usually present at birth but may become more prominent during early childhood.

▪ Diagnosis
The common lesions (salmon patches, stork bites) over the eyelids, nape of neck, and forehead are usually pale pink, fade progressively with time, and are not associated with underlying disease. Lesions in a trigeminal distribution (*Sturge-Weber syndrome*) may become deep purple and develop purple papules within the lesion. Sturge-Weber syndrome is associated with glaucoma, cerebral angiomatosis (calcification on x-ray), convulsions, and mental retardation. In *Klippel-Trénaunay-Weber syndrome*, a port-wine stain over the limb may be associated with deeper vascular malformations and hemihypertrophies. *Proteus syndrome*, characterized by gigantism of hands, feet, or limbs and associated with lipomas, hemangiomas, lymphangiomas, and nevi, has been confused with neurofibromatosis.

▪ Treatment
Laser.

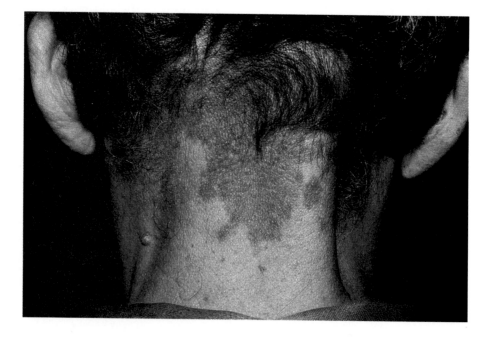

Posterior Nail Fold Telangiectasia

■ **Morphology**
Best seen with magnifying lens: Prominent dilated vessels with their long axes parallel to the axes of the digits are seen on the posterior nail folds of patients with systemic lupus erythematosus, progressive systemic sclerosis, dermatomyositis, rheumatoid arthritis, and Raynaud's syndrome. The presence of these vessels requires evaluation of the patient for these diseases.

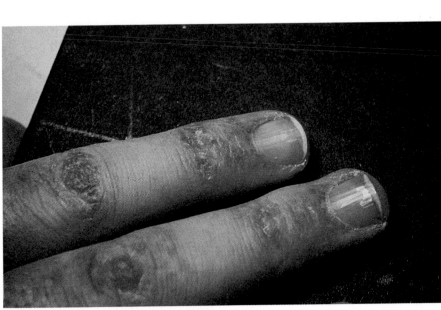

Dermatomyositis

Scleroderma

▪ Morphology
Square, oval, or polyangular, 1- to 6-mm telangiectatic macules that may have an eccentric punctum. Other signs of scleroderma are usually present.

▪ Distribution
Oral mucosa, face, palms, soles, nose, and subungual areas.

▪ Patient Profile
Patients often have hyperpigmentation in sun-exposed areas, calcinosis cutis, Raynaud's phenomenon, esophageal involvement, and sclerodactyly.

▪ Diagnosis
Biopsy demonstrates loss of skin appendages, increased collagen, and fibrosis of the subcutaneous fat. Laboratory studies that can confirm the diagnosis include positive antinuclear antibody (nucleolar or speckled pattern), abnormal esophageal motility, and decreased carbon monoxide diffusion capacity.

▪ Treatment
Laser for cosmetic effects.

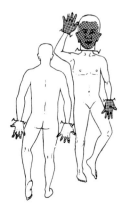

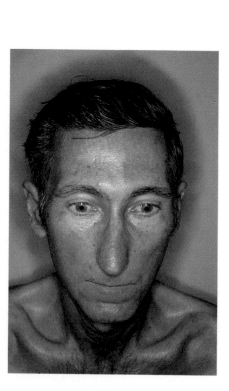

Telangiectasia Macularis
Eruptiva Perstans
(Mastocytosis)

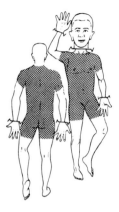

■ **Morphology**
Small red macules and groups of telangiectases with some hyperpigmentation.

■ **Distribution**
Trunk.

■ **Patient Profile**
Rubbing lesions causes hives to form (Darier's sign).

■ **Diagnosis**
Biopsy reveals infiltration of the skin with mast cells.

■ **Treatment**
Psoralens plus ultraviolet A, topical corticosteroids with occlusion. Antihistamines may decrease urtication. Lasers.

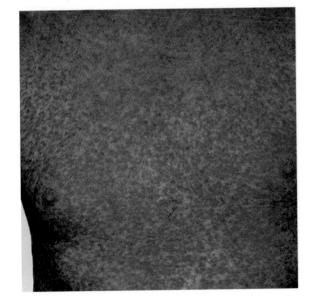

Telangiectasla with Other Skin Changes

Telanglectasia may be a prominent feature of certain skin diseases that are associated with atrophy.

Actinically damaged skin exhibits prominent telangiectasia purpura, yellow wrinkling, and hyperpigmentation.

Atrophy from systemic or topical administration of corticosteroids: Thinning of the skin, purpura, and telangiectasia characterize this lesion.

Dermatomyositis: Small telangiectatic vessels are seen in atrophic papules over the interphalangeal joints, elbows and knees, and diffusely around the eyelids.

Goltz's syndrome (focal dermal hypoplasia): Atrophy, bone and eye defects, and telangiectasia are the clinical features.

Lupus erythematosus: Frequently hyperkeratosis in addition to atrophy and telangiectasia. Neonatal lupus may have prominent telangiectasia.

Necrobiosis lipoidica diabeticorum: Discrete plaques with thinning of the skin, dilatation of blood vessels, and a characteristic yellow-orange color characterize this lesion.

Poikiloderma atrophicans vasculare: Lesions are similar to those of radiodermatitis with atrophy, hyperpigmentation, and hypopigmentation. The lesion is frequently associated with dermatomyositis or mycosis fungoides.

Radiodermatitis: Thinning of the skin, prominent dilated vessels, and hyperpigmentation and hypopigmentation are present in a lesion with a geometric border corresponding to an x-ray beam.

Rare childhood diseases with atrophy, telangiectasia, and hyperpigmentation: These diseases include xeroderma pigmentosum, Rothmund-Thomson syndrome, and dyskeratosis congenita. Patients with Cockayne's syndrome exhibit dwarfism, subcutaneous atrophy and telangiectasia on face, and photosensitivity.

Rosacea: Telangiectases are associated with red papules or pustules. Lesions are prominent over the cheeks, nose, and chin.

Scleroderma: Skin atrophy, sclerosis, and telangiectases are most prominent on face and hands but may involve all the skin.

Telangiectasia and prominent hyperpigmentation.

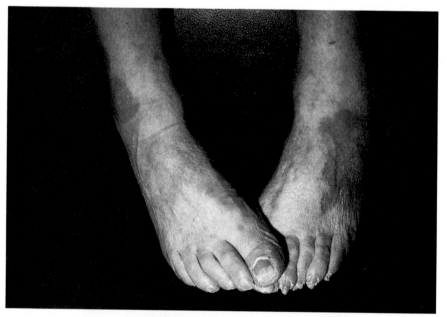

Necrobiosis lipoidica diabeticorum

Transient Red Macules

Cholinergic urticaria
Erythromelalgia
Flushing syndromes: carcinoid syndrome, pheochromocytoma, mastocytosis, nervous system diseases, Riley-Day syndrome
Juvenile rheumatoid arthritis (Still's disease)
Raynaud's phenomenon
Rheumatic fever
Transient erythemas of the newborn
Urticaria

Cholinergic Urticaria

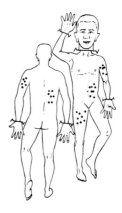

▪ **Morphology**
Flat, red base that may manifest small, minimally elevated, grouped white papules.

▪ **Distribution**
Anywhere, except on palms, soles, or mucous membranes.

▪ **Patient Profile**
Usually young adults of both sexes. Lesions are pruritic. Disease lasts for 1 to 3 hours.

▪ **Diagnosis**
Lesions are precipitated by heat, exertion, or emotional stress. Intradermal injections of methacholine (0.01 mg/0.5 mL saline) reproduce the lesion and pruritus.

▪ **Treatment**
Antihistamine 30 to 60 minutes before the activity that precipitates the lesions.

Erythromelalgia

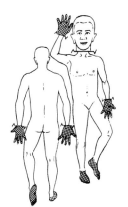

■ **Morphology**
Sharply marginated, erythematous, warm plaques on palms and soles.

■ **Distribution**
Hands and feet.

■ **Patient Profile**
Adults of both sexes. Attacks are triggered by warm environment, exercise, local heat, or standing. Disease may be primary or secondary to occlusive vascular disease, polycythemia, heavy metal poisoning, neurologic disease, lupus erythematosus, and gout. Acral erythema can be seen after bone marrow transplant, in graft-versus-host reaction, and after drug administration, especially doxorubicin (Adriamycin).

■ **Diagnosis**
Biopsy not diagnostic. Blood and platelet counts comfirm the diagnosis.

■ **Treatment**
Idiopathic form sometimes responsive to aspirin and NSAIDs.

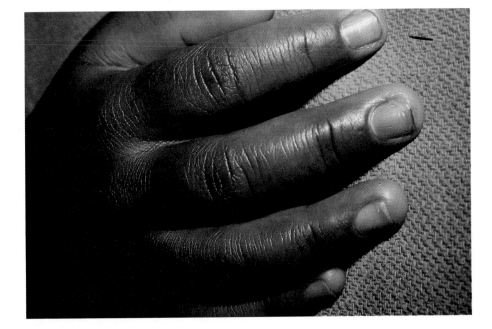

Flushing Syndromes

Red flushing on the head and neck is often provoked by emotional stress or stimuli such as menopause, drugs (amyl nitrite and nicotinic acid), and alcohol (especially in the presence of Antabuse, metronidazole [Flagyl], and vancomycin). Patients with rosacea have a tendency to flush. Asians and Native Americans have low levels of alcohol dehydrogenase or alcohol aldehyde dehydrogenase and are more susceptible to alcohol-induced flushing. Percutaneous absorbed thiram (in the rubber industry) has an Antabuse-like effect.

Organic causes of flushing are:

Carcinoid syndrome: Ileus, diarrhea, tachycardia, or asthma may accompany the flush. The flush is most prominent on the face and upper trunk. Flushing may be induced by ingestion of food and alcohol. Telangiectases, purple color, and scaling may occur around the eyes. 5-Hydroxyindoleacetic acid is increased in the urine.

Mastocytosis: Alcohol, polymyxin, or codeine may precipitate the flushing attack. The flush may last 15 to 30 minutes and can be associated with a vascular headache. Flushing may occur in patients without skin lesions who have GI mastocytomas. Biopsy reveals increased number of mast cells in the bone marrow. Urinary histamine metabolites and serum tryptase may be increased.

Nervous system diseases: Disorders of the trigeminal nerve may be associated with localized areas of swelling, redness, warmth, pain, and tearing.

Pheochromocytoma: Goose bumps, hyperhidrosis, and hypertension may accompany flushing attacks. Patients with flushing should have their blood pressure measured during a flushing episode. Elevated urinary catecholamine levels diagnose this condition.

Riley-Day syndrome: Erythema of the face and trunk, cyanosis of the extremities, corneal anesthesia, hyperhidrosis, hypertension, and absence of tearing are common features.

▪ Treatment

Treatment of underlying causes when found. Clonidine may benefit patients who experience idiopathic flushing attacks. Antihistamines (H_1 and H_2 blockers) may be useful for patients with mastocytosis.

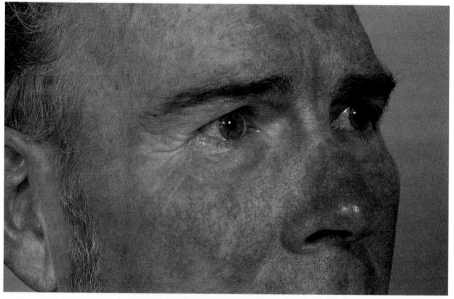

Carcinoid syndrome

Juvenile Rheumatoid Arthritis
(Still's Disease)

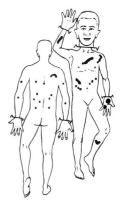

▪ Morphology
Discrete, small erythematous macules and papules that clear centrally and are induced by rubbing, scratching, or hot baths.

▪ Distribution
Trunk and proximal extremities but may occur on face, palms, and soles.

▪ Patient Profile
Children or young adults of both sexes. Rash occurs coincident with fever and may precede polyarthritis, lymphadenopathy, and splenomegaly by years.

▪ Diagnosis
Diagnosis is made on a clinical basis because routine rheumatoid factor tests may be negative in Still's disease.

▪ Treatment
Systemic evaluation before therapy is instituted.

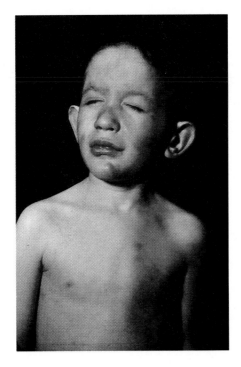

Raynaud's Phenomenon

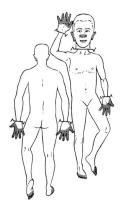

▪ Morphology
Cold, white areas of skin that become purple (cyanotic) and then red within several minutes. Periungual telangiectases, ulcers, and scars of digit tips may occur.

▪ Distribution
Fingers, toes, ear lobes, and nose.

▪ Patient Profile
Adults, more common in women than men. Asymmetric lesions or digital ulceration should suggest that the Raynaud's is secondary to an underlying disease. Diseases causing Raynaud's phenomenon include collagen vascular diseases, especially scleroderma; cryoglobulinemia or dysproteinemia; ingestion of ergots, heavy metals; exposure to vinyl chloride; thoracic outlet syndromes; or exposure to vibrating machines, such as jackhammers or chain saws.

Raynaud's phenomenon of more than 2 years' duration without an underlying cause is known as Raynaud's disease.

▪ Diagnosis
The sequence of episodic blanching, purple suffusion, and erythema after exposure to cold or emotional stress suggests the diagnosis of Raynaud's phenomenon. Erythromelalgia is characterized by red, warm skin.

▪ Treatment
Protective clothing, including two-layered gloves and gloves with battery-operated warmers. Topical nitroglycerin and some oral calcium channel blocking agents (e.g., nifedipine) are helpful. Biofeedback.

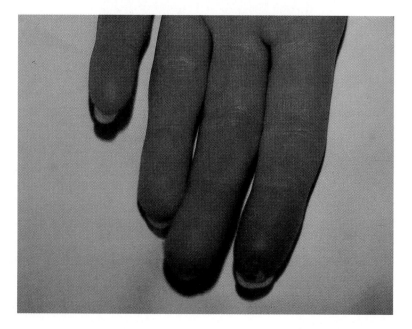

Rheumatic Fever
(Erythema Marginatum)

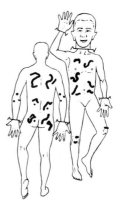

■ Morphology
Extremely evanescent, light pink to red. Arciform and oval nonscaly, hivelike lesions that may move from hour to hour.

■ Distribution
Trunk, axillae, and proximal extremities. Small, hivelike lesions occur over extensor aspect of elbows and knees.

■ Patient Profile
Children or young adults of both sexes with history of streptococcal sore throat, carditis, chorea, polyarthritis, or rheumatic fever nodules.

■ Diagnosis
This lesion is one of the major diagnostic criteria of rheumatic fever. Biopsy is not diagnostic.

■ Treatment
Antibiotics and NSAIDs.

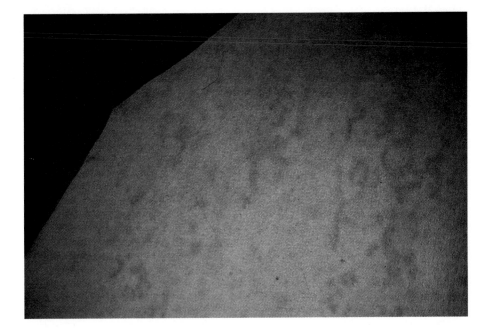

Transient Erythemas
of the Newborn

Erythema of the newborn: Transient erythema or harlequin color change is seen in the first few days of life. It may persist longer in premature infants.

Erythema toxicum neonatorum: Transient, often large, red urticarial lesions appear on the second or third day of life and may be surmounted by tiny vesicles containing eosinophils common in newborns.

Incontinentia pigmenti (p. 300): Transient erythema in arcuate or linear patterns may precede the vesicular lesions.

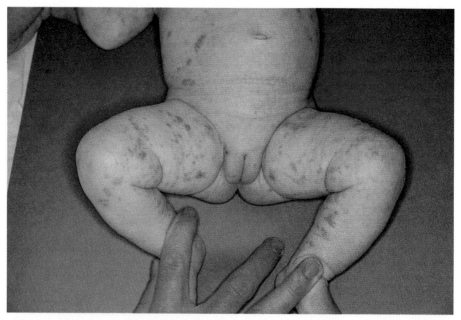

Incontinentia pigmenti

Urticaria (Hives)

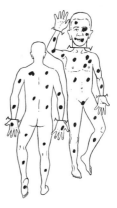

▪ Morphology
Erythematous, sharply circumscribed flat or elevated lesions. There is frequently a surrounding pale halo, and lesions do not scale. Lesions may range in size from 1 mm to many centimeters. They may be circular, annular, arciform, polycyclic, or geographic. Individual lesions last <24 hours.

▪ Distribution
Anywhere on body, including lips and tongue (angioedema).

▪ Patient Profile
Any age, both sexes. Lesions are frequently very itchy. Urticaria may be associated with ingestion of drugs (especially aspirin and penicillin), preservatives in foods (dyes and tartrazine), fish, nuts, and berries. Other common causes are acute infections, including infectious hepatitis, intestinal infestation, collagen vascular disease, insect bites, and physical factors such as heat or exercise, pressure, sunlight, cold, and water. Most cases are self-limited and disappear spontaneously. Patients with chronic urticaria should be carefully evaluated. Angioedema is characterized by diffuse swelling with minimal erythema.

▪ Diagnosis
Numerous transient lesions that come and go suggest this diagnosis. Cholinergic urticaria clears in 30 minutes to 4 hours. Acute: <6 weeks' duration. Chronic: >6 weeks' duration. Biopsy usually reveals dermal edema, vasodilatation, and sparse, perivascular round-cell infiltration. In patients with urticarial vasculitis, the individual hivelike lesions persist for more than 24 hours, and vasculitis may be seen on biopsy. These patients should be evaluated for hypocomplementemia.

▪ Treatment
Identification and elimination of the underlying cause. If respiratory distress is present, emergency treatment includes subcutaneous 1:1000 epinephrine (0.3 to 0.5 mL) and respiratory support. A short course of systemic corticosteroids (3 to 5 days) may be necessary. Daily antihistamines may be necessary for weeks to months. Chronic urticaria will require empiric trials of antihistamines and possibly allergen elimination.

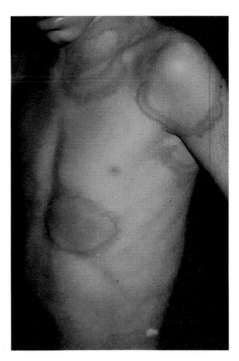

WHITE MACULES

DIAGNOSTIC OBSERVATIONS

To diagnose hypopigmented or depigmented skin lesions, note: age of onset, especially presence of lesions at birth; number of lesions; distribution of lesions, especially whether generalized or localized; and presence of associated lesions such as atrophy, scaling, other skin lesions, or changes in pigment of hair. The patient should also be examined with a Wood's light (black light) in a completely dark room. The Wood's light accentuates the decrease or absence of pigmentation and is especially helpful in evaluating patients with a fair complexion. It is also helpful in distinguishing conditions with partial depigmentation from those with complete depigmentation, because the latter condition shows milk-white fluorescence.

MAJOR CATEGORIES

Congenital or Genetic

Generalized
Albinism: Chédiak-Higashi syndrome, phenylketonuria, vitiligo

Localized
Nevus anemicus
Piebaldism: Waardenburg's syndrome, deafness, and piebaldism syndromes
Tuberous sclerosis
Other causes of hypopigmentation: dyskeratosis congenita, incontinentia pigmenti achromians, nevus depigmentosus

Acquired

Nonatrophic
Halo nevus
Pityriasis alba
Postinflammatory hypopigmentation: arsenical hypopigmentation, chemical depigmentation, idiopathic guttate hypomelanosis, leprosy, pinta, kwashiorkor, sarcoidosis
Tinea versicolor
Vitiligo

Atrophic
Discoid lupus erythematosus
Lichen sclerosus et atrophicus
Malignant atrophic papulosis
Poikiloderma vasculare atrophicans
Potent topical steroid use (atrophy)
Scleroderma, morphea
Sclerosis, scar, morphea
X-ray dermatitis

Generalized Congenital or Genetic White Macules

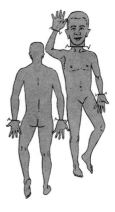

Albinism

■ **Morphology**

Total body depigmentation. White or golden hair is common, as are light blue irises that transilluminate and nystagmus.

■ **Distribution**

Entire skin.

■ **Patient Profile**

Congenital, both sexes, all racial groups. Patients are easily sunburned, and there is an increased incidence of skin cancers. Nystagmus, photophobia, and decreased vision are common. Albinism may be associated with deafness.

■ **Diagnosis**

Generalized depigmentation present at birth and associated with iris translucence is diagnostic of albinism. Examination with a Wood's light shows milk-white fluorescence. Hemorrhagic phenomenon may be seen in the rare Hermansky-Pudlak syn-drome. Inheritance is autosomal dominant or autosomal recessive. The molecular defect in tyrosinase and in tyrosine transporter proteins has been described. Patients may be true homozygotes for the same allele or compound heterozygotes for two mutant alleles. Biopsy reveals melanocytes that are devoid of melanin.

Among other rare causes of generalized hypopigmentation, the physician should consider:

Chédiak-Higashi syndrome: Moderate generalized hypopigmentation, gray

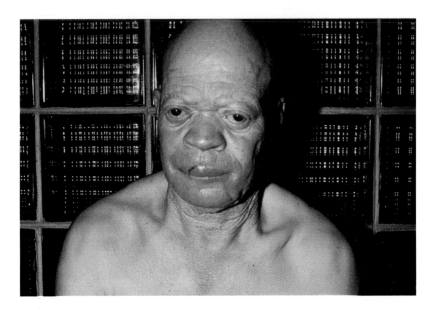

hair, recurrent infections, and hepato-splenomegaly characterize this syndrome. Giant granules are seen in cells.

Phenylketonuria: Moderate generalized hypopigmentation with eczema, seizures, and decreased mental and motor development characterize this condition. Positive urine test for phenylpyruvic acid with ferric chloride establishes this diagnosis.

Vitiligo: Generalized vitiligo can mimic albinism, but vitiligo is acquired, whereas albinism is congenital.

▪ Treatment
Sun-protective clothing and potent UVA and UVB sunscreens or opaque sun-protective screens. Routine visits for early diagnosis and treatment of malignant and premalignant lesions.

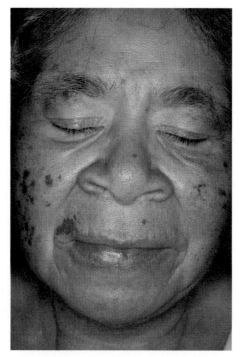

Vitiligo

Localized Hypopigmented Lesions

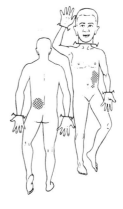

Nevus Anemicus

■ **Morphology**
Flat, usually single hypopigmented lesion with a jagged outline.

■ **Distribution**
Trunk is most commonly involved.

■ **Patient Profile**
Lesions present from childhood but often not recognized until adulthood. Asymptomatic.

■ **Diagnosis**
This hypopigmented area does not become red after rubbing, application of an ice cube, or injection of 0.1 mL of 1:1000 histamine. Biopsy is completely normal, and the lesion is due to vasoconstriction.

■ **Treatment**
Usually not necessary.

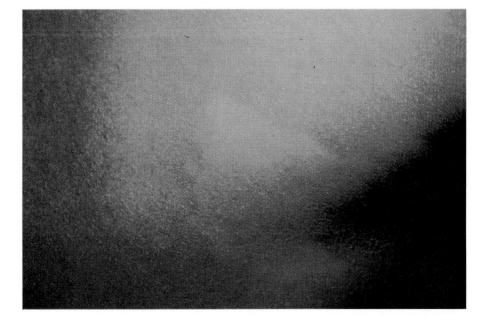

Piebaldism

▪ Morphology
Single or multiple symmetric, flat, stark white areas with jagged or geographic borders. The lesions may be from 1 cm to many centimeters in size. Localized areas of hypopigmented hairs (poliosis) may be present.

▪ Distribution
Lesions are frequently symmetric and located on face, scalp, back, and proximal extremities. There is almost always a stripe of normal pigmentation down the center of the back.

▪ Patient Profile
Congenital disease. Both sexes. Involved areas may sunburn easily.

▪ Diagnosis
White macules, present at birth, often in a symmetric pattern associated with a white forelock on the scalp suggest this diagnosis. Biopsy reveals a lack of melanocytes in affected skin. The presence at birth distinguishes it from vitiligo and postinflammatory hypopigmentation. Prenatal diagnosis possible based on molecular defect in c-*kit* oncogene.

Waardenburg's syndrome: Piebaldism, white forelock, neurosensory deafness, widening of the bridge of the nose with apparent lateral displacement of eyes, and heterochromia of the iris are seen in this autosomal dominant syndrome.

Deafness and piebaldism syndromes: X-linked, autosomal recessive, and autosomal dominant syndromes have been reported.

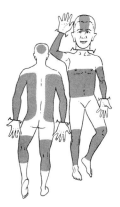

▪ Treatment
Early diagnosis of hearing disorder is important for adequate education. Lesions can be covered with cosmetic preparations or tattooing. Monobenzyl ether of hydroquinone can be used to depigment the remaining normal skin in those with extensive disease.

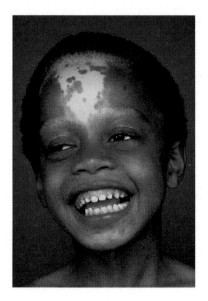

Tuberous Sclerosis

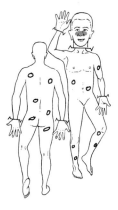

■ **Morphology**
Small (0.5 to 3.0 cm), flat hypopigmented areas with an oval or circular outline or numerous confetti-like hypopigmented lesions characterize this disease. Multiple, small, flesh-colored to red papules around the nasolabial fold (adenoma sebaceum) appear around the time of puberty. Raised, flesh-colored papules or plaques with accentuated skin markings (shagreen plaques) on the back and raised lesions on the forehead with epidermal accentuation may be present. Papules in the paronychial area are also seen. Poliosis (white hairs) may occur.

■ **Distribution**
Anywhere, but most commonly on trunk.

■ **Patient Profile**
Children of both sexes. White macules are present at birth. Seizures (hypsarrhythmia), mental retardation, and hamartomas in heart and kidney are common. Autosomal dominant, with frequent new mutations.

■ **Diagnosis**
Multiple hypopigmented lesions, present at birth, that are more prominent under Wood's light but do not show milk-white fluorescence suggest this diagnosis. Biopsy reveals normal numbers of melanocytes with decreased numbers of melanosomes. This lesion reddens with rubbing, whereas nevus anemicus (see p. 113) demonstrates no change in color with rubbing.

■ **Treatment**
None necessary for hypopigmented lesions.

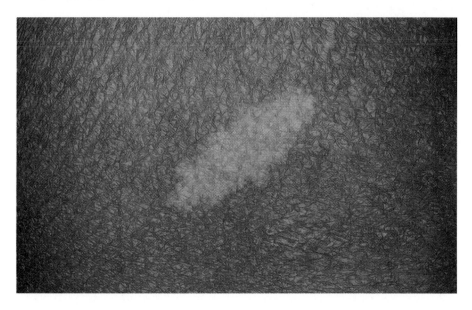

Ash leaf spot

Other Causes of Hypopigmentation

Dyskeratosis congenita: Hypopigmented oval to circular macules associated with hyperpigmentation, nail atrophy, scaling of the palms, lacrimal duct dysplasia, tearing, oral leukoplakia, and aplastic anemia characterize this syndrome. It occurs more frequently in males than in females.

Incontinentia pigmenti achromians (Ito): Large, hypopigmented areas in a swirl-like or geographic distribution appear at birth. They may be associated with underlying bony defects. Mental retardation and chromosomal abnormalities have been found.

Nevus depigmentosus: Large areas of hypopigmentation in a linear dermatome-like distribution appear at birth but may not be noticed until later in childhood.

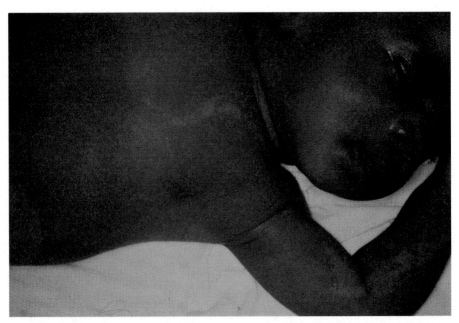

Incontinentia pigmenti achromians

Nonatrophic Acquired White Macules

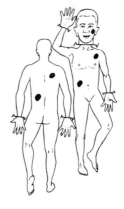

Halo Nevus

■ Morphology
One or more hypopigmented to white lesions that contain a red, brown, or black nevus in the center. Nevus regresses over several months and pigmentation returns.

■ Distribution
Anywhere, but most commonly on trunk and face.

■ Patient Profile
Any age but most common in adolescence; both sexes.

■ Diagnosis
Biopsy shows a dense lymphocytic infiltrate, melanocytes, and nevus cells. Rarely, malignant melanomas regress in a similar manner. In an adolescent with a typical halo nevus, biopsy usually is not necessary.

■ Treatment
Usually none necessary. Surgical excision may be necessary for diagnosis.

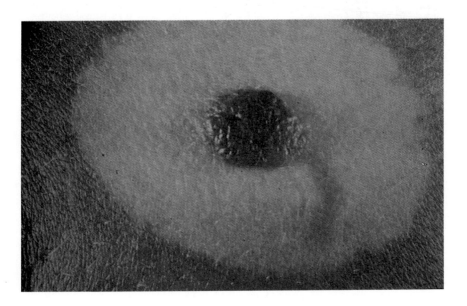

Pityriasis Alba

■ **Morphology**
Sparse, discrete, flat, scaling, hypopigmented areas with a poorly circumscribed
circular or oval outline.

■ **Distribution**
Most common on face and neck.

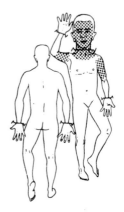

■ **Patient Profile**
Common in childhood. May be pruritic.
Associated with atopy.

■ **Diagnosis**
Biopsy is nonspecific. The location, seasonal incidence, and age of the patient
help to establish the diagnosis.

■ **Treatment**
Low-potency topical steroids, topical ketoconazole. Gradual repigmentation possible with sun exposure.

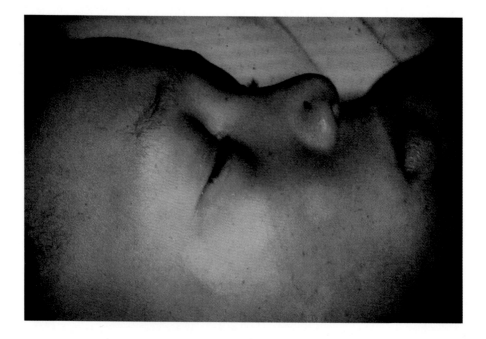

Postinflammatory Hypopigmentation

Many inflammatory dermatoses interfere with normal melanocyte function and produce macular areas of hypopigmentation with the distribution and shape of the original dermatoses. A Wood's light examination does not reveal milk-white depigmentation. For example, in syphilis, psoriasis, and atopic dermatitis, the hypopigmentation may persist for several months after the original lesion has cleared.

Arsenical hypopigmentation: This dermatosis is seen with chronic arsenic ingestion and consists of poorly marginated, pale areas on a hyperpigmented background. The back is most commonly involved and the lesions resemble "raindrops on a dusty road."

Chemical depigmentation: Exposure to monobenzyl ether of hydroquinone and phenolic compounds (especially cleaning solutions), topical corticosteroids, hydrogen peroxide, or catechols causes irregular hypopigmentation and depigmentation. Differentiation from vitiligo is often very difficult.

Idiopathic guttate hypomelanosis: This lesion is very common, especially in blacks. Extremities are most commonly involved with numerous small, polygonal lesions, many of which are a stark white. Hypopigmented macules of similar shapes are also present; their etiology is unknown.

Leprosy: Hypopigmented macules in tuberculoid or indeterminate leprosy will be anesthetic and do not develop an axon flare after histamine injection.

Kwashiorkor: This condition causes generalized hypopigmentation and decreased skin color. Evidence of protein malnutrition is present.

Pinta (p. 46): This infection causes mottled hypopigmentation; most patients are from Central and South America.

Sarcoidosis: The hypopigmentation may be present without other skin lesions. In patients with systemic involvement, biopsy of hypopigmented lesion may reveal granuloma.

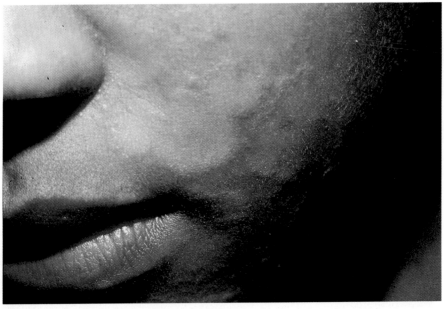

Sarcoidosis

Tinea Versicolor

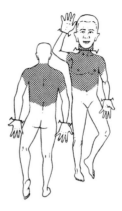

▪ Morphology
Flat to slightly elevated brown papules and plaques that scale when rubbed. Areas of hypopigmentation may be seen.

▪ Distribution
Upper trunk, shoulders, neck, proximal arms, occasionally face, and, rarely, below waist.

▪ Patient Profile
Common in adolescents and young adults of both sexes. Lesions may be slightly pruritic.

▪ Diagnosis
Lesion scrapings tested with potassium hydroxide preparation reveal large spores and thick hyphae.

▪ Treatment
Topical antifungals, short course of oral ketoconazole, selenium sulfide lotion to entire skin. Physician should advise that normal pigmentation returns slowly.

Vitiligo

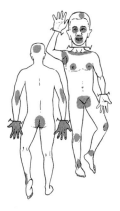

■ Morphology
Milk-white, nonscaly, variably sized flat lesions. Confluence of lesions may produce polycyclic arcs. As the vitiliginous lesion spreads into normal skin, the border is convex. Lesions may be red from ultraviolet light exposure. Hair in lesions of vitiligo may be white.

■ Distribution
Periorbital, perigenital, and dorsum of hands but may occur anywhere. Examination with Wood's lamp determines the extent of disease. This is especially important in lightly pigmented patients.

■ Patient Profile
Young adults and children of both sexes. Patients may have associated diabetes, hypothyroidism, Addison's disease, pernicious anemia, or candidiasis. Vitiligo may occur around nevi (halo nevus) or melanoma. A combination of vitiligo, uveitis, dysacousia, alopecia, and poliosis is called the *Vogt-Koyanagi-Harada syndrome.*

■ Diagnosis
Biopsy reveals absent melanocytes.

■ Treatment
A trial of high-potency topical steroids on selected lesions (class II or III) for several months is warranted, but not on lesions of the face or genitalia. Natural sunlight or PUVA therapy. Cosmetics to camouflage lesions. In extensive cases, monobenyzl ether of hydroquinone for complete depigmentation.

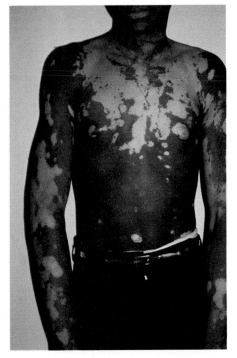

Atrophic Acquired White Macules

Lichen Sclerosus et Atrophicus ˋ

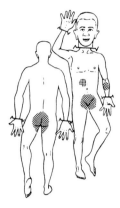

▪ **Morphology**
Grouped, sharply marginated, small, white spots that scale. Purpura may be present. Subtle thinning of epidermis with fine wrinkling.

▪ **Distribution**
Anywhere, but genitals most common.

▪ **Patient Profile**
Older adults, but this disease also occurs in children. More common in females than in males. Genital lesions may be pruritic. Increased incidence of carcinoma in genital lesions.

▪ **Diagnosis**
Biopsy is diagnostic and shows marked edema of the papillary dermis, sclerotic collagen, and loss of appendages.

▪ **Treatment**
High-potency topical corticosteroids. Application of 2% topical testosterone has been used with some success, as well as intensive PUVA therapy.

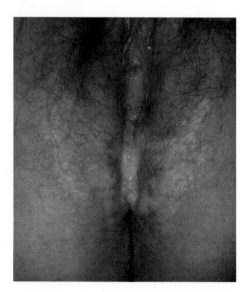

Malignant Atrophic Papulosis
(Degos' Disease)

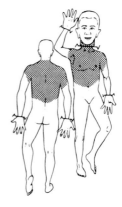

■ Morphology
Sharply circumscribed, porcelain-white atrophic lesions with a red rim. Lesions may begin as papules.

■ Distribution
Trunk, but can occur anywhere.

■ Patient Profile
Most common in adult men. Patients have abdominal pain and bowel infarction.

■ Diagnosis
Biopsy reveals thrombosis of dermal blood vessels and cutaneous infarction.

■ Treatment
None proven effective.

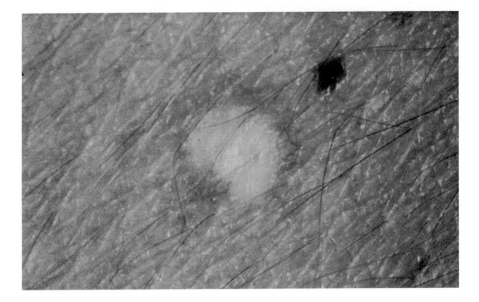

Scleroderma and Morphea

▪ Morphology
Droplike, small hypopigmented macules occur around hair follicles, producing a salt-and-pepper pattern. Cutaneous sclerosis, telangiectasia, hyperpigmentation, and ulcers also occur.

▪ Distribution
Anywhere, especially face and dorsum of hands.

▪ Patient Profile
Early lesions may be a sign of scleroderma and precede other cutaneous manifestations. Plaques of morphea (see p. 386) may be hypopigmented. They may also be seen in mixed connective tissue disease.

▪ Diagnosis
Biopsy shows increased collagen surrounding eccrine glands and increased dermal thickness. Careful examination for systemic stigmata of scleroderma is necessary. Tests for serum antinuclear antibodies, especially scl-70 and anticentromere antibodies, are frequently positive.

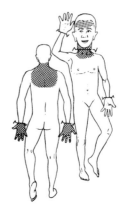

▪ Treatment
Penicillamine, systemic steroids, and photopheresis have been used with some success.

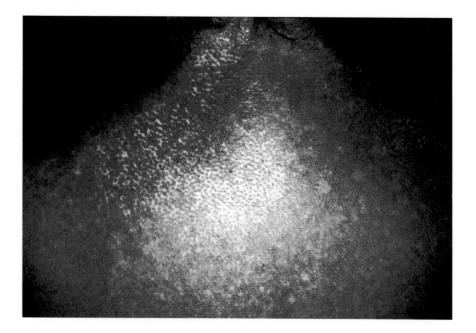

Chapter 4

■ ■ ■ ■ ■ ■ ■ ■ ■ ■ ■ ■ ■ ■ ■ ■ ■ ■ ■ ■

Diffuse Scaling Diseases

DIAGNOSTIC OBSERVATIONS

Diffuse scaling diseases are characterized by poorly circumscribed, diffuse scaling of the skin. The scale is usually white to brown. Scaling can easily be distinguished from crusting. Crusting or scabbing is the result of transudation of fluid and migration of leukocytes into the stratum corneum. Diseases causing sharply circumscribed areas of scaling over flat, red lesions are discussed in this section on red macules. Diseases causing sharply circumscribed areas of scaling over elevated red lesions are discussed in the section on red scaly papules (see Chapter 5, pp. 235–265).

Observe:

Color of scale

Size of scale

Location of scale, especially presence on palms and soles

Any family history of scaling

Generalized fine scaling may be seen during the resolution of a number of dermatoses, especially measles, sunburn, scarlatiniform drug eruption, and toxic epidermal necrolysis. It is common after scarlet fever and Kawasaki's disease; in those diseases, sheets of skin may be shed from palms and soles.

DIFFUSE SCALING OF PALMS AND SOLES

Arsenical keratoses (see p. 275)

Hereditary keratodermas (see p. 278)

Scaling without discrete papules (see p. 276)

Tyrosinemia II (see p. 280)

GENERALIZED SCALING

Epidermolytic hyperkeratosis

Erythema craquelé

Exfoliative dermatitis: acquired immunodeficiency disease, drug reaction, eczematous dermatitis, idiopathic dermatitis, lymphoma, mycosis fungoides, pityriasis rubra pilaris, psoriasis, seborrheic dermatitis.

Ichthyosis vulgaris

Lamellar ichthyosis

X-linked ichthyosis

Xerosis

Generalized Scaling

Epidermolytic Hyperkeratosis

▪ Morphology
Diffuse scaling and redness with wartlike papules, which may be arranged in rows, in the flexural areas. Vesicles and crusts may be seen.

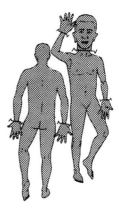

▪ Distribution
Generalized; accentuated in flexures and on palms and soles. Minimal involvement of face. No ectropion or oral lesions.

▪ Patient Profile
Present at birth; lifelong. Autosomal dominant with high spontaneous mutation rate. Mutations in keratins 1, 2, 9, and 10.

▪ Diagnosis
Scaling, redness, and blisters suggest this diagnosis. Biopsy is diagnostic with hyper-keratosis and foamlike cells within the granular and spinous layer. Prenatal molecular diagnosis is possible.

▪ Treatment
Increasing relative humidity in environment (e.g., bedroom at night); applying moisturizing agents (e.g., Aquaphor, propylene glycol; lactic-acid–containing preparations) after hydration of skin. Systemic retinoids can be used in postpubertal patients.

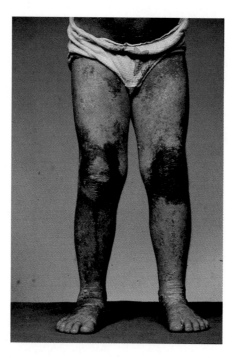

Erythema Craquelé

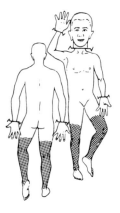

■ Morphology
Polygonal, large scales with sharp margins and redness between the scales simulating mosaic tile or cracks in dry mud.

■ Distribution
Anywhere, but usually most pronounced on the legs.

■ Patient Profile
Older adults. Lesions often pruritic. Common in winter when there is decreased relative humidity.

■ Diagnosis
Biopsy is not diagnostic.

■ Treatment
Increasing relative humidity in environment (e.g. bedroom at night); applying moisturizing agents (e.g. Aquaphor, propylene glycol; lactic-acid–containing preparations) after hydration of skin. High- to medium-potency topical corticosteroid ointments (class II to IV) may be necessary.

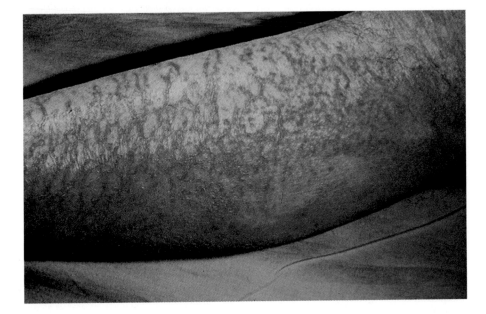

Exfoliative Dermatitis

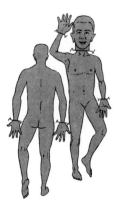

▪ Morphology
Generalized redness, warmth, and scaling. Alopecia (complete or partial), ectropion, subungual debris, and malformations of the nail plate may be present.

▪ Distribution
Symmetric. Generalized, including palms and soles. Mucous membranes uninvolved.

▪ Patient Profile
Usually adults of both sexes. Lesions often very pruritic. Patients may have adenopathy, chills, fever, poor temperature control, tachycardia, peripheral edema, gynecomastia, and high-output heart failure.

▪ Diagnosis
Generalized redness and scaling suggest this diagnosis. Presence since birth suggests the diagnosis of lamellar ichthyosis, epidermolytic hyperkeratosis, or congenital psoriasis. The multiple causes of exfoliative dermatitis include:

Drug reaction: Gold, penicillin, barbiturates, phenytoin (Dilantin), allopurinol are common. Any drug may be a cause.

Eczematous dermatitis: Atopic or chronic contact dermatitis (see pp. 243, 284).

Idiopathic dermatitis: Many patients with erythroderma may be followed up for many years without a specific cause being established.

Lymphoma (see p. 220).

Mycosis fungoides (see p. 253) cutaneous T-cell lymphoma.

Pityriasis rubra pilaris (see p. 256).

Psoriasis (see p. 258).

Seborrheic dermatitis (see p. 260).

Patients with the diagnosis of exfoliative dermatitis need a complete evaluation. Biopsy shows thickened epidermis with parakeratotic stratum corneum. Biopsy is not diagnostic of the etiology, except when the patient has mycosis fungoides.

▪ Treatment
Rapid control of condition is important to decrease systemic effects. Treatment of underlying disease. Corticosteroids (class I or II) under occlusion cause cutaneous vasoconstriction and a decrease in cutaneous blood flow, in turn decreasing cardiovascular strain. Systemic retinoids if psoriasis or pityriasis rubra pilaris is the underlying cause.

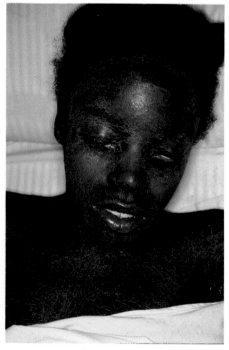

Drug reaction

Ichthyosis Vulgaris

■ **Morphology**
Fine, small, flaky, white scales with minimal underlying erythema. Increased palmar markings, scaling and fissures of the palms and soles are common.

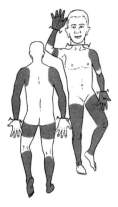

■ **Distribution**
Generalized with prominent lesions on the extensor aspects of limbs. Lesions often spare flexors. Palms and soles may have persistent, painful fissures.

■ **Patient Profile**
Very common disease. Usually starts in childhood, but rarely before the first 6 months of life; life-long. Worse in winter. Familial, with autosomal dominant inheritance. May be associated with atopic disease. Onset after the age of 30 is suggestive of acquired ichthyosis, which may be associated with malignancy and especially lymphoma. Patients with acquired ichthyosis require evaluation for internal malignancy and infection with human immunodeficiency virus.

■ **Diagnosis**
Onset during childhood, seasonal variation, presence of palm and sole fissures in a patient with fine, white scaling on the extremities strongly suggest this diagnosis. Biopsy shows a marked decrease or absence of the granular layer.

■ **Treatment**
Increasing relative humidity in environment (e.g., bedroom at night); applying moisturizing agents (e.g., Aquaphor, propylene glycol, lactic-acid–containing preparations) after hydration of skin.

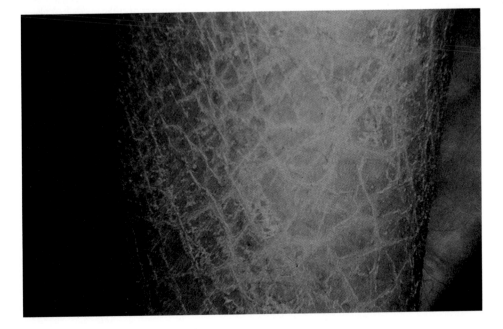

Lamellar Ichthyosis

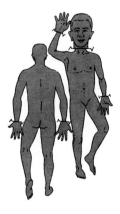

▪ **Morphology**
Generalized redness and scaling. Scales may be up to 3 cm in diameter and are detached at the periphery. Sclerodermatous tightening of the fingers with nail thickening and ectropion may be present.

▪ **Distribution**
Generalized but often worst on legs and scalp. Patients may have alopecia with scarring. Mucous membranes are normal.

▪ **Patient Profile**
Disease present at birth (collodion baby); life-long. Both sexes. Nonpruritic lesions. Autosomal recessive inheritance.

▪ **Diagnosis**
Presence of large, generalized red scales at birth suggests lamellar ichthyosis. Biopsy reveals marked hyperkeratoses, acanthosis, and normal granular layer. Many cases with deficient epidermal transglutaminase 1 because of gene mutations. Rarer forms of ichthyosis with this general appearance include:
Netherton's syndrome: Lamellar ichthyosis associated with broken-off bamboo hairs and atopy, including atopic dermatitis.

Nonbullous ichthyosiform erythroderma: Thinner epidermis, redder skin, milder ectopics than lamellar ichthyosis. No systemic effects.
Sjögren-Larssen syndrome: Lamellar ichthyosis associated with spastic diplegia and mental retardation.

▪ **Treatment**
In addition to aggressive hydration with thick emollients, postpubertal patients respond to systemic retinoids.

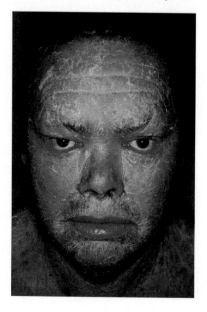

X-Linked Ichthyosis

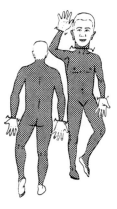

▪ Morphology
Circular, dirty-brown scales, 0.5 to 3 cm in diameter, that are attached centrally and detached peripherally.

▪ Distribution
Neck, shoulders, trunk, and extremities. Palms and soles may have hyperkeratosis.

▪ Patient Profile
Males. Disease begins during first year of life, afflicting most in the first month; life-long. X-linked. Worse in winter and may completely clear in summer. Patients should be evaluated for descent of the testes.

▪ Diagnosis
Biopsy reveals hyperkeratosis and a normal granular layer. Asymptomatic corneal opacities may be associated with this disease. Deficiency of cholesterol sulfatase in cultured fibroblasts confirms the diagnosis. Fast-migrating α-lipoprotein seen on lipoprotein electrophoresis.

▪ Treatment
Increasing relative humidity in environment (e.g., bedroom at night); applying moisturizing agents (e.g. , Aquaphor, propylene glycol, lactic-acid–containing preparations) after hydration of skin.

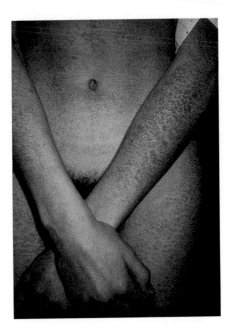

Xerosis

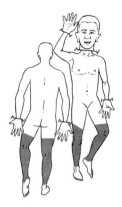

■ **Morphology**
Irregular areas of scale varying in size from 1 mm to a few centimeters.

■ **Distribution**
Anywhere, but most prominent on extremities, especially lower legs.

■ **Patient Profile**
Any age, but usually older adults. Disease most common in winter. Pruritic scales.

■ **Diagnosis**
Mosaic-like tile pattern of scaling without erythema associated with pruritus points to this diagnosis.

■ **Treatment**
Increasing relative humidity in environment (e.g., bedroom at night); applying moisturizing agents (e.g., Aquaphor, propylene glycol, lactic-acid–containing preparations) after hydration of skin.

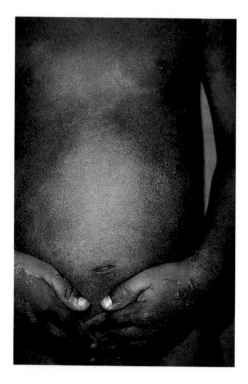

CHAPTER 5

■ ■ ■ ■ ■ ■ ■ ■ ■ ■ ■ ■ ■ ■ ■ ■ ■ ■ ■ ■

Papules

DIAGNOSTIC OBSERVATIONS

Papules are lesions that are raised above the skin. Plaques are papules or groups of papules >1 cm in diameter. Papules are differentiated from nodules by the observation that nodules are deep in the skin and the skin can be moved over the lesions, called the *iceberg phenomenon.*

Observe papules for the following characteristics:

Number

Color

Surface irregularities, especially scaling

Density of small lesions

Abrupt onset (over hours to several days) or gradual onset

Response to compression

MAJOR CATEGORIES

Blue-black

Brown

Flesh-colored, including linear and painful papular lesions

Purpuric papules

Smooth, red papules with abrupt onset

Smooth, red papules with gradual onset

Scaling papules

Yellow papules

Palm and sole papules with scaling disease

BLUE-BLACK PAPULES

DIAGNOSTIC OBSERVATIONS

These lesions are blue to blue-black in color.

Single
Atypical Nevi (see p. 149)
Blue nevus
Ecthyma gangrenosum
Foreign bodies
Giant comedone
Malignant melanoma

Multiple (Including Vascular Lesions)
Angioma (see p. 212)
Fabry's disease
Hemangioma (see p. 217)
Kaposi's sarcoma
Lichen planus
Malignancy (lymphoma, leukemia, mycosis fungoides)
Malignant melanoma (see p. 146)
Open acne comedones
Venous lakes and blue rubber bleb nevus syndrome

Single Blue-Black Papule

Blue Nevus

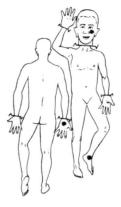

■ Morphology
Sharply circumscribed, slightly raised, blue papule up to several centimeters in size with a regular surface. Lesions are usually single.

■ Distribution
Face, lower arm, and hand, but may be anywhere.

■ Patient Profile
Both sexes. The lesion is asymptomatic and usually appears in children and young adults.

■ Diagnosis
Biopsy reveals normal-appearing dermal melanocytes, which differentiates this lesion from abnormal melanocytes of melanoma.

Giant comedones: Appear as blue-black papules. Pressure on sides of lesions extrudes a firm black mass and establishes the diagnosis.

Foreign bodies: Have a bluish hue and are minimally elevated. Sometimes history of trauma. Cutaneous osteomas may simulate these lesions but can be differentiated on biopsy.

■ Treatment
Excision is necessary if in doubt about diagnosis. Small, regular lesions on hands are usually benign and can be observed periodically.

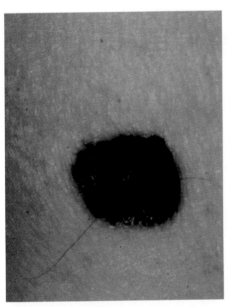

Blue nevus

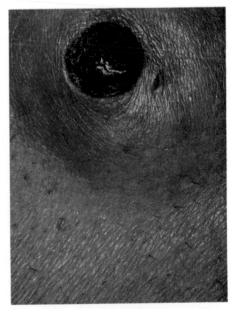

Giant comedone

Ecthyma Gangrenosum

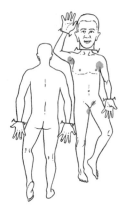

▪ **Morphology**
Bluish-gray, slightly elevated painless lesion. A blue-black eschar eventually develops on the surface of the lesion. Often single, sometimes multiple.

▪ **Distribution**
Often axillary or anogenital area.

▪ **Patient Profile**
Infants or adults with urinary tract abnormalities, hematologic malignancies, or immunosuppression.

▪ **Diagnosis**
Culture of the lesion is positive for the causative agent *Pseudomonas aeruginosa*. Biopsy of the lesion demonstrates a vasculitis and presence of gram-negative rods.

▪ **Treatment**
Systemic antibiotics.

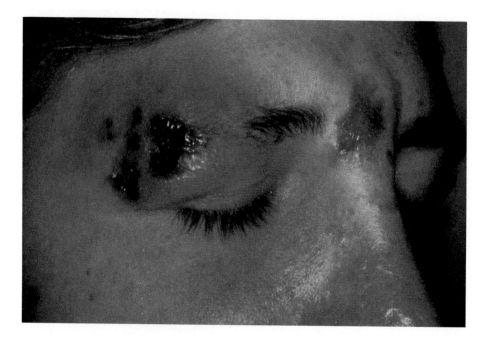

Malignant Melanoma

▪ **Morphology**
Irregularly pigmented blue-black papule with flecks of brown, red, and white pigment. The borders of the lesions are irregular and may be notched. Skin markings are altered. Examination with a hand lens often reveals irregularity of surface. Older lesions ulcerate and form nodules. Metastatic lesions may be multiple.

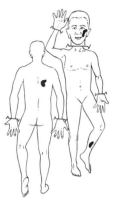

▪ **Distribution**
Anywhere.

▪ **Patient Profile**
Usually older patients of both sexes. Uncommon in blacks.

▪ **Diagnosis**
A raised, pigmented lesion with variation in color and border or alteration of skin markings requires a biopsy. Histologic examination demonstrates melanoma. Look for the ABCD changes associated with malignant melanoma: **a**symmetry, **b**order irregularity, **c**olor variegation (red, blue, white), and **d**iameter >4 to 6 mm.

▪ **Treatment**
Excisional biopsy. Prognosis is directly related to thickness of the lesions, determined microscopically. Patients with lesions <0.76 mm thick have over a 99% 5-year survival. Lesions <1 mm thick should be removed, with a 1-cm margin.

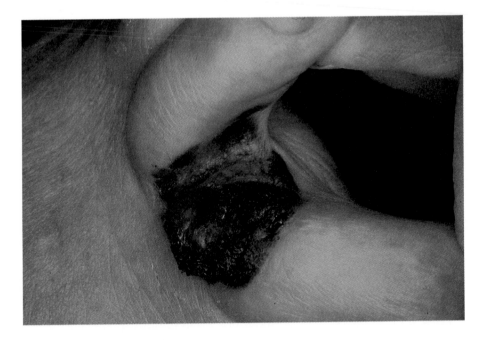

Multiple Blue-Black Papules (Including Vascular Lesions)

Kaposi's Sarcoma

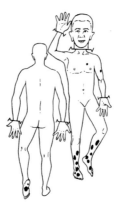

▪ Morphology
Purple-blue to red papules that decrease in size on firm pressure and return to original size over a period of 10 to 15 seconds. Lesions may have mild scaling, and they often go on to ulceration and bleeding. Lesions may be linear and arise rapidly in patients with AIDS.

▪ Distribution
Lower extremity in older patients. Anywhere, including the face and trunk, in HIV-positive patients.

▪ Patient Profile
Most common in older men and HIV-positive patients. Older patients often have bilateral edema of legs, adenopathy, gastrointestinal (GI) hemorrhage, and leukemia. In Africa, occurs in young adults. Immunosuppression in non-HIV patients can lead to Kaposi's lesions. Classic Kaposi's is more common in males and associated with leg edema and GI hemorrhage. Lesions grow slowly over months and persist if untreated.

▪ Diagnosis
Biopsy reveals proliferation of blood vessels with neoplastic endothelial cells. In older lesions, angiomatous proliferation or proliferation of neoplastic spindle-shaped cells is seen. Lymphangiosarcoma, malignant angioendothelioma, hemangiopericytoma, and multiple glomus tumors may mimic Kaposi's sarcoma. HIV testing recommended for all patients with this histologic diagnosis.

▪ Treatment
Cryotherapy, intralesional bleomycin, or radiotherapy is effective.

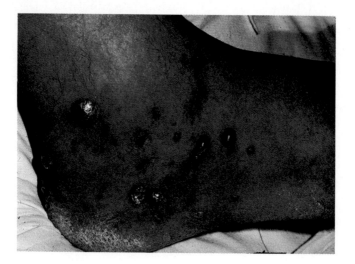

Lichen Planus

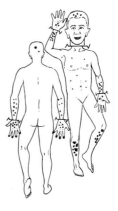

■ Morphology
Blue to purple papules that are discrete or confluent and that have reticulate white areas (Wickham's striae) and little or no scale. There may be diffuse hyperkeratosis on palms and soles. Hyperpigmentation, hypopigmentation, and atrophy also occur. Rarely, vesicles are present. There may be ulcers on palms, soles, and the oral and genital mucosa.

■ Distribution
Lesions are symmetric, on flexure surfaces, and are frequently linear or annular. Mucosal lesions (erosions or hyperkeratosis) are frequent in the mouth and less common on genitalia. Nails may have pits or grooves. Scalp may have scarring alopecia.

■ Patient Profile
Usually adults of both sexes. Duration of several months to several years. Pruritus (often severe) is common. Trauma or scratching may precipitate lesions (*Koebner's phenomenon*).

■ Diagnosis
Biopsy is diagnostic and shows hyperkeratosis, thickening of the granular layer, basal cell liquefaction, basement membrane thinning, and a bandlike lymphocytic and histiocytic upper dermal infiltrate.

■ Treatment
Class I or II topical corticosteroid can be used on skin and mucosal lesions. Severe generalized disease may require 3 to 6 weeks of oral corticosteroids until lesions have arrested, followed by tapering of steroids. UVB can control pruritus. PUVA therapy, isotretinoin (Accutane) useful for severe disease.

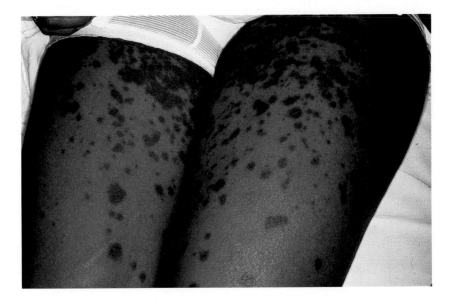

Malignancy
(Lymphoma, Leukemia, Mycosis
Fungoides, Metastatic Melanoma)

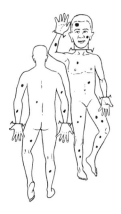

■ **Morphology**
Purple-blue papules, initially with normal
skin markings. Usually multiple. Scaling,
erosion, or ulceration may be present.

■ **Distribution**
Anywhere.

■ **Patient Profile**
Adults of both sexes. Lesions often erupt
in crops, grow rapidly, and persist if untreated. Stigmata of underlying neoplasm
(such as purpura), constitutional symptoms, organomegaly, and adenopathy often present.

■ **Diagnosis**
Diagnosis by biopsy with histology, depending on primary process. Febrile neutrophilic dermatoses (Sweet's syndrome)
and erythema elevatum diutinum may
resemble lymphoma.

■ **Treatment**
Systemic therapy of underlying diseases is
beyond the scope of this text.

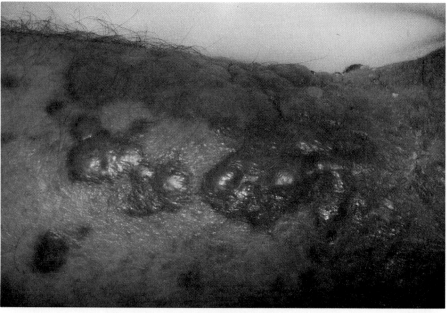

Lymphoma

Open Acne Comedones

■ **Morphology**
Small, blue-black, volcano-shaped papules. Lateral compression expresses cheesy, keratinous material. Papules, pustules, cysts, and oily skin are present.

■ **Distribution**
Face and upper trunk.

■ **Patient Profile**
Adolescents and young adults with acne. Elderly men have comedones associated with elastotic skin changes periorbitally (Favre-Racouchot syndrome). Open comedones are prominent in acne associated with greasy cosmetics and exposure to industrial oils. Often, deep black pigmentation of acne lesions after minocycline therapy.

■ **Diagnosis**
Blue-black lesions that exude material on lateral compression in patients with severe acne are open comedones.

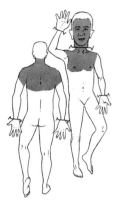

■ **Treatment**
Comedonal acne can be treated with topical antibiotics and desquamating agents (benzoyl peroxide gels 2.5% or 10% bid) and topical retinoic acid. Acne surgery.

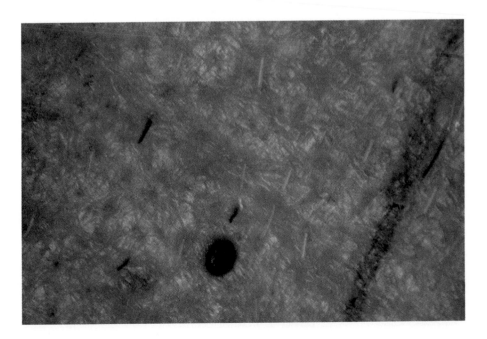

Venous Lakes

▪ Morphology
Blue papules, 5 mm to several centimeters in size. Lesions are compressible and lose their color and substance with pressure. Multiple or single.

▪ Distribution
Lips, face, anywhere on skin.

▪ Patient Profile
Very common in older patients. In younger patients, multiple lesions may be associated with GI lesions and bleeding. This is the blue rubber bleb nevus syndrome.

▪ Diagnosis
Biopsy reveals venous ectasia.

▪ Treatment
Often unnecessary. Electrodesiccation, laser, or excision may be used in selective cases.

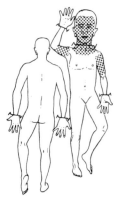

Venous lakes

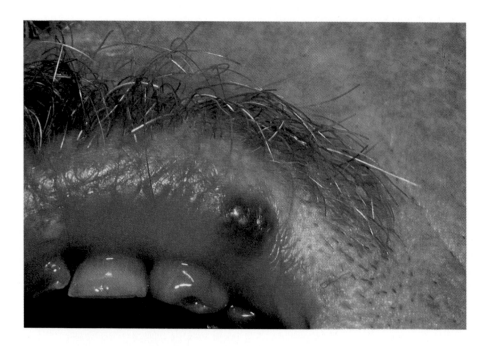

BROWN PAPULES

DIAGNOSTIC OBSERVATIONS

These lesions are definitely brown. Inflammatory red papules often fade to a red-brown color. Reddish-brown lesions are described in the red papule section (see pp. 189, 211). Multiple brownish-red papules of various sizes may be seen in a variety of diseases with dermal inflammation. Lesions often start as red papules. The epidermis is often intact. Biopsy with cultures, special stains, and a complete evaluation of the patient are necessary.

Single

Basal cell carcinoma
Dermatofibroma
Malignant melanoma
Mastocytoma

Multiple

Acanthosis nigricans
Atypical nevi
Cat scratch disease (see p. 460)
Deep fungal disease (see p. 459)
Foreign body disease (see p. 401)
Histiocytosis X
Lichen amyloidosis (see p. 265)
Leishmaniasis (see pp. 204, 423)
Mastocytosis (urticaria pigmentosa) (see p. 44)
Mycobacterial disease: including tuberculosis, atypical mycobacterial disease, and swimming pool granuloma (see p. 459)
Nevi
Porokeratosis
Sarcoidosis (see p. 170)
Seborrheic keratoses
Syphilis and yaws (see pp. 50, 461)
Tinea versicolor

Single Brown Papule

Basal Cell Carcinoma

▪ Morphology
Raised, translucent, brown-flecked papules that have dilated blood vessels around
the rim of the lesions. Ulcerations, flecks of
brown-blue pigmentation, scarring, or
slight scaling may be present. Normal skin
markings are lost. Some lesions have a
distinct, threadlike border. May be single
or multiple.

▪ Distribution
Usually sun-exposed areas, especially face
and neck, but may be anywhere.

▪ Patient Profile
Both sexes, usually beginning in middle
age. Basal cells are common in fair-skinned
individuals with outdoor occupations. Lesions are chronic and progressive. Rare in
blacks and Asians. Xeroderma pigmentosum and basal cell nevus syndrome are
two diseases with a tendency for increased
numbers of these lesions in young people.

▪ Diagnosis
This common lesion should be considered
in the differential diagnosis of all small
telangiectatic papules on sun-damaged
skin. All lesions should be blanched by
diascopy or the skin should be stretched to
demonstrate the translucent character and
demarcate the border of the tumor. Clini-

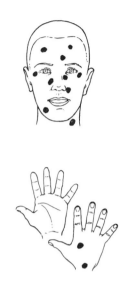

cally must be differentiated from an atypical fibroxanthoma. Biopsy shows proliferation of basal cells, stromal proliferation,
and retraction of the epithelium from the
stroma.

▪ Treatment
After biopsy, treatment with surgical excision, curettage and electrodesiccation, or
Mohs' surgery. Mohs' surgery is indicated
for recurrent lesions, lesions with morpheaform histology, lesions >10 cm, and tumors in areas of high recurrence rates,
such as the nose and nasolabial folds.
Radiotherapy is useful in selected cases.

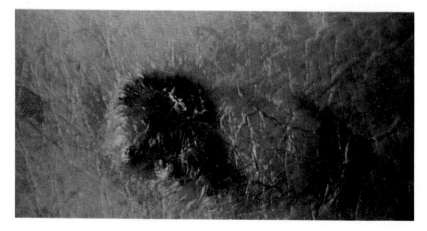

Dermatofibroma

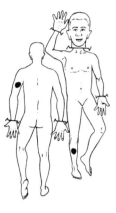

▪ Morphology
Firm, flat, rough hyperpigmented papules up to 2 cm in diameter. Compression around the lesion causes retraction beneath the skin (Fitzpatrick's sign).

▪ Distribution
Usually single, often 2 to 3 scattered lesions, rarely multiple. Extremities most common but may occur anywhere.

▪ Patient Profile
Adults. Very common lesion. Usually asymptomatic. History of trauma or preceding insect bite.

▪ Diagnosis
Biopsy reveals nonencapsulated, benign histiocyte, and fibroblastic proliferation with epidermal hyperplasia.

▪ Treatment
Liquid nitrogen, excision, intralesional steroids.

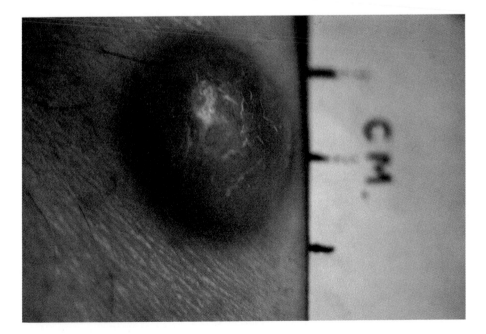

Malignant Melanoma

▪ Morphology
Irregularly pigmented papule with areas of brown, red, white, and blue. Usually single. The borders of the lesions are irregular and there may be notches. Skin markings are altered. Careful examination with a hand lens often reveals irregularity of surface. Older lesions ulcerate and form nodules.

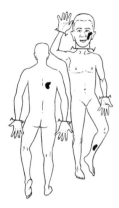

▪ Distribution
Anywhere. More common in females.

▪ Patient Profile
Usually older patients of both sexes. Uncommon in blacks.

▪ Diagnosis
A raised, pigmented lesion with variation in color and border or alteration of skin markings requires a biopsy. Histologic examination demonstrates melanoma. Look for the ABCD changes associated with malignant melanoma: **a**symmetry, **b**order irregularity, **c**olor variegation (red, blue, white), and **d**iameter >4 to 6 mm.

▪ Treatment
Excisional biopsy. Prognosis is directly related to thickness of the lesions, determined microscopically. Patients with lesions <0.76 mm thick have over a 99% 5-year survival. Lesions <1 mm thick should be removed, with a 1-cm margin.

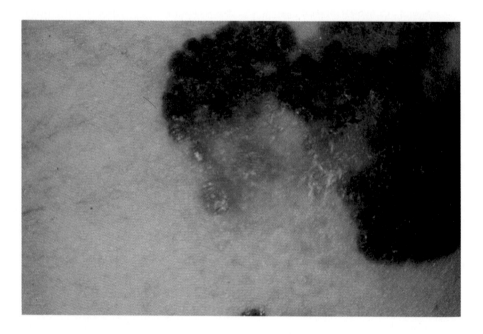

Mastocytoma

▪ **Morphology**
Brown, slightly raised papule that becomes swollen and red with rubbing. May blister in early childhood. Rarely associated with the development of multiple lesions.

▪ **Distribution**
Anywhere, commonly on the extremities.

▪ **Patient Profile**
Infants to children 3 years old. Histamine release from the lesion may cause tachycardia, blanching, or hypotension.

▪ **Diagnosis**
Production of erythema and edema within a few minutes in a brownish papule by stroking is diagnostic (Darier's sign). Biopsy shows toluidine-blue–positive intradermal mast cells.

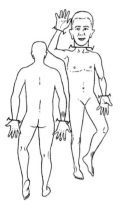

▪ **Treatment**
Ultra-high-potency topical steroids with occlusion overnight for 6 weeks. Intralesional steroids. Excision. Systemic antihistamines may be needed.

Multiple Brown Papules

Acanthosis Nigricans

▪ Morphology
Brown to black plaques with prominent skin markings, giving a velvetlike appearance. Skin tags associated.

▪ Distribution
Symmetric; axillae, neck, knuckle, and elbows. Oral or palmar hyperkeratosis suggests an associated malignancy.

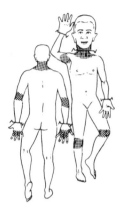

▪ Patient Profile
In younger age group, associated with obesity, endocrinopathy, and insulin resistance. In older patients, associated with adenocarcinoma (gastrointestinal tract). Syndromes associated with acanthosis nigricans include Lawrence-Seip, Rud's, Crouzon's, Bloom, Wilson's, Prader-Willi, ataxia-telangiectasia, and polycystic ovary disease.

▪ Diagnosis
Biopsy is nondiagnostic and demonstrates acanthosis of the epidermis. Patient should be studied for associated conditions.

▪ Treatment
Treatment of underlying disease. Topical 12% lactic acid or Retin-A.

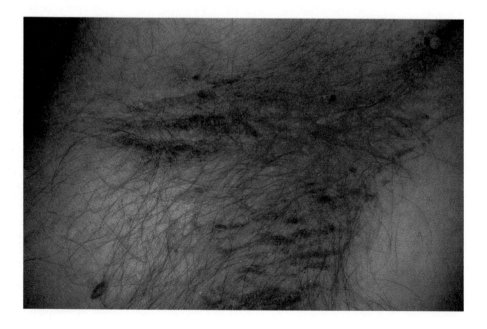

Atypical Nevi

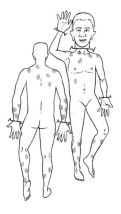

▪ Morphology
Sharply circumscribed brown to black macules and papules. Lesions may be a few millimeters to 1 to 2 cm in largest diameter. Often marked variation in color and irregular borders. Lesions usually multiple and more than 50 lesions frequently present.

▪ Distribution
Anywhere, but more on sun-exposed areas.

▪ Patient Profile
Both sexes. Lesions begin in childhood or adolescence. Lesions are usually symptomatic. They may be precursors of melanoma. Frequent family history of melanoma.

▪ Diagnosis
Lesions are present for years and have a sharply circumscribed border, normal surface, and uniform color. Biopsy reveals nests of nevus cells.

▪ Treatment
Patients should be taught to monitor lesions for ABCD: **a**symmetry, **b**order irregularity, **c**olor variegation (red, white, blue), **d**iameter >4 to 6 mm. Change in a nevus requires an excisional biopsy to exclude melanoma.

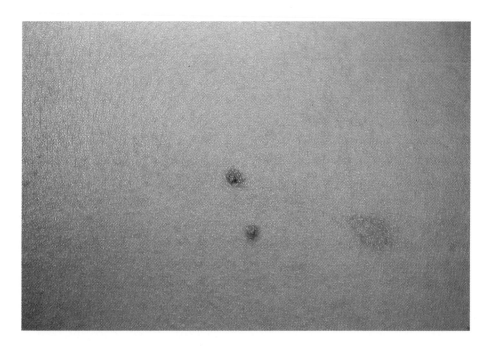

Histiocytosis (Histiocytosis X)
(Letterer-Siwe Disease)

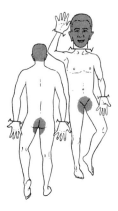

■ Morphology
Papules are yellow-brown, minimally scaly, but may develop crusts. Individual papules may become pruritic or very crusted. A diffuse, seborrheic dermatitis-like eruption with redness and scaling is frequently found in histiocytosis X.

■ Distribution
Frequently on the trunk, axilla, groin, scalp, face, or retroauricular areas.

■ Patient Profile
Usually children younger than 4 years of age who may be systemically well at the time of onset of skin lesions. Fever, malaise, weight loss, hepatosplenomegaly, anemia, and persistent infection frequently occur later in the disease. This disease may be fatal. Benign forms of histiocytic infiltration exist.

■ Diagnosis
Purpuric papules in a child with a scaling eruption suggest this serious diagnosis, and biopsy is mandatory. Biopsy shows histiocytes that invade the epidermis. Scabies can mimic this serious disease and should be excluded by scraping the lesions and searching for mites.

■ Treatment
Systemic chemotherapy for malignant form.

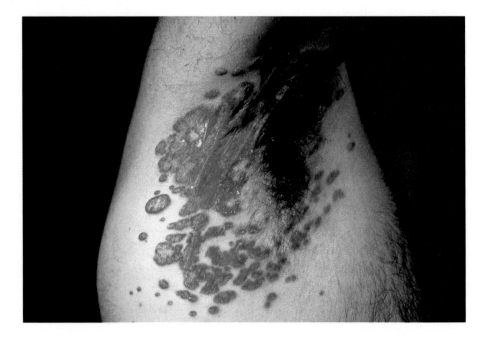

Nevi
(Moles)

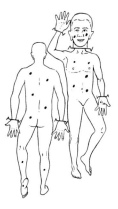

▪ Morphology
Sharply circumscribed, uniformly tan, brown, or flesh-colored papules. The surface may be slightly irregular, and coarse hairs may be present. May be single or multiple. Usually multiple, giant hairy nevi are present at birth and may involve large surface areas. Occasionally a white ring surrounds the nevus (halo nevus).

▪ Distribution
Anywhere, including palms, soles, and mucosae.

▪ Patient Profile
Both sexes. Very common and noticed most frequently in children and young adults. Large nevi that are present at birth, and especially giant hairy nevi, have a potential of developing malignant melanoma. Nevi may become darker during pregnancy.

▪ Diagnosis
Change in the appearance of a nevus requires biopsy to rule out melanoma. These extremely common lesions are present for years and have a sharply circum-scribed border, normal surface, and uniform color. Biopsy reveals nests of nevus cells.

▪ Treatment
Follow-up for the ABCD changes: **a**symmetry, **b**order irregularity, **c**olor variegation (red, white, blue), **d**iameter >4 to 6 mm. Patients with more than 100 lesions often represent those having the atypical mole syndrome and should be followed up every 6 to 12 months for potential melanoma. Complete surgical excision of suspected lesions.

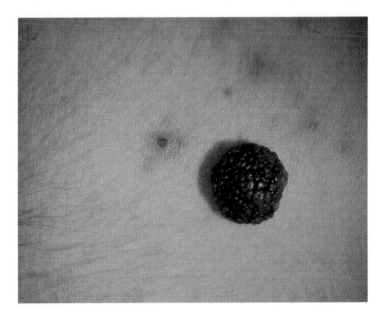

Porokeratosis

▪ **Morphology**
One or more brown, slightly raised papules with a well-demarcated, double-edged scaling border. The center of the lesion may appear atrophic. A linear arrangement of individual lesions may be seen (linear porokeratosis).

▪ **Distribution**
Anywhere, but may have a sun-exposed distribution (disseminated superficial actinic porokeratosis [DSAP]) or palm or sole distribution (porokeratosis palmaris et plantaris disseminata).

▪ **Patient Profile**
Variants of porokeratosis often begin in childhood, except for DSAP, a disease of adults. Basal cell and squamous cell carcinomas may arise in lesions of porokeratosis.

▪ **Diagnosis**
Biopsy of a lesion demonstrates a tightly packed column of parakeratotic epidermal cells called a *coronoid lamella*, which repre-

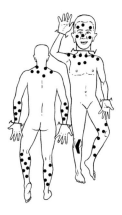

sents the double-edged border of the lesion.

▪ **Treatment**
Excision or destruction with cryotherapy or electrodesiccation; topical retinoic acid.

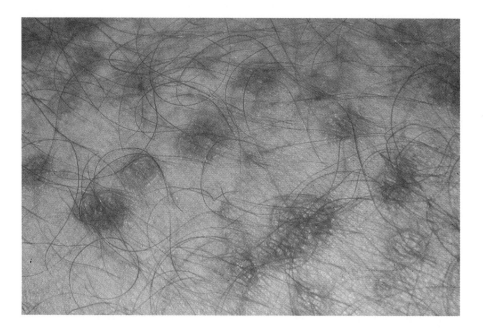

Seborrheic Keratoses

▪ Morphology
These are sharply circumscribed, elevated, pasted-on-appearing, brown to black papules (a few to several centimeters). The surface is irregular, slightly scaly, and rough. The lesions are often multiple, sometimes pedunculated, and, if irritated, they have a red base and associated tenderness.

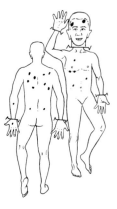

▪ Distribution
Trunk, but may be anywhere, including the face.

▪ Patient Profile
Both sexes. Lesions usually begin to appear during the fourth decade and increase in prevalence with age. Usually asymptomatic. Rarely familial. Eruptive seborrheic keratoses rarely may be a sign of underlying malignancy.

▪ Diagnosis
This very common lesion grows slowly and persists. The color of an individual lesion is uniform. The pasted-on appearance is characteristic. Scraping the surface produces brownish debris. The onset of multiple seborrheic keratoses may follow an inflammatory dermatosis or, rarely, may be a sign of internal malignancy. Sudden enlargement of seborrheic keratoses may occur in pityriasis rubra pilaris. Multiple seborrheic keratoses may be seen on the faces of blacks in their second and third decades (dermatosis papulosa nigra). Biopsy of seborrheic keratoses shows hyperkeratosis, papillomatosis, and acanthosis of benign cells.

▪ Treatment
Light liquid nitrogen, electrodesiccation, removal of excess scale with lactic-acid–containing medications.

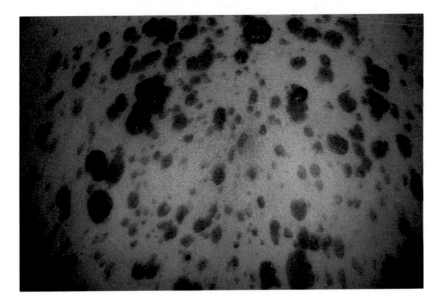

Tinea Versicolor

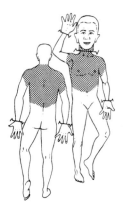

▪ Morphology
Minimally elevated tan to brown papules and plaques that scale on rubbing. Hypopigmentation may be seen.

▪ Distribution
Upper trunk, shoulders, neck, proximal arms; occasionally face; rarely below waist.

▪ Patient Profile
Usually adolescents or young adults of both sexes. Lesions may be slightly pruritic.

▪ Diagnosis
Lesion scrapings tested with potassium hydroxide preparation (see p. 115) reveal large spores and thick hyphae.

▪ Treatment
Topical antifungals, short course of oral ketoconazole, Selsun shampoo to affected skin. The patient should be advised that normal pigmentation returns slowly.

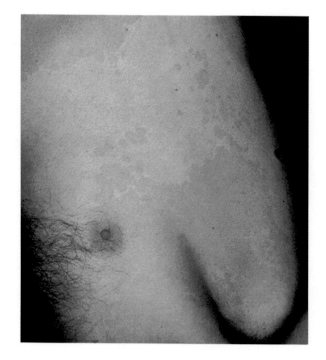

FLESH-COLORED PAPULES

DIAGNOSTIC OBSERVATIONS

These lesions have a normal surface and are flesh-colored to slightly pink. They often require biopsy for diagnosis. Certain lesions are pedunculated, with a stalk-like lesion whose base is narrower than the body (e.g., some neurofibromata and nevi and most skin tags). Some of these lesions have central expressible cores (acne comedone, milia, and molluscum contagiosum). Some are extremely pruritic (e.g., Fox-Fordyce disease, lichen planus, prurigo nodularis).

Linear papular lesions and painful papular lesions are included in this section. Tables of uncommon facial and general body papules are included (see pp. 174, 178).

Acne comedone
Actinic elastosis
Basal cell carcinoma: often single
Condyloma acuminatum: usually very irregular surface (see p. 242)
Dermatofibroma: often single
Fox-Fordyce disease
Granuloma annulare
Keloids: history of trauma
Lichen nitidus: small (<1 mm)
Lichen planus (see p. 251)
Lymphangioma circumscriptum
Metastatic tumors (see pp. 220, 408)
Milia
Molluscum contagiosum
Neurofibromata
Nevi
Pretibial myxedema
Prurigo (see pp. 257, 410)
Sarcoidosis
Skin tags
Warts
Rare, single, flesh-colored papules
Rare, small, persistent, flesh-colored papules around the eyes (see Table 5-1)
Rare, small, persistent, flesh-colored papules anywhere (see Table 5-2)

Acne Comedone
(Whitehead)

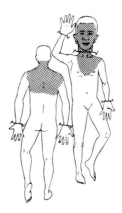

■ Morphology
Flesh-colored to hypopigmented papule associated with red papules, open comedones (blackheads), cysts, and pustules.

■ Distribution
Face, upper chest, upper back.

■ Patient Profile
Adolescents and adults of both sexes. Common condition. Made worse by oil-containing cosmetics.

■ Diagnosis
Nicking the papule releases cheesy material. Biopsy reveals hyperkeratosis and blocking of follicular apparatus. Single lesions resemble milia.

■ Treatment
Topical Retin-A, antibiotics, benzoyl peroxide. Often requires nicking and expression with a comedo extractor.

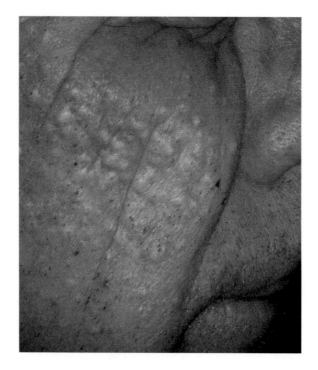

Actinic Elastosis

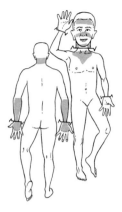

■ **Morphology**
Coarse wrinkling of skin resulting in flesh-colored papules and nodules. Pigmented macules (lentigines) and telangiectases frequently seen.

■ **Distribution**
Sun-exposed areas: face, neck, upper chest, extensor arms, and dorsum of hands.

■ **Patient Profile**
White patient with extensive history of extensive sun exposure. Very common in southern United States. Similar changes on the face have been reported in heavy smokers.

■ **Diagnosis**
Clinical lesions and distribution are diagnostic. Biopsy shows nodular aggregations of amorphous material in the papillary dermis, ectatic vessels, and altered pigmentation.

■ **Treatment**
Sunscreens and topical retinoic acids.

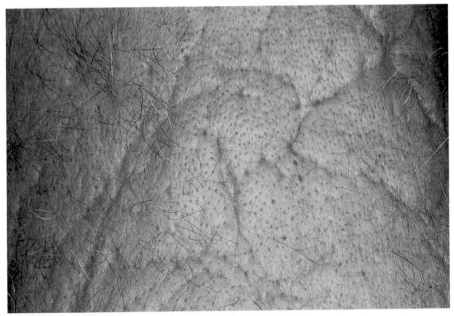

Cutis rhomboidalis nuchae

Basal Cell Carcinoma

▪ **Morphology**

Raised, translucent or skin-colored papule with dilated blood vessels around its rim. Ulcerations, flecks of brown-blue pigmentation, scarring or slight scaling may be present. Normal skin markings are lost. Some lesions have a distinct threadlike border. Lesions may be single or multiple.

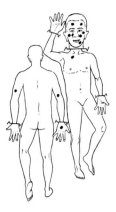

▪ **Distribution**

Usually sun-exposed areas, especially face and neck, but may be anywhere.

▪ **Patient Profile**

Both sexes, usually beginning in middle age. Common in fair-skinned individuals with outdoor occupations. Lesions are chronic and progressive. Rare in blacks and Asians. Two diseases that predispose young people to increased numbers of basal cell carcinomas are xeroderma pigmentosum and basal cell nevus syndrome.

▪ **Diagnosis**

This common lesion should be considered for all small, telangiectatic papules on sun-damaged skin. Lesions should be blanched by diascopy or the skin should be stretched to demonstrate translucency and demarcate the border of the tumor. Must be differentiated from an atypical fibroxanthoma. Diagnosis is confirmed by biopsy, which shows proliferation of basal cells, stromal proliferation, and retraction of the epithelium from the stroma. Tumors of other adnexal structures often resemble basal cell carcinomas clinically but can be distinguished by biopsy. Some of these adnexal tumors are multiple or painful.

▪ **Treatment**

Biopsy establishes the diagnosis. Treatment with excision, curettage and electrodesiccation, or Mohs' surgery. Mohs' surgery is indicated for recurrent lesions, lesions with morpheaform histology, lesions >1 cm, and tumors in areas of high recurrence (e.g., the nose and nasolabial folds). Radiotherapy in selected cases.

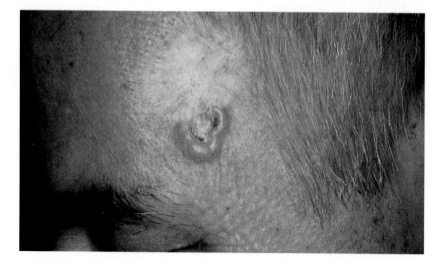

Dermatofibroma

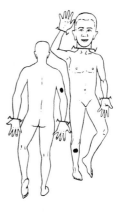

▪ Morphology
Firm, flat, skin-colored or hyperpigmented papules up to 2 cm wide. Compression around the lesion causes retraction beneath the skin (Fitzpatrick's sign).

▪ Distribution
Usually single. Most common on lower extremities, but may occur anywhere.

▪ Patient Profile
Adults, especially women; very common lesion. Usually asymptomatic. History of trauma or preceding insect bites.

▪ Diagnosis
Biopsy reveals nonencapsulated, benign histiocytic and fibroblastic proliferation with epidermal hyperplasia.

▪ Treatment
Liquid nitrogen, excision, intralesional corticosteroids.

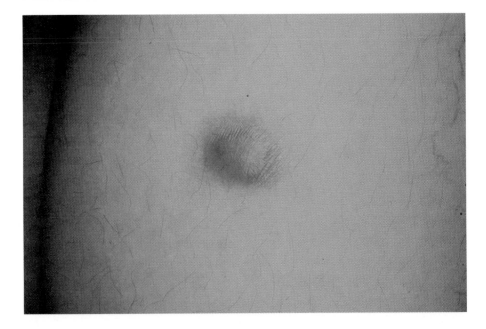

Fox-Fordyce Disease

■ Morphology
Multiple, small (3 to 5 mm), round, smooth, flesh-colored perifollicular papules.

■ Distribution
Axillae, areola, and pubic area are primarily involved.

■ Patient Profile
Women predominantly; onset after puberty. Very pruritic lesions. Condition clears during pregnancy. Decreased axillary sweating and odor.

■ Diagnosis
Multiple pruritic axillary lesions in postpubertal women suggest this diagnosis. Biopsy is diagnostic and shows intraepidermal apocrine duct rupture and apocrine gland destruction.

■ Treatment
Class II or III topical corticosteroid, topical Retin-A, systemic antihistamines for itch; oral birth control pills.

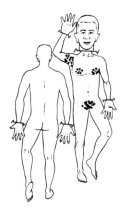

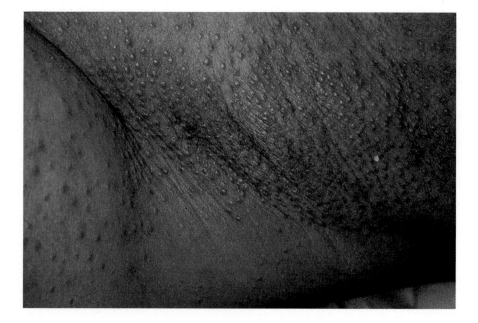

Granuloma Annulare

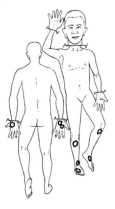

▪ Morphology
Groups of small (1 to 5 mm) flesh-colored papules coalesce to form rings. Lesions may be slightly pink, violaceous, or, rarely, scaly. Lesions spread peripherally, clear centrally, and resolve without atrophy over months. Subcutaneous nodules (1 to 5 cm in diameter) may be present near joints.

▪ Distribution
Dorsum of hands and feet. Extensor aspect of extremities near joints. Some patients will develop generalized disease.

▪ Patient Profile
More frequent in women. Young adults and children most commonly affected. Lesions rarely pruritic. Patients younger than 10 years, older than 40 years, immunosuppressed, or HIV-positive more likely to develop generalized disease.

▪ Diagnosis
Flesh-colored papules arranged in rings near joints are highly suggestive of this diagnosis. The papular nature of the border can be emphasized by stretching the lesion. Older women with diabetes mellitus may have disseminated granuloma annulare. Biopsy shows necrobiotic degeneration of collagen and a chronic inflammatory infiltrate.

▪ Treatment
Topical steroids (class II or III) may hasten resolution. Niacinamide (1000 to 1500 mg) and isotretinoin have been used for severe cases.

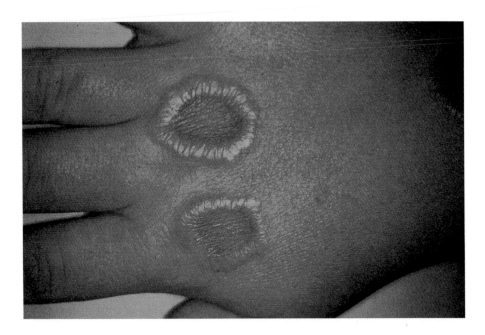

Keloids

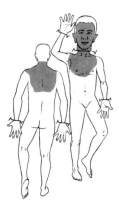

▪ Morphology
Firm, smooth, shiny, usually flesh-colored papules of various sizes. The lesions are sharply circumscribed and may be pedunculated or irregular in outline. Lesions are often single but may be multiple, depending on the nature of previous trauma.

▪ Distribution
Lesions may occur anywhere. Face, ears, chin, posterior neck (acne keloidosis), and upper chest are the most common sites.

▪ Patient Profile
Young adults, commonly women. Blacks and other hyperpigmented individuals have a predisposition to keloids. Lesions may continue to grow for months after trauma. May be pruritic or painful.

▪ Diagnosis
Progressive, slow-growing lesions without epidermal change following trauma are characteristic. Keloids extend beyond the borders of the site of trauma; hypertrophic scars do not. Biopsy shows thickened collagen bundles, differentiating this lesion from hypertrophic scars.

▪ Treatment
Intralesional corticosteroids repeated monthly until resolved. Surgical excision with injection of steroids into the base can be helpful.

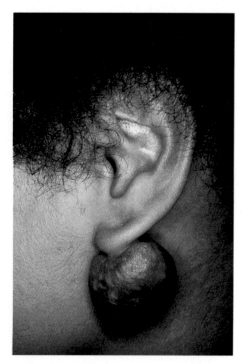

Lichen Nitidus

■ **Morphology**

Pinpoint (1 mm) flat-topped, white to skin-colored, closely grouped, nonscaling papules. May be linear (Koebner's phenomenon).

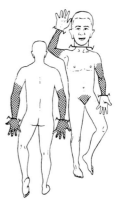

■ **Distribution**

Penis (glans and shaft), forearms are most common sites, but lesions may be anywhere.

■ **Patient Profile**

Both sexes; more common in adults. Frequent in blacks. Nonpruritic lesions.

■ **Diagnosis**

The lesions may coexist with lichen planus (see p. 139). Biopsy is diagnostic and shows tiny granulomas without caseation below a hyperkeratotic and parakeratotic epidermis.

■ **Treatment**

Topical steroids (class II or III; class IV or V on genitals).

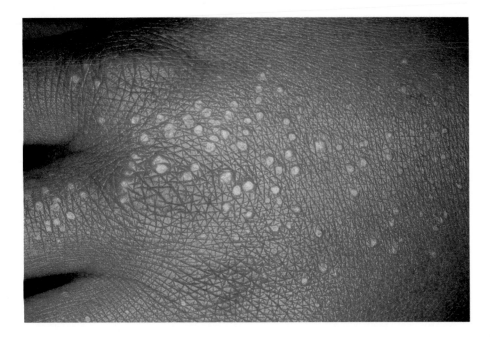

Lymphangioma Circumscriptum

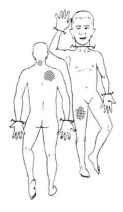

▪ Morphology
Papules are grouped, hyperkeratotic, wart-like, and arise over deep vesicles. Vesicles are small, deep, and may be tan in color.

▪ Distribution
Trunk, shoulder, neck, and proximal limbs are most common sites but can occur anywhere. Oral mucous membranes may be involved.

▪ Patient Profile
Lesions present at birth or appear during early childhood in both sexes. Life-long duration. Nonpruritic, may bleed or exude lymph fluid with local trauma.

▪ Diagnosis
The early age of onset, yellow-brown color, and grouping of this lesion are diagnostic. Biopsy reveals dilated, thin-walled lymphatic vessels.

▪ Treatment
Excision, including deep component, or laser for destruction. Smaller lesions often respond to electrodesiccation. May recur despite surgical procedure.

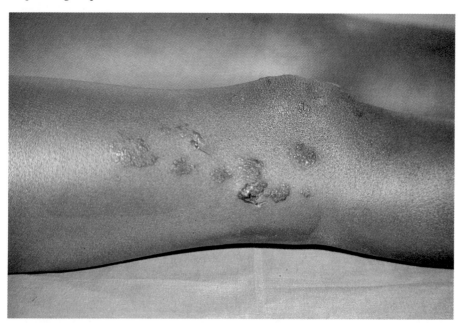

Milia

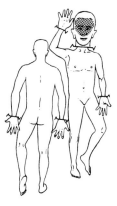

■ **Morphology**
Small, slightly raised, smooth, white to flesh-colored papules, 1 to 2 mm in diameter. Usually multiple.

■ **Distribution**
Most common on face, especially around eyelids, but may occur anywhere.

■ **Patient Profile**
All ages, both sexes. Asymptomatic.

■ **Diagnosis**
When nicked with a scalpel, a white core can be expressed. Subepidermal bullous diseases may produce milia, especially epidermolysis bullosa and porphyria cutanea tarda.

■ **Treatment**
Nicking surface and expressing with a comedo extractor. Topical Retin-A.

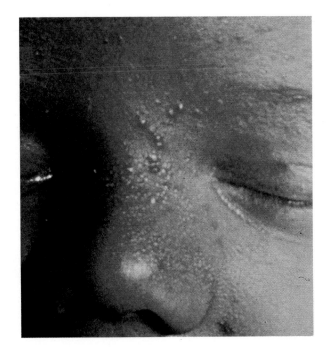

Molluscum Contagiosum

■ **Morphology**

Smooth, skin-colored to pink, dome-shaped papules (1 mm to 1.5 cm in diameter) with a central dimple or umbilication. A central keratotic plug can be expressed by nicking the papule and compressing the sides. There may be redness and scaling around the lesions.

■ **Distribution**

Anywhere. Face common in children and immunosuppressed patients, especially with HIV. Genitals and anogenital areas common in adults.

■ **Patient Profile**

Both sexes; common in children, young adults, and immunosuppressed patients, including those who are HIV-positive. Disease may be spread by sexual contact in adults. Multiple and recalcitrant nongenital lesions in an adult are suggestive of HIV infection.

■ **Diagnosis**

A smooth, umbilicated papule with an expressible keratotic core is diagnostic.

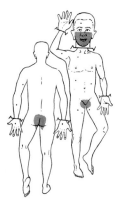

Examination of the keratotic debris reveals eosinophilic molluscum (about 25 µg in diameter). Biopsy reveals diagnostic eosinophilic intracytoplasmic inclusions.

■ **Treatment**

Extrusion, light freeze with liquid nitrogen; topical cantharone.

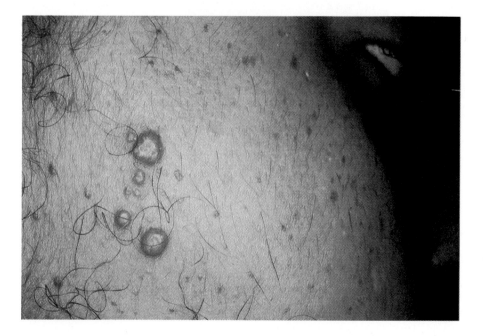

Neurofibromatosis

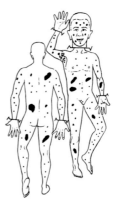

■ Morphology
Multiple soft, flesh-colored papules, several millimeters to several centimeters in size. The smaller lesions can be pushed back into the skin through an apparent space (buttonhole sign). Large, pedunculated lesions and subcutaneous plexiform neuromas may be present. Café au lait spots and axillary freckling are frequently present.

■ Distribution
Anywhere, including mucosae, palms, and soles. Lesions may be grouped in dermatomes. May be confused with Proteus syndrome (gigantism of hands, feet, or limbs, with lipomas, hemangiomas, lymphangiomas, and nevi).

■ Patient Profile
Any age, both sexes. Papules usually appear in late childhood or early adulthood. Mental retardation, premature puberty, acoustic neuromas, pheochromocytoma, bone lesions, scoliosis, and localized gigantism may be present. Autosomal dominant inheritance or spontaneous mutation.

■ Diagnosis
Soft papules with a positive buttonhole sign strongly suggest this diagnosis. Con-firmed by café au lait spots and other associated clinical features. Iris hamartomas (gray-white spots, Lisch nodules) can be seen by direct examination in all patients by age 16. Similar lesions limited to the lips suggest the multiple neuroma syndrome, which is associated with calcitonin-secreting parathyroid tumors and pheochromocytomas. Biopsy reveals wavy neuronal tissue with elongated spindle cells and presence of mast cells.

■ Treatment
Genetic counseling; regular follow-up for internal manifestations. Prenatal diagnosis often possible. Surgical removal of isolated lesions possible, but they may recur.

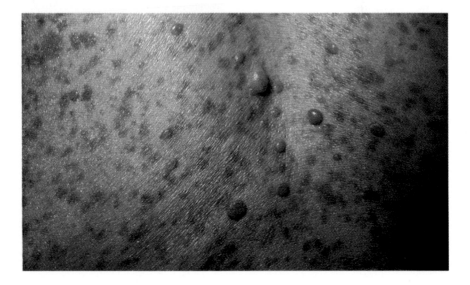

Nevi
(Moles)

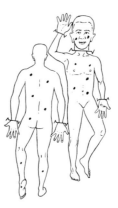

▪ Morphology
Sharply circumscribed, usually pigmented, but can be flesh-colored to light pink or tan papules. Surface may be slightly irregular, and coarse hairs may be present. Lesions may be multiple. Occasionally a white ring surrounds the lesion (halo nevus).

▪ Distribution
Anywhere, including palms, soles, and mucosae.

▪ Patient Profile
Both sexes. Very common; most begin in childhood or adolescence. Lesions are usually asymptomatic and last for years. May become more prominent during pregnancy.

▪ Diagnosis
These extremely common lesions are present for years and have a sharply circumscribed border, normal surface, and uniform color. Biopsy reveals nests of nevus cells. Spitz nevus (juvenile melanoma) is a benign lesion that demonstrates streaming of melanocytes into the dermis. Change in nevus requires a biopsy to rule out possibility of melanoma.

▪ Treatment
Surgical removal.

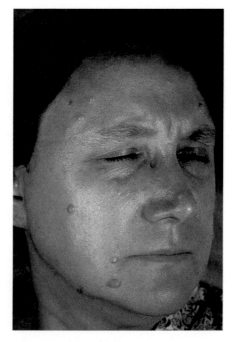

Pretibial Myxedema

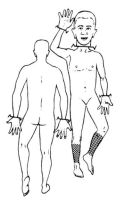

▪ Morphology
Firm, nonpitting, flesh-colored to slightly hyperpigmented lesions (1 to 20 cm) with coarse hair and a cobblestone appearance. Often coalesce into plaques.

▪ Distribution
Symmetric; most common on lower legs.

▪ Patient Profile
Adults of both sexes. Asymptomatic, chronic condition. Patient with thyroid dysfunction; exophthalmos and clubbing may be present.

▪ Diagnosis
Biopsy shows mucin deposition in dermis.

▪ Treatment
Topical class I corticosteroids with occlusion or intralesional corticosteroids.

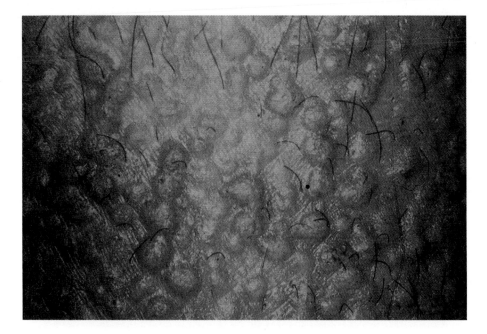

Sarcoidosis

▪ Morphology
Multiple flesh-colored papules of various sizes (0.5 to 10 cm). The surface of the lesions is usually smooth, but fine telangiectasia, slight scaling, or minimal atrophy may be seen. Lesions may appear in ring-like annular grouping. Erythema nodosum (see p. 421) may occur.

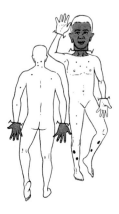

▪ Distribution
Small papules may be anywhere, but most common on the face (especially ears and nose) and extremities. Large plaques with dilated vessels are most common on the face, especially around ears and nose. Sarcoid papules often occur in scars. Erythema nodosum is found on pretibial areas (see p. 421).

▪ Patient Profile
Any age but most common in 20- to 50-year-old group. More common in women and American blacks. Dyspnea, cough, and hilar adenopathy. Uveitis, parotid and lacrimal gland enlargement, organomegaly, generalized lymphadenopathy, and neuropathy are frequent.

▪ Diagnosis
Multiple dermal papules with minor surface change associated with systemic signs and symptoms suggest this diagnosis. Biopsy is mandatory and shows discrete, noncaseating granulomas that often contain giant cells with inclusion bodies. Sarcoidlike granulomas may be induced by beryllium, silica, talc, quartz, zirconium, and mercury. A careful history and polarizing microscopy usually will eliminate these causes.

▪ Treatment
Ultrapotent topical steroids (class I), or intralesional corticosteroid monthly. Oral corticosteroids often will eliminate skin lesions and may be necessary for systemic involvement. Methotrexate, chloroquine sometimes helpful.

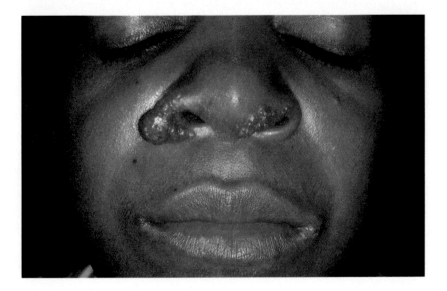

Skin Tags
(Acrochordons)

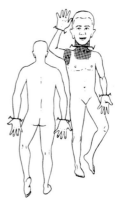

▪ Morphology
Multiple, small, stalk-like lesions without thickening at the base. Lesions are skin-colored or brown with slightly wrinkled surfaces. Irritation may cause redness.

▪ Distribution
Neck, axillae, and upper chest are most common sites.

▪ Patient Profile
Middle-aged adults of both sexes. Usually asymptomatic. Lesions may be associated with acromegaly or acanthosis nigricans.

▪ Diagnosis
Biopsy reveals benign epidermal papilloma.

▪ Treatment
Shave excision.

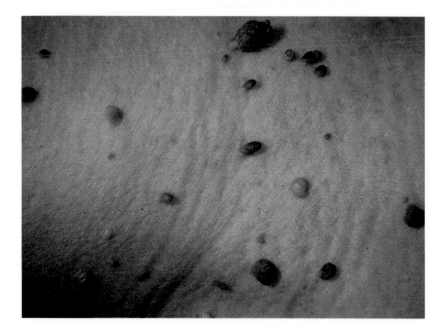

Warts

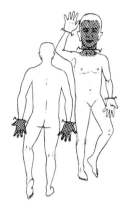

▪ Morphology
Multiple, discrete, skin-colored to pink flat-topped papules (2 to 10 mm) with irregular surfaces; linear arrangement or grouped. Common warts (see p. 241) may also occur.

▪ Distribution
Face, neck, and back of hands are most common sites.

▪ Patient Profile
Children and young adults. Nonpruritic lesions.

▪ Diagnosis
Flesh-colored flat papules with minimal surface change suggest flat warts. Lichen planus has similar morphology but is usually purple (see p. 251). Biopsy shows acanthosis, hyperkeratosis, and vacuolated cells in malpighian layer. Rapid onset of multiple lesions raises possibility of HIV.

▪ Treatment
Light liquid nitrogen, cantharone, topical Retin-A.

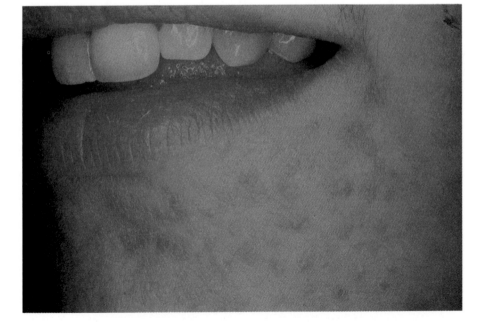

Rare, Single, Flesh-Colored Papules

There are many papular lesions of the skin. Biopsy is necessary for diagnosis in all of the following:

Amelanocytic melanoma: Usually pigmented but may be flesh-colored.

Apocrine hidrocystoma: Single dome-shaped bluish lesion on the face that releases brownish fluid with puncture.

Calcifying epithelioma of Malherbe: Usually solitary papule or nodule (0.5 to 2 cm in diameter) on face, scalp, neck, or upper trunk. Lesions may be cystic with an irregular surface and whitish yellow flecks. Multiple lesions are associated with myotonic dystrophy. Occurs in children and adults.

Connective tissue nevi: Beginning in childhood, 0.5 to 5 cm, and composed of one or many closely grouped skin-colored to yellow papules with a cobblestone pattern and no epidermal change. May be associated with tuberous sclerosis (see p. 115) or osteopoikilosis.

Hidradenoma papilliferum: Solitary vulvar lesion up to 1 cm in size.

Mastocytoma (see p. 147): Rarely flesh-colored.

Merkel cell tumor: Neuroendocrine tumor, most common on head, neck, and extremities.

Metastatic tumors (p. 408): Often nodular and may be erythematous.

Pilonidal sinus.

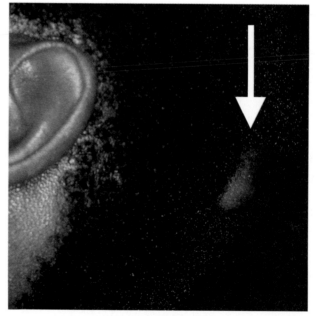

Calcifying epithelioma

Rare, Small, Persistent, Flesh-Colored Papules

TABLE 5–1. **Uncommon Causes of Multiple, Small, Persistent, Nonscaling, Flesh-Colored Papules on the Face***

Disease	Characteristics	Location	Age of Onset/Genetics
Acne	1–3-mm smooth papules with tiny plug	Face, neck upper back.	Late childhood to any age.
Amyloidosis	Papules coalesce into plaques (purpuric with slight trauma)	Body folds, periorbitally.	Adults.
Basal cell nevus syndrome	3–6-mm flesh-colored papules	Face, back.	Childhood. Autosomal dominant.
Colloid milium	Translucent to slightly yellow 1–2-mm papules	Sun-exposed areas: face periorbitally, nose, ears, back of hands.	Any age but usually middle-aged adults. Occurs in childhood.
Cowden disease	1–5-mm shiny or slightly hyperkeratotic lesions	Face, palms, tongue, and oral mucosa.	Childhood, puberty. Autosomal dominant.
Eccrine hidrocystomas	1–3-mm opaque to bluish papulovesicles	Face, periorbitally.	Older adult women.
Lipoid proteinosis	Smooth papules, plaques	Periorbital, forehead.	Adult.
Sarcoid	Smooth papules, plaques	Face, periorbital, forehead.	Adult.
Syringomas	5-mm to several cm white to pink lesions	Face, especially around eyes; upper chest.	Puberty.
Trichoepitheliomas	2–5-mm lesions	Face, especially nasolabial folds, upper lip, eyelids.	Childhood. Autosomal dominant.
Tuberous sclerosis	1–3 mm with telangiectasia (adenoma sebaceum)	Face, nasolabial folds. Upper lip usually spared.	Late childhood. Autosomal dominant.

	Associated Findings	
Skin	*Systemic*	*Histology*
Blackheads.		Cyst dilation of follicle.
Alopecia, urticaria, angio-edema. Leonine facies, enlarged tongue.	Multiple myeloma, nephrotic syndrome, neuropathy, weakness, fatigue	Amorphous eosinophilic material in upper dermis and in blood vessel walls. Deposits stain with Congo red.
Pits of palms and sole, lipomas.	Jaw cysts; rib abnormalities; early calcification of falx, hypertelorism, frontal bossing, short fourth meta-carpal	Resembles basal cell carcinoma, with overgrowth of basal-like cells.
		Amorphous eosinophilic material with entrapped vessels and fibroblasts in upper dermis.
Angiomas, lipomas.	Fibrocystic disease, gastric polyps, carcinomatosis, mental retardation	Facial lesions are tricholem-momas.
Accentuated by heat.		Cystic cavity with two layers of small, cuboidal cells.
Scarring, dorsum of hands.	Hoarseness, oral lesions	Deposition of hyaline material in skin.
Plaques, nodules, ery-thema nodosum.	Adenopathy, pulmonary dis-ease, hepatosplenomegaly	Noncaseating granuloma.
	Frequent in patients with Down syndrome	Ducts lined by two rows of epi-thelial cells. Commalike tails resembling tadpoles common.
Cylindroma of scalp fre-quently associated.		Horn cysts, surrounded by basi-loma cell. Rudimentary hairs.
Fibrous papules of nail folds, gingiva, trunk. Hypopigmented macules.	Convulsions, retardation, renal eye hamartomas	Sclerotic collagen surrounding atrophied appendages and dilated capillaries.

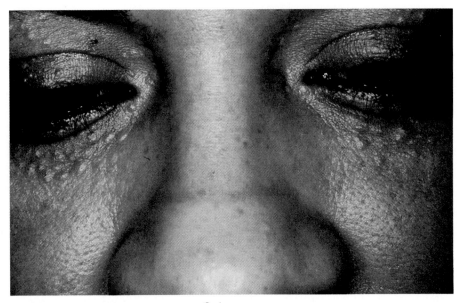

Syringomas

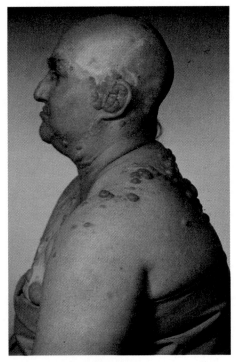

Cylindromas

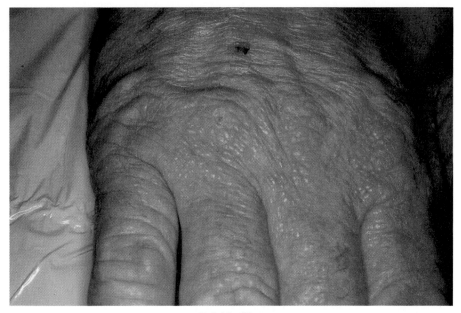

Colloid millium

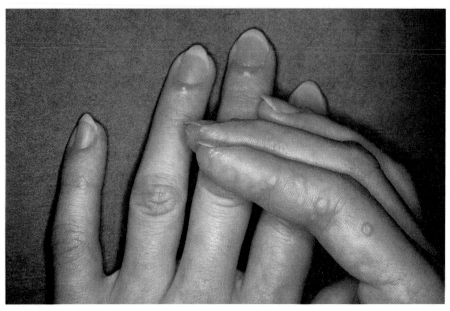

Multicentric reticulohistiocytosis

TABLE 5–2. **Uncommon, Multiple, Persistent, Flesh-Colored Papules (Anywhere)***

Disease	Characteristics	Location	Age of Onset/Genetics
Adnexal tumors (cylindroma, syringoma)	Multiple pink to flesh-colored papules.	Scalp, face, rest of body.	Adulthood.
Amyloidosis	Papules coalesce into plaques (purpuric with slight trauma).	Body folds, periorbitally.	Adulthood.
Connective tissue nevus	Smooth, flesh-colored, firm nodule(s).	Low back and extremities.	Birth or childhood.
Colloid milium	Translucent to slightly yellow 1–2-mm papules.	Sun-exposed areas: face periorbitally, nose, ears, back of hands.	Any age but usually middle-aged adults. Occurs in childhood.
Degos' disease	Pink to gray papules (in crops) that umbilicate and develop white porcelain-like centers.	Trunk, extremities, mucosae.	Adulthood.
Generalized eruptive histiocytosis	Symmetric, hundreds to thousands of lesions. Skin-colored to reddish blue.	Trunk, proximal extremities.	Adulthood.
Hunter's syndrome	3–5 lesions.	On trunk, on back, between scapular and postaxillary line.	Childhood, X-linked.
Knuckle pads	Flesh-colored thickening over interphalangeal joints.	Interphalangeal joints.	Young adulthood.
Lichen amyloidosis	Multiple groups of yellow to brown papules that may be scaly.	Extensor aspect of legs, arms, presacral.	Middle-aged adults.
Multicentric reticulohistiocytosis	Skin-colored, firm, yellowish to red papulonodules.	Face, hands, nail folds, mucosae.	Most frequently in adult women.
Multiple cysts (hair cysts, steatocystoma multiplex)	Multiple pink to flesh-colored papules with central dimple.	Axillae, anterior chest, groin, arms.	Young adulthood.
Papular mucinosis (lichen myxedematosus)	Soft, pale to yellow small papules. Lesions may be linear. Diffuse thickening of skin (scleromyxedema) may occur.	Axillae, extensor forearms.	Adulthood.
Xanthogranuloma (juvenile nevoxanthoendothelioma)	Skin-colored to yellow papules. Generalized. May be single.	Scalp, face, trunk, mouth.	Childhood, including infancy.
Xanthoma disseminatum	Yellow to brown papules or plaques.	Flexural areas, axillae, groin, popliteal and axillary fossae, neck, mucosae.	5–25 yr, more common in males.

*Biopsy often necessary for diagnosis.

	Associated Findings	
Skin	Other	Histology
		Nodules of adnexal epithelial cells
Alopecia, urticaria, angio-edema. Leonine facies, enlarged tongue.	Multiple myeloma, nephrotic syndrome, neuropathy, weakness, fatigue.	Amorphous, eosinophilic material in upper dermis and in blood vessel walls. Deposits stain with Congo red.
		Biopsy shows increased collagen and elastin.
		Amorphous eosinophilic material with entrapped vessels and fibroblasts in upper dermis.
	Abdominal pain, weight loss, intestinal perforation.	Subendothelial fibroplasia within vessels.
		Monomorphous histiocytes that have a pale cytoplasm.
Hirsutism.	Corneal opacification, mental retardation, organomegaly.	Metachromatic material between collagen bundles.
Leukonychia, keratoderma.	Deafness.	
Hyperkeratosis.		Homogeneous amyloid limited to papillary dermis.
Leonine facies.	Deforming polyarthritis. Tendon sheath swelling, fever, weight loss.	Large, multinucleated cells with granular cytoplasm. Cells are positive for glycoproteins and lipids.
		Hair cysts, sebaceous cysts.
		Mucin deposited in upper third of dermis.
	Lesions on iris.	Giant cells with wreathlike nuclei are characteristic.
	Diabetes insipidus, respiratory obstruction.	Sheets and cluster of foam cells. Rare giant cells.

Linear Papular Lesions and Painful Papules

DIAGNOSTIC OBSERVATIONS
Certain diseases may produce a linear band of lesions in a dermatome-like distribution. The papules maintain the basic morphology of the disease. Linear lesions are most frequent on the extremities. Biopsy is required for definitive diagnosis. Linear nodules suggest malignancy or deep infection with fungi or mycobacteria. Painful papules, on the other hand, are often single.

Causes of Linear Papular Lesions
Darier's disease (see p. 245)
Focal dermal hypoplasia (see p. 273)
Herpes zoster (see p. 86)
Incontinentia pigmenti (see p. 300)
Lichen nitidus (see p. 163)
Lichen planus (see p. 251)
Lichen striatus
Molluscum contagiosum (see p. 166)
Papular mucinosis (see p. 178–179)
Psoriasis (see p. 258–259)
Sarcoidosis (see p. 170, 223)
Warts (see p. 241)

Causes of Painful Papules
Angiolipoma: soft, deep, usually multiple lesions, 0.5 cm in diameter, that are flesh-colored or slightly blue. The underlying skin is normal.
Blue rubber bleb nevus.
Chondrodermatitis nodularis chronica helicis: single red papule, indurated and extremely tender, on outer helix of ear. Patients will awake from sleep if they roll on lesion.
Chordoma cutis.
Dercum's disease.
Eccrine spiradenoma: single lesion, flesh-colored or slightly blue, usually <1 cm in diameter, that occurs on face and trunk.
Endometrioma.
Glomus tumor: usually a single red to blue papule up to 1 cm in diameter near tips of digits. Lesions may be under nails. Bone erosions may be seen on x-ray in the latter location. Temperature change and pressure cause marked pain with proximal radiation. A familial form with multiple, nontender lesions also exists.
Leiomyomas: single or grouped, multiple flesh-colored to yellow-brown lesions on extensor aspect of arms, anterior trunk, areola of nipple, and scrotum. Lesions extend deeply into skin. Piloleiomyoma a variant.
Neurilemoma.
Neuroma: traumatic neuromas that are 0.1- to 1-cm painful papules, usually on the trunk or proximal extremities in areas of previous trauma.

Purpuric Papules

Causes of Palpable Purpura

Atheroembolism
Consumption coagulopathy
Coumadin necrosis
Leukocytoclastic vasculitis: drug-related, Schönlein-Henoch purpura, allergic vasculitis, collagen vascular disease, rheumatoid arthritis, dysproteinemia, thrombotic thrombocytopenic purpura, idiopathic
Rocky Mountain spotted fever
Septicemia
Subacute bacterial endocarditis

Atheroembolism

▪ **Morphology**
Sparse, large, purpuric papules that progress to infarction and ulceration.

▪ **Distribution**
Lower extremities.

▪ **Patient Profile**
Older patients with atherosclerosis who frequently have received anticoagulants and suddenly develop one or more large lesions on the lower extremity.

▪ **Diagnosis**
Cholesterol clefts are seen in biopsies fixed in ethanol. Tumor emboli may cause palpable purpuric lesions in a patient with advanced metastatic disease.

▪ **Treatment**
Surgical treatment of underlying plaques.

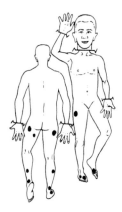

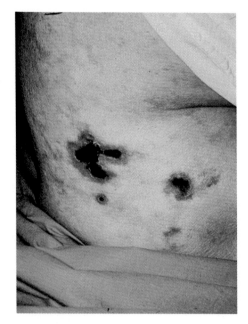

Consumption Coagulopathy
(Purpura Fulminans)

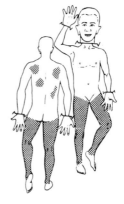

▪ Morphology
Large, geometric, polyangulated, non-blanching, minimally elevated, red-purple to gray-blue plaques.

▪ Distribution
Anywhere, but more common on dependent areas.

▪ Patient Profile
Severely ill patient with fever, coma, and shock. This syndrome is associated with septicemia, drug ingestion (especially coumadin), tumors, or infection.

▪ Diagnosis
There is a decrease in platelets and clotting factors in the blood. Fibrin degradation products are seen in the blood and urine, and biopsy reveals vasculitis.

▪ Treatment
Supportive therapy, heparinization, treatment of underlying condition.

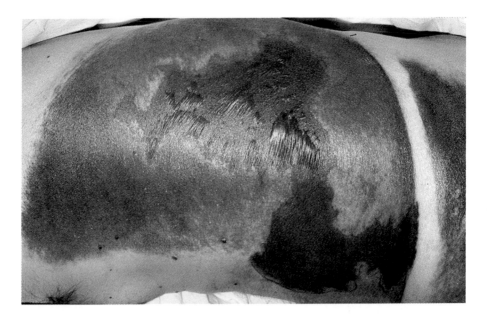

Coumadin Necrosis

▪ **Morphology**
Purpura that evolves to skin necrosis and black eschar formation.

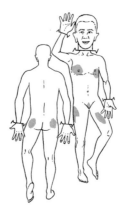

▪ **Distribution**
Breasts, buttocks, thighs, and penis most commonly involved.

▪ **Patient Profile**
Lesions usually begin within 3 to 5 days of initiating coumadin therapy. More common in females. Many patients have an associated protein C deficiency. Similar lesions may be seen in patients with decreased levels of protein S.

▪ **Diagnosis**
Clinical history and presentation strongly suggest the diagnosis. A biopsy of the involved area demonstrates thrombosis of superficial and deep vessels with associated epidermal and dermal necrosis.

▪ **Treatment**
Discontinuing coumadin; initiating surgical debridement and local wound care.

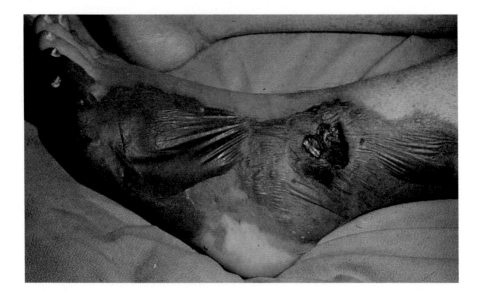

Leukocytoclastic Vasculitis

■ Morphology
Vasculitis presents with multiple, elevated, purpuric lesions of various sizes. Lesions may blister, infarct, and ulcerate. Early lesions may appear hivelike. Lesions heal with residual hyperpigmentation.

■ Distribution
Lesions are distal and common in dependent areas such as lower legs and feet. Mucosal lesions uncommonly occur. Lesions may occur in straight lines under areas of pressure (e.g., garters, watchbands).

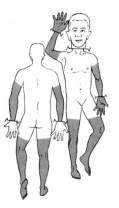

■ Patient Profile
Allergic vasculitis: Renal disease and arthritis may occur with this disease.

Collagen vascular disease: Systemic lupus erythematosus, rheumatoid arthritis, Wegener's granulomatosis, and mixed connective-tissue disease may present with cutaneous vasculitis.

Drug-induced cutaneous vasculitis: Occurs in both sexes at any age. Careful drug history is mandatory.

Dysproteinemia: Macroglobulins and cryoglobulins that fix complement may produce leukocytoclastic vasculitis.

Idiopathic disease: Many adults have leukocytoclastic angiitis without discernible cause.

Rheumatoid arthritis: Severe rheumatoid arthritis, often with neuropathy, high titers of rheumatoid factor, rheumatoid nodules. Corticosteroid doses often are altered before vasculitis occurs.

Schönlein-Henoch purpura: Usually in children after streptococcal infections. Associated with abdominal pain, with or without intussusception, arthritis, renal disease.

Thrombotic thrombocytopenic purpura: May present with cutaneous vasculitis; associated with thrombocytopenia, hemolytic anemia, fever, central nervous system disease, and hepatosplenomegaly.

■ Diagnosis
Biopsy reveals leukocytoclastic angiitis, and immunofluorescent biopsy reveals deposition of immunoglobulin and complement in vessels.

■ Treatment
Systemic steroids or antimetabolites often necessary. Systemic corticosteroids in therapy of idiopathic disease still controversial.

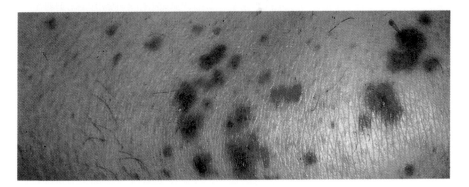

Rocky Mountain Spotted Fever

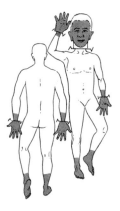

▪ Morphology
Numerous small purpuric lesions that often begin as red, hivelike papules.

▪ Distribution
Lesions begin at wrists, ankles; spread to palms, soles, and face before trunk. Mucosal lesions uncommon.

▪ Patient Profile
All ages, both sexes. Three to 12 days after being bitten by a tick, the patient develops fever, headache, photophobia, and myalgia. There is associated meningoencephalitis. Predominant in southeastern United States.

▪ Diagnosis
Rocky Mountain spotted fever is diagnosed by clinical presentation or immunofluorescent study of a frozen skin biopsy using antibodies to *Rickettsia rickettsii*. The diagnosis is confirmed by specific serologues and a positive Weil-Felix reaction to OX-2 and OX-19. Typhus has a similar presentation, but the rash begins on the trunk, spreads peripherally, and is confirmed by a positive OX-19 reaction. An identical clinical picture to Rocky Mountain spotted fever occurs after exposure to measles virus in a patient previously immunized with killed measles vaccine and in patients infected with coxsackievirus A5 or B3. These diagnoses are confirmed serologically. Meningococcemia begins acrally with fewer and larger lesions and is diagnosed by demonstrating organisms in spinal fluid, blood, or throat.

▪ Treatment
Systemic tetracycline or chloramphenicol for patients younger than 10 years of age.

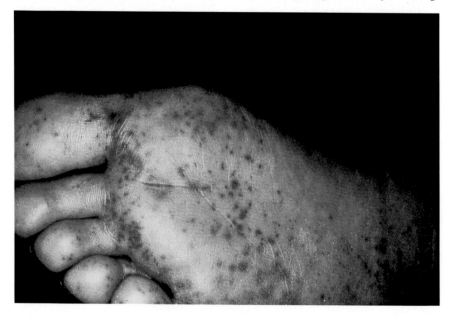

Septicemia

Lesions are sparse purpuric papules that may be tender. Lesions are from several millimeters to several centimeters in size. They may blister, form pustules, and infarct. Any infectious agent can produce this syndrome; the most common organisms are listed on Table 5–3.

TABLE 5–3. **Organisms Associated with Septicemias**

Organism	Location	Fever	Associated Findings	Presence of Gram's Stain of Lesions
Gonococcus	Distal	+	Tenosynovitis, oligoarticular arthritis of large joint, urethritis, proctitis, pharyngitis.	Difficult to demonstrate
Meningococcus	Distal	+	Pharyngitis, nausea and vomiting, headache, meningitis, polyarthritis.	Common
Pseudomonas	Groin, lower abdomen, axilla	+	Immunosuppressed host or patient with tumor or burn. Any organ may be involved.	Numerous organisms demonstrable
Staphylococcus	Distal lesions become pustular	+	Pneumonia, meningitis, carditis, arthritis.	Common
Candida, Trichosporon, Malassezia	Distal lesions, usually several centimeters in size	+	Diabetes, indwelling venous catheter, immunosuppression, oral lesions, pneumonitis, nephritis.	Numerous hyphal elements in Gram's stain
Mucor	Anterior chest or abdomen	+	Diabetes, sinusitis, orbital involvement, meningitis.	Numerous organisms demonstrable

+ Often prominent, may be chief complaint.

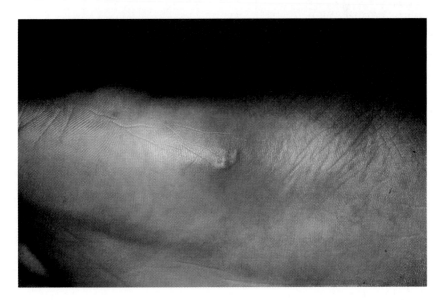

Subacute Bacterial Endocarditis

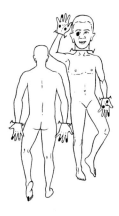

▪ Morphology
Sparse, acral, palpable purpuric lesions, several millimeters in diameter, associated with splinter hemorrhages under nails.

▪ Distribution
Tips of fingers and toes. Similar lesions may be seen on mucosa, especially conjunctivae.

▪ Patient Profile
Any age, both sexes. Patients may have heart murmurs, fever, proteinuria, and arthralgias. Tender digital lesions are often related to streptococcal disease and are referred to as *Osler's nodes.* Nonpainful palmar lesions are associated with staphylococci and are called *Janeway lesions.*

▪ Diagnosis
Blood cultures demonstrate organisms. Skin biopsy reveals inflammation of the glomus in Osler's nodes and leukocytoclastic angiitis in staphylococcal disease.

▪ Treatment
Systemic antibiotics for underlying infectious agent.

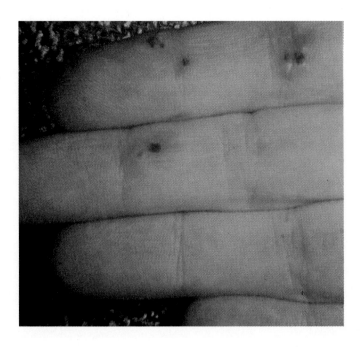

SMOOTH, RED PAPULES WITH ABRUPT ONSET

DIAGNOSTIC OBSERVATIONS
These lesions appear abruptly over minutes to days and often fade rapidly over days to weeks. The exanthems (see Tables 3–3 to 3–5, pp. 68–73) should be considered in this differential diagnosis.

MAJOR CATEGORIES

Grouped
Contact dermatitis
Folliculitis
Insect bites
Herpes infection
Miliaria

Multiple
Autoeczematization
Bacillary angiomatosis
Drug-induced eruption
Erythema multiforme
Graft-versus-host disease (GVHD)
Pityriasis rosea (see p. 255)
Polymorphous light eruption (see p. 233)
Psoriasis (see pp. 258–259)
Secondary syphilis (see p. 262)
Systemic lupus erythematosus
Vasculitis

Single
Coma induced (see p. 319)
Erysipelas
Fixed drug reaction
Leishmaniasis

Transient (Appear and Disappear within Hours to Days)
Burns: chemicals, heat, sunlight, ultraviolet irradiation (see p. 81)
Cholinergic urticaria
Goose bumps (cutis anserina)
Grover's disease
Jellyfish sting
Juvenile rheumatoid arthritis
Urticaria

Grouped Smooth, Red Papules, Abrupt Onset

Contact Dermatitis

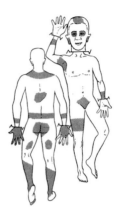

▪ Morphology
Papules and plaques are red, hivelike, and sharply circumscribed. Within days, vesicles usually develop.

▪ Distribution
Anywhere but more frequent in exposed areas. Lesions are grouped to correspond to the area of contact; linear or other geometric lesions, which correspond to exposure, are frequently seen.

▪ Patient Profile
Any age, both sexes. Lesions appear 12 to 48 hours after contact with allergen and last 12 to 14 days. Usually pruritic.

▪ Diagnosis
The configuration and location of the dermatitis are the most important clues to diagnosis. See page 18 for details of patch testing and specific contactants.

▪ Treatment
Topical soaks for oozing and crusted lesions. Antihistamines for pruritus, class I or II steroids bid. Systemic corticosteroids beginning with 60 mg prednisone and tapering over 10 to 14 days may be necessary for severe facial or genital edema.

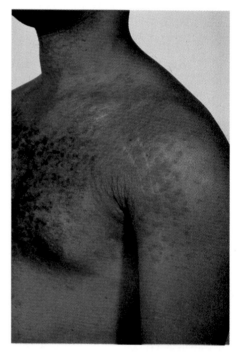

Folliculitis

▪ **Morphology**
Small red papules in hair follicles; may often become pustular.

▪ **Distribution**
Hairy areas, especially face, neck, scalp, chest, and back.

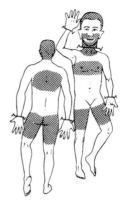

▪ **Patient Profile**
Adults, more common in men. Lesions may itch. Bacterial and *Pityrosporum* folliculitis frequently occur in HIV-positive patients. A nonbacterial folliculitis characterized by numerous eosinophils on skin biopsy (eosinophilic folliculitis) also occurs in AIDS patients.

▪ **Diagnosis**
Nicking the lesion may release pus. Bacteria and fungi may cause folliculitis; scrapings for fungus and culture for bacteria should be obtained. *Pityrosporum ovale*, which is not routinely cultured, may cause folliculitis in HIV-positive patients.

▪ **Treatment**
Bacterial folliculitis: erythromycin or Keflex for a month, topical mupirocin ointment bid into nares to decrease nasal carriage of staphylococci. *Pityrosporum* folliculitis responds to topical ketoconazole. For eosinophilic folliculitis, treatment with UVB, topical corticosteroids, and antihistamines.

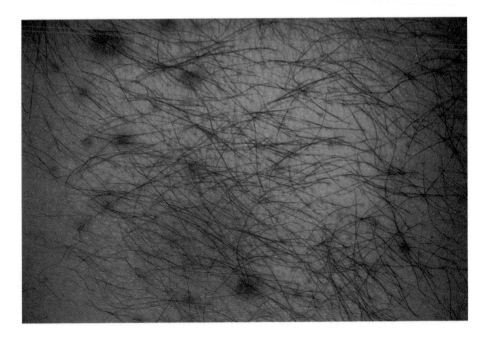

Insect Bites

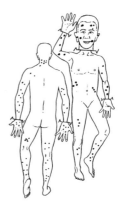

▪ Morphology
Papules are red, hivelike, and often excoriated. There may be a central punctum and pinpoint purpura. Vesicles and purpura may occur.

▪ Distribution
Anywhere but most frequent on exposed areas. Lesions erupt simultaneously and are often grouped. No oral lesions.

▪ Patient Profile
Any age, both sexes. Lesions appear acutely, but patients may be bitten recurrently for months.

▪ Diagnosis
This diagnosis may be difficult because insects such as mites and fleas can live in upholstered furniture, in carpets, or on pets. Cercaria or nonhuman schistosomes cause similar lesions, which appear after the patient has been in infected water. Scabies has a more gradual onset but should also be considered in this differential diagnosis. Biopsy shows polymorphonuclear leukocytic infiltration early. Dense lymphohistiocytic infiltrate associated with eosinophils occurs later.

▪ Treatment
Class I or II topical steroids bid; lesions may take weeks to resolve.

Miliaria

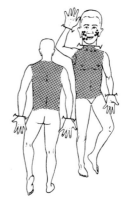

■ Morphology
Small, multiple flesh-colored to red papules at the orifice of sweat glands, with a regular distribution. Tiny vesicles or pustules may be present.

■ Distribution
Sides of neck, face, upper chest, back, and groin.

■ Patient Profile
Newborn infants and young children are most commonly affected but can occur in any age group and especially in hot, humid weather.

■ Diagnosis
The sudden onset of multiple, regularly spaced small lesions after heat exposure suggests miliaria. Biopsy reveals occlusion and inflammation of the sweat ducts.

■ Treatment
Class III or IV steroids if lesions are pruritic. Cool water or saline soaks bid. Place in cool environment.

Multiple Smooth, Red Papules

Autoeczematization

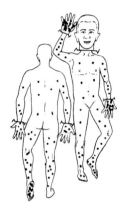

▪ Morphology
Papules are multiple, small, and red. Vesicles or vesicopapules may be associated with these lesions.

▪ Distribution
Symmetric but often generalized; involves extremities, palms, and soles.

▪ Patient Profile
Any age, both sexes. Pruritic lesions that evolve over days and may persist for 2 to 4 weeks.

▪ Diagnosis
This generalized eruption is secondary to a preexisting active inflammatory dermatitis. Fungal infections, contact dermatitis, or stasis dermatitis are common causes. The absence of a local inflammatory dermatitis makes this diagnosis unlikely.

▪ Treatment
Class IV topical steroids; oral antihistamines; and often oral corticosteroids, prednisone tapered to zero over a 2- to 3-week course.

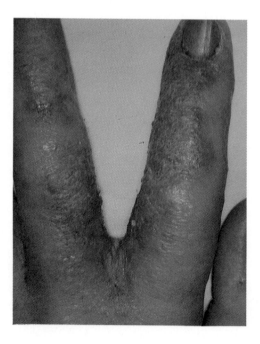

Bacillary Angiomatosis

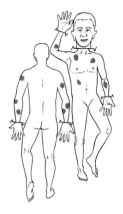

■ Morphology
Red to violaceous dome-shaped papules that may resemble angiomas. Lesions may be tender.

■ Distribution
Any site, but palms, soles, and mouth usually spared.

■ Patient Profile
Immunosuppressed patient, usually HIV-positive. Has been rarely described in patients with normal immune system.

■ Diagnosis
Demonstration of pleomorphic rickettsial bacilli (*Rochalimaea henselae*) on Warthin-Starry silver stain of lesional skin biopsy.

■ Treatment
Erythromycin or doxycycline.

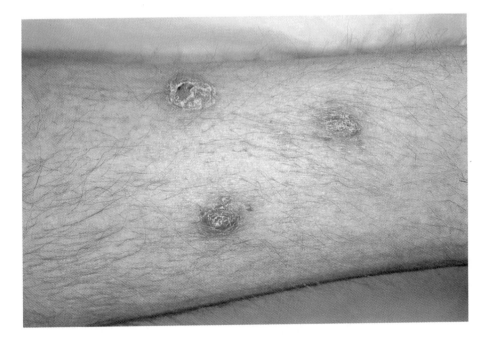

Drug-Induced Eruption

▪ Morphology
Multiple, symmetric, raised red papules.

▪ Distribution
Symmetric. Lesions usually progress over days. Oral lesions may be found.

▪ Patient Profile
Any age, both sexes. Lesions may itch. Drug eruptions most often occur soon after beginning a drug; they may occur in patients taking a drug for months to years. May take 4 to 6 weeks to clear after stopping drug.

▪ Diagnosis
Clearing of eruption after discontinuing drug, followed by recurrence of eruption with readministration of drug, is diagnostic. Biopsy is not diagnostic but may show increased number of eosinophils.

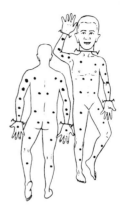

▪ Treatment
Elimination of the offending agent is curative. Systemic antihistamines for symptomatic relief. A course of systemic steroids beginning with 60 mg prednisone qd and tapering over 2 to 3 weeks may be necessary with severely symptomatic patients. Topical steroids (class I or II) may be helpful.

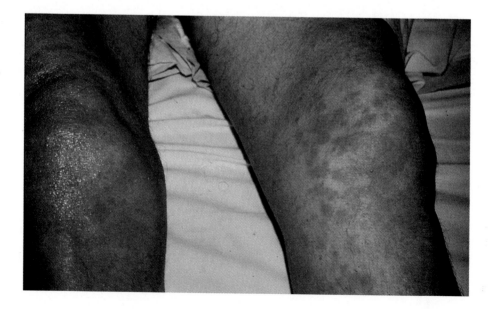

Erythema Multiforme

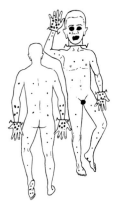

▪ Morphology
Papules and plaques are red and hivelike. Target lesions have a central red area, a rim of pallor, and an outermost rim of erythema. Vesicles and bullae may occur.

▪ Distribution
Generalized, symmetric, with accentuation over extensor aspects of distal limbs, including palms and soles. Mucosal erosions are common.

▪ Patient Profile
Usual ages 3 to 30, less common in infants and patients older than age 50. Both sexes. Disease evolves over several days and usually lasts 2 to 3 weeks. May be recurrent. Lesions may itch or burn.

▪ Diagnosis
Disease is precipitated by numerous causes, most commonly drugs, herpes simplex and other viral infections, primary atypical pneumonia, streptococcal infection, and systemic lupus erythematosus. Chilblains are cold-induced, hivelike lesions that may appear as erythema multiforme and last 1 to 2 weeks; lesions often appear on toes, fingers, nose, and ears. Biopsy reveals a dense, perivascular, lymphohistiocytic infiltrate in the upper papillary dermis and isolated epidermal cell necrosis. Subepidermal bullae may also occur. Rarely, bullous pemphigoid (see p. 291), dermatitis herpetiformis (p. 287), and pityriasis lichenoides et varioliformis acuta (see p. 221) will have only red papules.

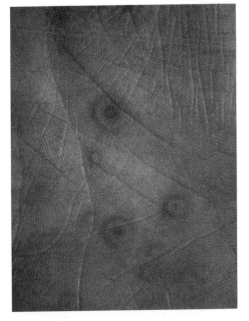

▪ Treatment
Pruritus should be treated with systemic antihistamines. Systemic corticosteroids have little benefit for the acute phase of this disease. Recurrent disease is often related to recurrent herpes simplex infection, which can be prevented with oral acyclovir.

Graft-versus-Host Disease (GVHD)

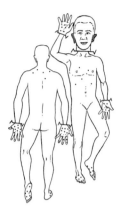

▪ Morphology
Acute GVHD lesions appear as erythematous papules. Blisters may occur but are less common. Edema and violaceous discoloration may be present on ears and periungual areas. Lesions of chronic GVHD are blue-purple papules that later may evolve into sclerotic plaques.

▪ Distribution
Acute and chronic GVHD lesions begin on the distal extremities but often become generalized.

▪ Patient Profile
Usually in patients receiving allogenic bone marrow transplants. Rarely a result of other organ transplants or blood transfusions. Chronic GVHD patients often have associated hair loss and anhidrosis.

▪ Diagnosis
Biopsy of acute lesions may reveal vacuolization of the basal cell layer and a sparse perivascular lymphocyte infiltrate, melanin incontinence, increased collagen deposition with loss of hair follicles and sweat glands.

▪ Treatment
Immunosuppressant agents and PUVA therapy.

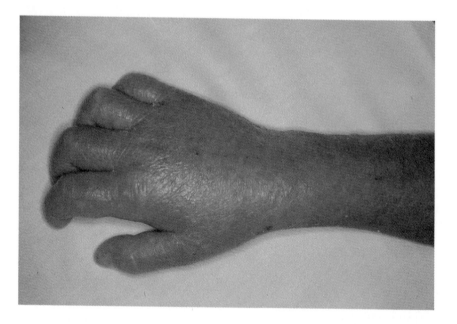

Systemic Lupus Erythematosus

▪ Morphology
Red papules and plaques that may have fine scaling, hyperpigmentation, hypopigmentation, telangiectasia, and atrophy.

▪ Distribution
Anywhere, but most frequently on the face or sun-exposed areas of the body, especially over both malar eminences (butterfly distribution). Asymptomatic palatal lesions may be present.

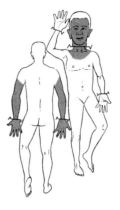

▪ Patient Profile
More common in females during the first three decades of life. Lesions are chronic and nonpruritic.

▪ Diagnosis
Presence of these lesions, which may be asymptomatic, in a patient with neurologic disease, arthritis, renal disease, or neuropsychiatric disturbances suggests the diagnosis. Serologic tests (Table 5-4), biopsy of skin lesions for routine histology, and immunofluorescence establish the diagnosis.

▪ Treatment
Complete evaluation for systemic manifestations is necessary. Antimalarials, systemic corticosteroids, and antimetabolites for patients with systemic involvement (renal, central nervous system, lung) often necessary. UVA and UVB sunscreens.

TABLE 5–4. **Serologic Tests for Systemic Lupus Erythematosus**

Serologic Test	% Positive	Significance
Antinuclear antibody	90+%	High sensitivity, low specificity
Anti-Sm	30%	Highly specific
Anti-histone	80% (drug induced)	Highly specific for drug-induced disease
Anti-Ro, anti-La	30%–40%	Photosensitivity

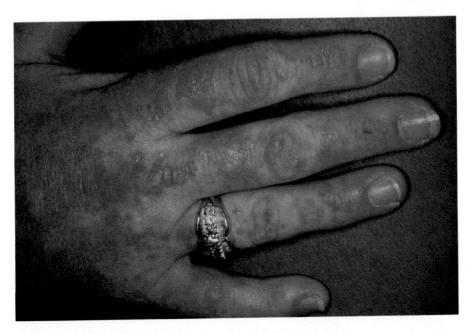

Vasculitis
(Allergic Vasculitis)

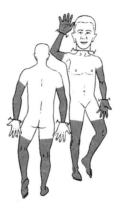

■ Morphology
Hivelike red papules are the first stage of the disease. Lesions then become purpuric and may blister.

■ Distribution
Symmetric, predominantly acral; frequently more lesions on lower extremities. Hundreds of lesions may be present. There may be accentuation of lesions under areas of pressure (e.g., beneath belts or tight clothing).

■ Patient Profile
All ages, both sexes. Usually sudden onset with acute forms lasting days to weeks. Chronic forms last months to years. Burning may precede eruption of lesions; usually nonpruritic. Disease may be associated with arthritis, abdominal pain, and renal disease.

■ Diagnosis
There are many causes of vasculitis; some classic groupings have been given special names:

Allergic cutaneous vasculitis: This form of vasculitis is seen at any age and frequently caused by drugs. Other causes of the syndrome include lupus erythematosus, rheumatoid arthritis, cryoglobulinemia, macroglobulinemia, infectious hepatitis, meningococcemia, and gonococcemia; appropriate tests for these diseases should be done. The existence of definitely palpable pruritic, symmetric lesions is the clinical clue to allergic

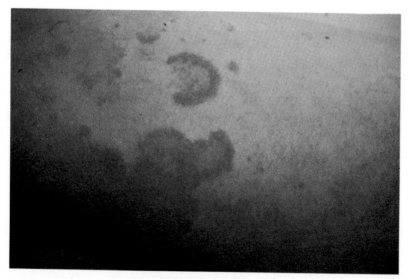

Urticarial vasculitis

vasculitis. Biopsy reveals leukocytoclastic angiitis.

Schönlein-Henoch purpura (anaphylactoid purpura): This disease of children and young adults is characterized by arthritis, abdominal pain, and skin lesions.

Septic vasculitis: When the number of primary lesions is limited, septic vasculitis (see p. 187) should be considered.

■ Treatment

If infectious, treatment of underlying cause. Systemic corticosteroid or cytotoxic agents may be necessary for GI, neurologic, or renal involvement.

Single Smooth, Red Papules, Abrupt Onset

Erysipelas

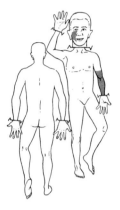

▪ Morphology
Red, warm to hot, sharply marginated, flat to slightly raised plaques of erythema that are indurated and may be painful. In more advanced lesions, purpura and vesicles may be seen.

▪ Distribution
Extremities, face

▪ Patient Profile
Adults or children. Patient may be systemically ill with high fever and toxicity. Lesions are nonpruritic and rapidly change in size within hours. Linear streaking from inflamed lymphatics may be present.

▪ Diagnosis
Erysipelas is a possible diagnosis for any rapidly progressing red, warm plaque. The lesion can progress to streptococcal gangrene or cavernous sinus thrombosis. The cause of this disease is *Streptococcus hemolyticus*. In children who have erysipelas-like lesions, *Haemophilus* cellulitis should be considered. In the immunosup-pressed patient, *Cryptococcus* may cause erysipelas-like eruption. Diagnosis is confirmed by demonstrating streptococci in aspirates of the lesion on Gram's stain and in culture. Biopsy shows acute inflammation and organisms. Erysipeloid caused by the gram-positive *Erysipelothrix rhusiopathiae* should be considered in hand lesions of people who have contact with fish or animals. In Central and South America, erysipelas-like lesions of the eyelid may be due to Chagas' disease.

▪ Treatment
Streptococcus or *Haemophilus* cellulitis often requires hospitalization for intravenous antibiotics.

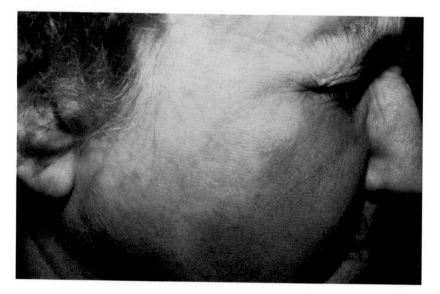

Fixed Drug Reaction

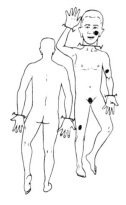

▪ Morphology
One or more sharply marginated red plaques that may blister and heal with marked hyperpigmentation.

▪ Distribution
Anywhere, but most commonly extremities and genitalia.

▪ Patient Profile
Usually adults of both sexes. Lesion occurs within several days of drug ingestion. Drugs commonly associated with fixed drug eruptions include phenolphthalein-containing laxatives, oral contraceptives, barbiturates, salicylates, NSAIDs, and tetracyclines.

▪ Diagnosis
Red lesions recur in exactly the same location with ingestion of a specific drug. Biopsy reveals basal cell vacuolization, incontinence of melanin, and perivascular mononuclear cell infiltrate.

▪ Treatment
Discontinuing precipitating agent. Class II (III on genitals) topical steroids bid until lesion resolves.

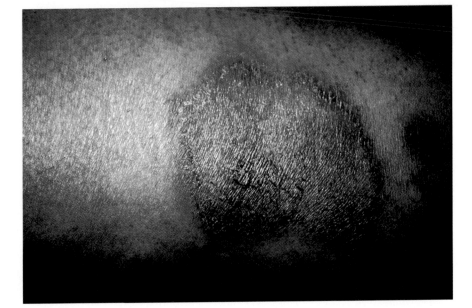

Leishmaniasis

▪ **Morphology**
Erythematous papule that slowly enlarges to become a crusted nodule. Satellite papules may be present. Ulcer formation occurs at the site of the lesion, followed by scar formation.

▪ **Distribution**
Lesion develops at the site of sandfly bite.

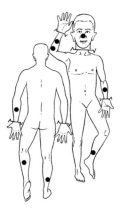

▪ **Patient Profile**
History of travel to Asia, Africa, and Middle East. Multiple lesions may occur with *Leishmania major*. Cutaneous leishmaniasis, diffuse cutaneous leishmaniasis (DCL), mucocutaneous leishmaniasis (MCL), and visceral leishmaniasis (VL) represent the different forms of the disease.

▪ **Diagnosis**
Diagnosis is established by demonstrating the parasite on direct smear from the lesion. Staining the smear with Giemsa shows pale-blue oval amastigotes within tissue macrophages.

▪ **Treatment**
Cutaneous leishmaniasis is self-limited; DCL, MCL, and VL may require intralesional sodium stibogluconate or systemic pentamidine.

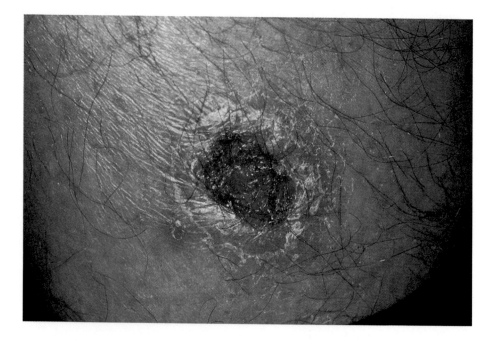

Transient Smooth, Red Papules, Abrupt Onset

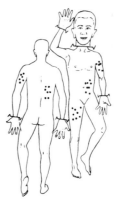

Cholinergic Urticaria

■ Morphology
Small (1 to 2 cm in diameter) white papules on a red base. Lesions are often closely grouped.

■ Distribution
Anywhere, except palms, soles, or mucous membranes.

■ Patient Profile
Any age, both sexes. Lesions are very pruritic and last 1 to 3 hours.

■ Diagnosis
Lesions are precipitated by heat, exertion, or emotional stress. Intradermal injections of methacholine (0.01 mg/0.5 mL saline) reproduce the lesion and pruritus.

■ Treatment
Antihistamines 30 to 45 minutes before activity that precipitates lesions.

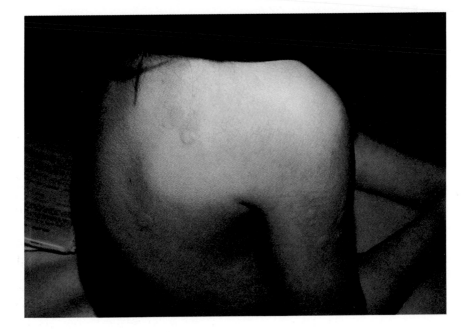

Grover's Disease

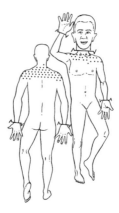

■ **Morphology**
Pruritic, erythematous papules. Vesicular lesions also may be present.

■ **Distribution**
Trunk, neck, and proximal extremities.

■ **Patient Profile**
Most common in white males older than 40 years. Lesions are extremely pruritic.

■ **Diagnosis**
Red papules and papulovesicles that are extremely pruritic are highly diagnostic. Biopsy of lesional skin shows acantholysis of epidermal cells resembling the histologic changes of Darier-White disease, pemphigus, and benign familial pemphigus.

■ **Treatment**
Ultraviolet B and PUVA therapy.

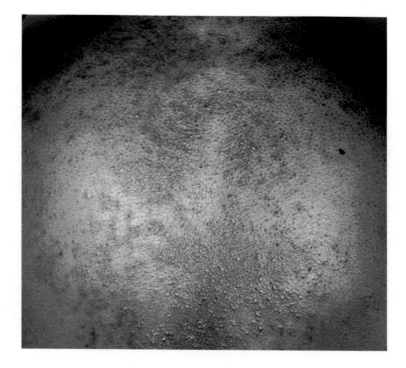

Jellyfish Sting

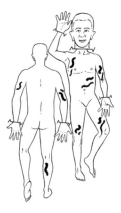

▪ Morphology
Erythematous, urticarial, painful papules in a linear pattern. Lesions may develop petechiae and postinflammatory hyperpigmentation.

▪ Distribution
Any anatomic site.

▪ Patient Profile
History of swimming in salt water preceding the eruption. Local skin eruption may be associated with systemic symptoms ranging from nausea and vomiting to muscle aches and weakness to anaphylaxis and cardiac and respiratory arrest.

▪ Diagnosis
Clinical history and skin eruption establish the diagnosis.

▪ Treatment
Supportive measures.

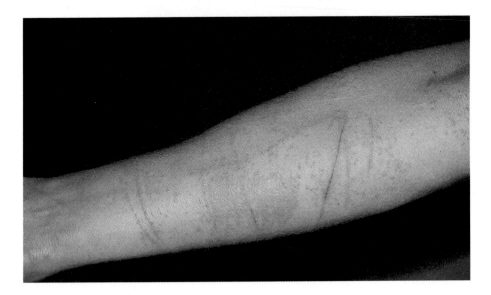

Juvenile Rheumatoid Arthritis

▪ Morphology
Discrete, small erythematous macules and papules with a tendency to central clearing. Linear, arciform lesions may occur. Lesions induced by rubbing, scratching, or hot baths.

▪ Distribution
Trunk, extremities, face, palms, and soles.

▪ Patient Profile
Children or young adults of both sexes. Rash is coincident with fever and lasts hours; may precede polyarthritis, lymphadenopathy, and splenomegaly by months to years.

▪ Diagnosis
Biopsy is not diagnostic. Rheumatoid factor tests may be negative. Difficult to distinguish from rheumatic fever.

▪ Treatment
See rheumatology text.

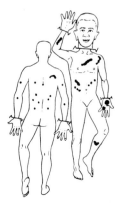

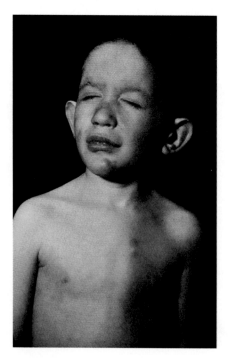

Urticaria
(Hives)

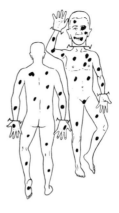

■ Morphology
Erythematous, sharply circumscribed, macular or papular lesions (1 mm to many centimeters). There is frequently a surrounding pale halo, and lesions do not scale. May be circular, annular, arciform polycyclic, or geographic.

■ Distribution
Anywhere on body, including lips and tongue (angioedema). Especially under areas of pressure.

■ Patient Profile
Any age, both sexes. Lesions are frequently very itchy. Lesions last hours and rarely more than a day. Lesions recurring for more than 6 weeks are categorized as chronic urticaria. Lesions can be induced by trauma, dermatographism. Urticaria may be associated with ingestion of drugs (especially aspirin and penicillin), preservatives in foods (dyes and tartrazine), fish, nuts, and berries. Other very common causes are infections, including infectious hepatitis, intestinal parasites, collagen vascular disease, insect bites, contactants, and exposure to physical agents such as pressure, sunlight, cold, heat, water, and vibration. The most common form of chronic urticaria is idiopathic. Urticaria in bathing suit area after sea bathing may be due to sensitization to marine animals (marine dermatitis, seabather's eruption). Urticarial dermatitis occurs on exposed portions of the body after being in water contaminated with fluke larvae. Most cases are self-limited and disappear spontaneously. Persistent urticarial lesions occur-

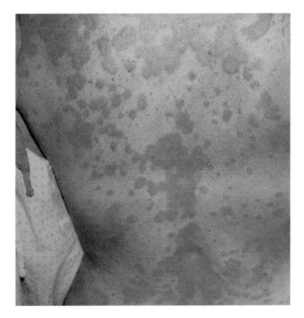

ring on the sides of the hands and feet have been described in patients with serum sickness secondary to immune serum therapy or drugs. Patients with persistent urticaria should be carefully evaluated for collagen vascular disease, hepatitis, hidden drug use.

▪ Diagnosis

Numerous transient lesions that come and go suggest this diagnosis. Biopsy usually reveals dermal edema, vasodilatation, and sparse, perivascular mononuclear cell infiltration. Leukocytoclastic vasculitis may be seen in urticarial vasculitis in which individual lesions persist more than a day; these patients should be evaluated for hypocomplementemia and C1-esterase deficiency.

▪ Treatment

Avoidance of aspirin, nonsteroidals, and opioids. Antihistamines on a regular basis. Agents include H_1 blockers and H_2 blockers.

SMOOTH, RED PAPULES WITH GRADUAL ONSET

DIAGNOSTIC OBSERVATIONS
These are red, raised lesions that have a gradual onset and last weeks to years. Certain lesions have characteristic locations. Many have minimal scale, but scale is not a major feature of the lesions in this category.

MAJOR CATEGORIES

Any Location
Angiokeratoma and cherry angiomas
Configurate erythema and Lyme disease
Erythema elevatum diutinum
Fabry's disease
Granuloma annulare
Granulomatous diseases
Hemangioma
Kaposi's sarcoma, bacterial angiomatosis, and malignant angioendothelioma (see p. 138, 195)
Kawasaki's disease
Leprosy
Leishmaniasis (see p. 204)
Lichen planus: usually blue-purple (p. 251)
Lymphomatoid papulosis
Malignancy: leukemia, lymphoma, metastatic carcinoma, mycosis fungoides
Molluscum contagiosum (see p. 166)
Pityriasis lichenoides et varioliformis acuta (PLEVA)
Pyogenic granuloma: often hemorrhagic
Sarcoidosis
Scabies
Syphilis: usually scaly (see p. 262)

Specific Locations

Digits
Glomus tumor: painful

Head and Neck
Acne vulgaris and rosacea
Follicular mucinosis
Granuloma faciale
Lupus erythematosus
Lymphocytic infiltrate
Lymphocytoma cutis
Perioral dermatitis (see p. 227)
Polymorphous light eruption
Relapsing polychondritis

Genitals
Erythroplasia of Queyrat

Smooth, Red Papules, Gradual Onset (Any Location)

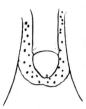

Angiokeratoma of Fordyce

Angiokeratoma and Cherry Angiomas

▪ Morphology
Red to purple small papules with minimal scale. Lesions may be grouped together (angiokeratoma circumscriptum). On occasion they may be up to several centimeters in size. Lesions do not blanch completely with pressure.

▪ Distribution
Under tongue; on scrotum (angiokeratoma of Fordyce), upper trunk (cherry angioma), thighs, and buttocks (angiokeratoma circumscriptum), but may be anywhere.

▪ Patient Profile
Very common. The number of lesions on the trunk and scrotum and under the tongue increases with age. Angiokeratoma circumscriptum is usually present at birth.

▪ Diagnosis
Biopsy reveals dilated vessels and hyperkeratosis.

▪ Treatment
Usually not necessary. Lesion often recurs after electrodesiccation. Cherry hemangiomas respond to laser therapy.

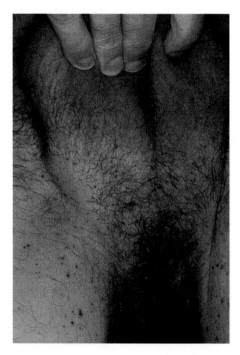

Configurate Erythema and Lyme Disease

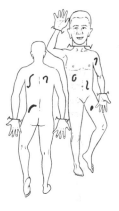

▪ Morphology
Erythematous ring-shaped and polycyclic lesions may scale slightly (erythema annulare centrifugum), spread by peripheral extension with central clearing. Occasionally, waves of erythema simulate tree bark (erythema gyratum repens).

▪ Distribution
Usually trunk; may involve entire skin.

▪ Patient Profile
Both sexes, any age; most frequent in young adults. Nonpruritic lesions. Lesions are associated with fungal infections, neoplasms, blood dyscrasias, drug sensitivity, and immunologic disturbances. Usually idiopathic.

Borrelial disease should be considered. On occasion, a single lesion spreads rapidly from a central punctum (erythema chronicum migrans). This may be associated with a tick bite and oligoarticular arthritis, neurologic disorders, fatigue, and cardiovascular signs and symptoms (Lyme disease). Residing in an epidemic region for *Ixodes* ticks is a clue for borrelial disease.

▪ Diagnosis
The clinical picture suggests the diagnosis. Biopsy reveals perivascular mononuclear cell infiltration, and is especially helpful in ruling out other possibilities, such as lymphoma, leukemia, sarcoid, tuberculosis, leprosy, leishmaniasis, mycosis fungoides, granuloma annulare, and lupus erythematosus.

▪ Treatment
In suspected borrelial disease, systemic antibiotics can decrease neurologic, arthritic, and cardiovascular complications. In children, penicillin or cephalosporin is indicated.

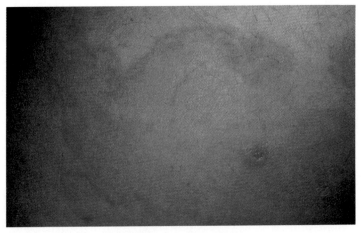

Erythema chronicum migrans

Erythema Elevatum Diutinum

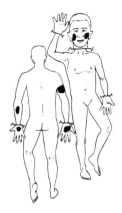

▪ Morphology
Red to purple papules and plaques that may develop ringlike configurations.

▪ Distribution
Symmetric; face, extensor aspect of hands and arms.

▪ Patient Profile
More common in men than in women. Older age group. Lesions are persistent.

▪ Diagnosis
Biopsy is diagnostic and reveals hyaline degeneration around proliferating and degenerating capillaries. There is a dense, inflammatory infiltrate with polymorphonuclear leukocytes and eosinophils.

▪ Treatment
Dapsone can arrest this disease. Long-term therapy is necessary. G6PD levels are required before beginning therapy, and hemoglobin and reticulocyte monitoring during therapy.

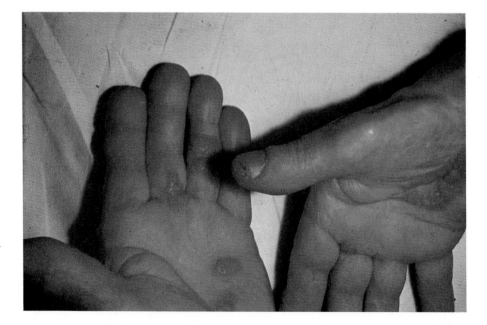

Granuloma Annulare

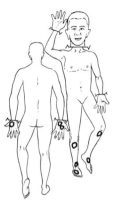

▪ Morphology
Groups of small (1 to 5 mm) pink to red papules coalesce to form rings. Lesions may be minimally scaly. Lesions spread peripherally, clear centrally, and resolve without atrophy over months. Subcutaneous nodules (1 to 5 cm in diameter) may be present near joints.

▪ Distribution
Dorsum of hands and feet. Extensor aspect of extremities near joints. Some patients will develop generalized disease.

▪ Patient Profile
More frequent in women. Young adults and children most commonly affected. Lesions rarely pruritic. Patients younger than 10 years and older than 40 years more likely to develop generalized disease. Seen also in immunosuppressed or HIV-positive patients.

▪ Diagnosis
Pink papules arranged in rings near joints are highly suggestive of this diagnosis. The papular nature of the ring can be emphasized by stretching the lesion. Older women with disseminated granuloma annulare may have diabetes mellitus. Biopsy shows necrobiotic degeneration of collagen and a chronic inflammatory infiltrate.

▪ Treatment
Usually not necessary but can respond to potent steroids. Topical steroids (II or III) may hasten resolution. Niacinamide (1000 to 1500 mg) and isotretinoin have been used for several cases.

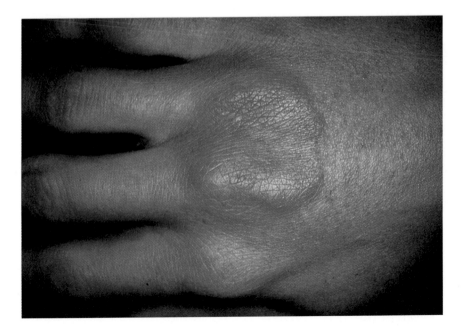

Granulomatous Diseases

Multiple brownish-red papules of various sizes may be seen in a variety of diseases with dermal inflammation. The epidermis is often intact. Biopsy with cultures and special stains and a complete evaluation of the patient is necessary in this differential diagnosis.

Cat scratch disease (see p. 460)
Deep fungal disease (see p. 459)
Foreign body disease (see p. 401)
Leishmaniasis (see p. 204)
Mycobacterial disease: including tuberculosis, atypical mycobacterial disease, and swimming pool granuloma (see p. 412)
Sarcoidosis (see p. 223)
Syphilis and yaws (see pp. 402, 461)

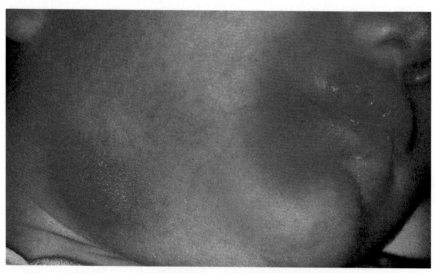

Tuberculosis

Hemangioma

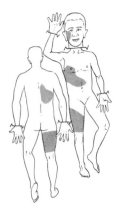

▪ Morphology
Single or multiple red to blue-purple plaques that blanch dramatically with pressure. Diffuse redness, increased hair growth, and scaling may occur over lesions.

▪ Distribution
Anywhere. Lesions may appear in dermatomal distribution.

▪ Patient Profile
Lesions may appear at birth and frequently increase in size during the first few months of life. Lesions may spontaneously regress and may be associated with underlying neurologic or skeletal abnormalities. Some infants will develop multiple hemangiomas that may or may not be associated with organ (liver, lung, GI tract, and CNS) hemangiomas. Development of purpura in the lesion and petechiae may result from thrombocytopenia due to sequestration of platelets in the hemangioma (Kasabach-Merritt syndrome).

▪ Diagnosis
A blue to purple plaque that blanches with pressure suggests the diagnosis of hemangioma. Biopsy reveals vascular proliferation. Lymphangioma may simulate hemangioma.

▪ Treatment
Laser often useful. Intralesional or systemic steroids and interferon alfa-2 in lesions interfering with function.

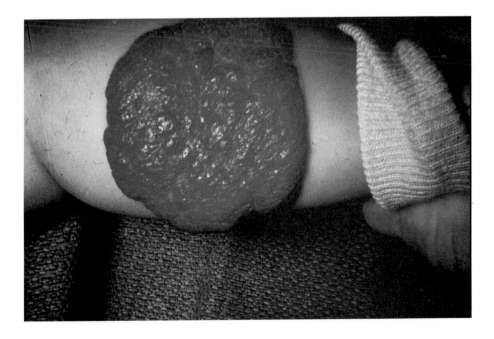

Kawasaki's Disease

▪ **Morphology**
Erythematous papules and macules.

▪ **Distribution**
Trunk and proximal extremities but can be more generalized.

▪ **Patient Profile**
Child with a fever, lymphadenopathy, oral involvement, and an exanthem. May have complicating cardiac involvement, arthralgia or arthritis, urethritis, aseptic meningitis, and GI complaints.

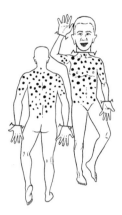

▪ **Diagnosis**
Child with fever for 5 or more days with 4 or 5 of the following: bilateral conjunctival injection, orophyarnx involvement (injected or fissured lips, injected pharynx, strawberry tongue), erythema of palms and soles, edema of hands or feet, periungual desquamation, polymorphous exanthem, and acute cervical lymphadenopathy. Must be differentiated from toxic shock syndrome, which is seen primarily in adults, associated with fever, generalized erythroderma, hypotension, and thrombocytosis.

▪ **Treatment**
Aspirin, IV immunoglobulin, symptomatic support.

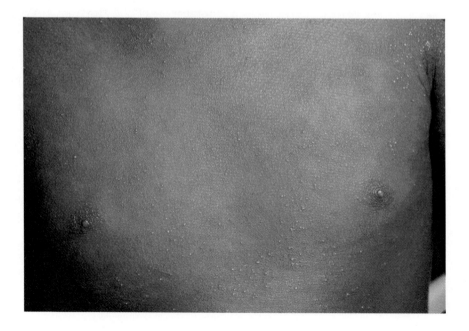

Leprosy

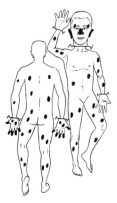

■ Morphology
Multiple red to flesh-colored symmetric papules, plaques, nodules, and macules. Lesions may vary from small papules to large plaques and may be annular or polycyclic.

■ Distribution
Face, especially tip of nose and ears; hands; arms; and buttocks. Lesions spare the skin over the spinal column.

■ Patient Profile
Any age, usually adults of both sexes. Patient has lived in endemic areas. This is a common subtropical and tropical disease. Lepromatous leprosy has peripheral neuropathy but the skin lesions have sensation. Borderline and tuberculoid leprosy have anesthetic lesions. Painless plantar ulcers are common. Anhidrosis and ichthyosis may occur. Eyes, bones, and joints may be involved.

■ Diagnosis
Biopsy shows diffuse infiltration of the dermis with foamy macrophages that contain acid-fast organisms. Nasal and earlobe scrapings may demonstrate *Mycobacterium leprae.* Granulomatous leprosy will have few, if any, organisms.

■ Treatment
See an infectious disease text.

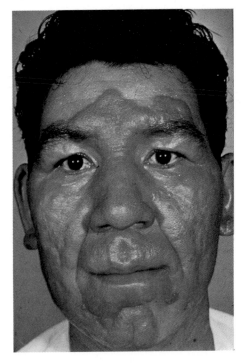

Malignancy
(Lymphoma, Leukemia, Metastatic
Carcinoma, Mycosis Fungoides,
Adnexal Tumor)

▪ **Morphology**
Red-brown to blue-purple papules and
plaques, initially with normal skin markings. Usually multiple. May scale, erode,
or ulcerate.

▪ **Distribution**
Anywhere. Asymmetric.

▪ **Patient Profile**
Both sexes, older age group. Lesions often
erupt in crops and grow rapidly. Patients
usually have stigmata of underlying neoplasm, such as purpura, constitutional
symptoms, organomegaly, and adenopathy. Lesions may develop over days and
persist if untreated.

▪ **Diagnosis**
This diagnosis requires biopsy; the histology depends on the primary process.

▪ **Treatment**
Treatment of underlying disease.

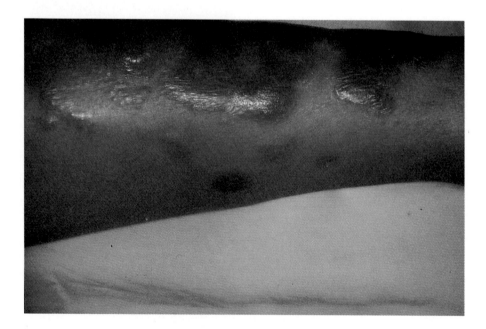

Pityriasis Lichenoides et Varioliformis Acuta (PLEVA)

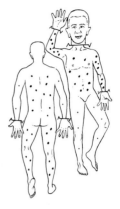

▪ Morphology
Papules evolve into vesicles and hemorrhagic crusts. Ulcers, depressed scars, and hypopigmentation common. Scaly red papules are the most common lesions, and intact vesicles are rare.

▪ Distribution
Trunk and flexor portions of arms and thighs most commonly affected. Lesions are scattered and not grouped. Mucosal lesions are very rare.

▪ Patient Profile
Both sexes; usually during late childhood and adolescence. Mild headache and malaise may accompany eruptions. Lesions may burn or irritate but do not itch. The disease lasts weeks to months.

▪ Diagnosis
The variety of lesions, papules, vesicles, and scars in a generally healthy young person suggests this diagnosis.

Toxoplasmosis is associated with this clinical picture; a Sabin dye test or indirect-fluorescent antibody study is indicated. Biopsy shows a lymphocytic perivascular infiltrate and edematous reaction with hemorrhage below and within the epidermis. The results of laboratory tests are negative.

▪ Treatment
Patients often respond to systemic antibiotics (1 g tetracycline or erythromycin per day). Methotrexate, 15 to 25 mg each week, has been used in refractory patients. PUVA therapy.

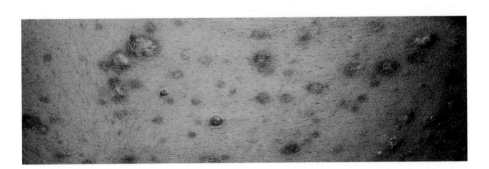

Pyogenic Granuloma

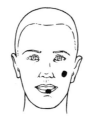
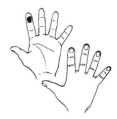

■ Morphology
A bright red to brown multiloculated (0.5 to 1 cm) papule that erodes and develops a hemorrhagic crust. Usually occurs singly and reaches maximum size in a few weeks.

■ Distribution
Anywhere, but common on face and fingers. On gingiva in pregnancy.

■ Patient Profile
Both sexes, any age, but more common in childhood; also seen during pregnancy. Trauma frequently precedes lesion. Lesion may bleed profusely if scratched. May be a complication of oral isotretinoin therapy.

■ Diagnosis
Biopsy shows capillary proliferation, swollen endothelial cells, and infiltration by inflammatory cells.

■ Treatment
Shave excision and laser or electrodesiccation of the base. Laser.

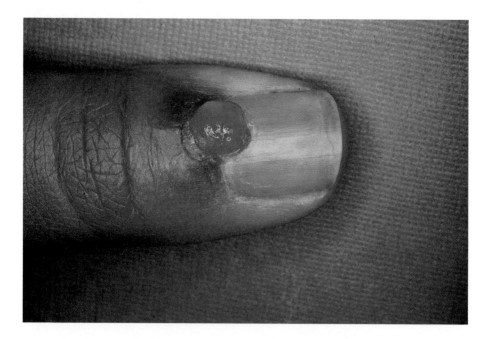

Sarcoidosis

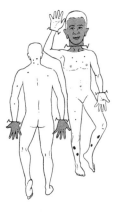

▪ Morphology
Multiple pink to red papules of various sizes (0.5 to 10 cm). The surface of the lesions is usually smooth, but fine telangiectasia, slight scaling, or minimal atrophy may be seen. Ringlike grouping of individual lesions may be seen. Erythema nodosum (see p. 421) may occur.

▪ Distribution
Small papules may be anywhere, but most common on the face and extremities. Large plaques with dilated vessels are most common on the face and especially around ears and nose. Sarcoid papules often occur in scars and can be follicular in distribution. Erythema nodosum is found on the legs (see p. 421).

▪ Patient Profile
Any age, most common in 20- to 50-year-old age group. More common in females and American blacks. Dyspnea, cough, and hilar adenopathy. Uveitis, parotid and lacrimal gland enlargement, organomegaly, generalized lymphadenopathy, and neuropathy are frequent.

▪ Diagnosis
Multiple dermal papules with minor surface change associated with systemic signs and symptoms suggest this diagnosis. Biopsy is mandatory and shows discrete, noncaseating granulomas that often contain giant cells with inclusion bodies. Sarcoidlike granulomas also may be caused by beryllium, silica, talc, quartz, zirconium, and mercury. A careful history and polarizing microscopy of biopsy will eliminate these causes.

▪ Treatment
Small lesions may respond to class I topical steroids or intralesional steroids. Deforming skin lesions may require hydroxychloroquine or, rarely, systemic steroids.

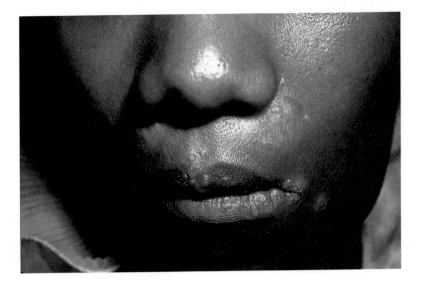

Scabies

▪ **Morphology**
Papules are small, hivelike, excoriated, and sometimes purpuric. Indurated nodules occur, especially on the genitalia.

▪ **Distribution**
Lesions are prominent on flexor aspects of wrists; between fingers; ulnar border of hand; anterior axillary fold; skin around nipple, groin, penis, umbilicus, and toe webs. Children may have lesions on palms and soles. No oral lesions.

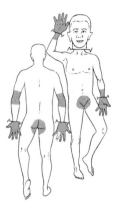

▪ **Patient Profile**
All ages but more frequent in young adults. Both sexes. Disease may last for months. Perirectal lesions may be seen in the elderly. Extremely pruritic lesions.

▪ **Diagnosis**
Scabies is transmitted by close personal contact. Patients should be questioned about similar problems among sexual contacts or family members. Diagnosis is established by demonstrating the mite. A fresh lesion, preferably on the hands or wrists, should be selected, the deepest part of the burrow scraped carefully and vigorously with a scalpel blade, and the material examined in mineral oil under the microscope (see p. 17).

▪ **Treatment**
Application of permethrin (Elimite) over the body from the neck down overnight is preferred. Lindane (Kwell) often effective. Pruritus may persist for several weeks after treatment and should be treated with topical steroids and systemic antihistamines. Postscabetic nodules may require treatment with class I or II topical corticosteroids or intralesional corticosteroids.

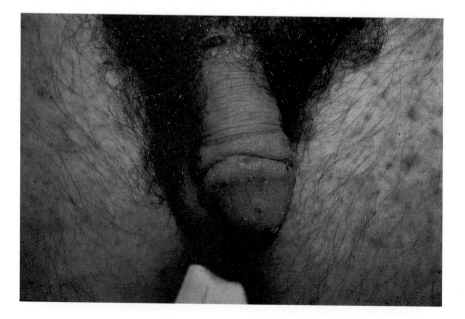

Smooth, Red Papules, Gradual Onset (Digits)

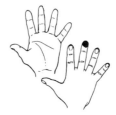

Digits

Glomus Tumor

■ **Morphology**
Single and occasionally multiple red papules, <1 cm in size.

■ **Distribution**
Tips of digits and possibly under nails.

■ **Patient Profile**
Adults. Glomus tumors under the nail are more common in women. Lesions are painful to touch or with temperature change. Multiple glomus tumors may be painless.

■ **Diagnosis**
Biopsy reveals encapsulated tumor with plump round cells containing clear cytoplasm arranged around vessels.

■ **Treatment**
Surgical excision.

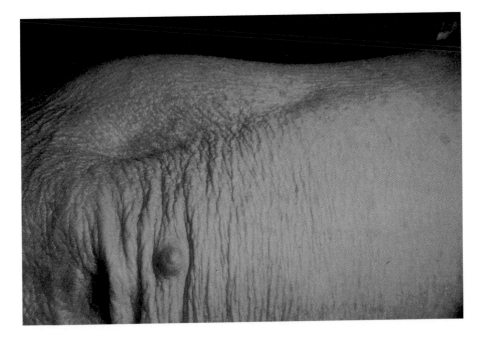

Genitals

Erythroplasia of Queyrat

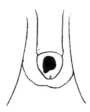

■ **Morphology**
Single, sharply circumscribed, smooth, red papule. Slightly raised red plaques. Lesions have a velvety surface.

■ **Distribution**
Glans penis and, rarely, labia.

■ **Patient Profile**
Most common in older, uncircumcised men but can occur in women. Slight burning or itching may be present.

■ **Diagnosis**
Biopsy is necessary for diagnosis and shows atypical epidermal hyperplasia.

■ **Treatment**
This is carcinoma in situ and should be treated with excision or topical 5-fluorouracil.

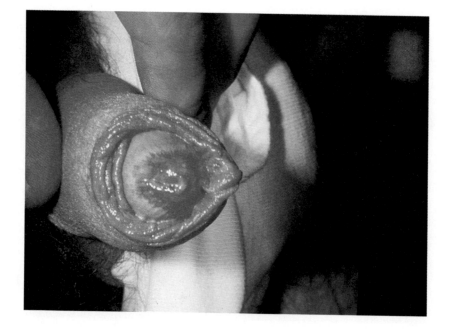

Head and Neck

Acne Vulgaris and Rosacea

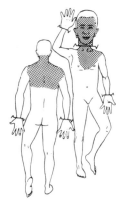

Morphology
Red papules that may be associated with open comedones (blackheads), closed comedones (whiteheads), and cysts.

▪ Distribution
Face, including eyelids, upper chest, and upper back.

▪ Patient Profile
Common among adolescents and young adults of both sexes. Lesions are exacerbated by greasy cosmetics, high humidity, and fluorinated topical steroids (perioral dermatitis). Sudden appearance of ulcerative acne often accompanied by fever is called *acne fulminans*. Most common in teenage males. Tender lesions on trunk that usually spare the face and neck and heal with scarring.

▪ Diagnosis
Acne papules of the middle third of face may be associated with thickening of skin on nose (rhinophyma) and telangiectasia in adults. This condition is known as *acne rosacea*.

▪ Treatment
Topical erythromycin or clindamycin; topical metronidazole. Systemic tetracycline or minocycline.

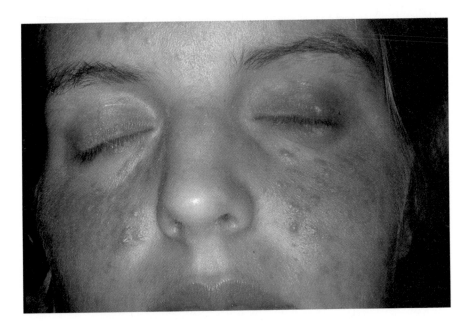

Follicular Mucinosis

▪ **Morphology**
Single or multiple red papules or plaques with hair loss.

▪ **Distribution**
Most common on scalp, forehead, neck, and shoulders.

▪ **Patient Profile**
All ages, both sexes. Nonpruritic lesions.

▪ **Diagnosis**
A plaque or perifollicular papule with prominent alopecia suggests this diagnosis. The disease is usually benign, but it may be associated with lymphoma, especially mycosis fungoides in adults. Biopsy is diagnostic and shows mucinous material in root sheaths of hair follicles.

▪ **Treatment**
Class I or II topical corticosteroids; intralesional corticosteroids.

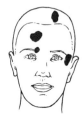

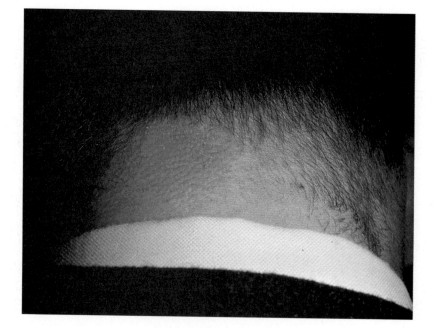

Granuloma Faciale

■ **Morphology**
Red to purple-brown plaques with follicular prominence and telangiectasia. Usually single, rarely multiple.

■ **Distribution**
Face, rarely elsewhere on body and hands.

■ **Patient Profile**
Older adults. Lasts for years, grows slowly, pruritic.

■ **Diagnosis**
Biopsy is necessary for diagnosis; it reveals dense, neutrophilic, and eosinophilic inflammatory infiltrate that spares uppermost papillary dermis. Similar lesions on nose and nasal mucosa are seen in rhinoscleroma.

■ **Treatment**
Cryotherapy, intralesional corticosteroids, or laser. Often very resistant to therapy.

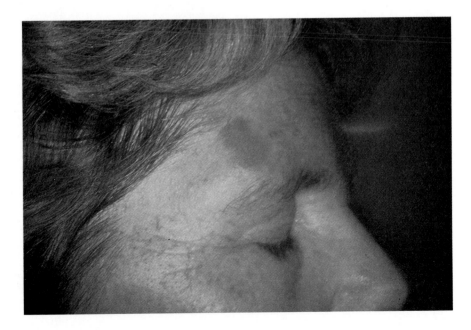

Lupus Erythematosus
(Acute)

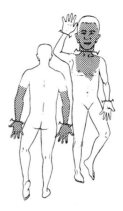

▪ Morphology
Red papules and plaques with fine scale.

▪ Distribution
Anywhere, but most common on face and other sun-exposed areas of body, malar eminences (butterfly distribution).

▪ Patient Profile
Mostly young adult women. Chronic disease. Nonpruritic lesions.

▪ Diagnosis
Patient is often febrile and ill. Presence of these skin lesions in patient with neurologic disease, arthritis, renal disease, or neuropsychiatric disturbances suggests the diagnosis. Serologic tests, skin biopsy for routine histology, and immunofluorescence establish the diagnosis.

▪ Treatment
Systemic corticosteroids useful in acute attack or flares. Hydroxychloroquine and sunscreens for chronic therapy.

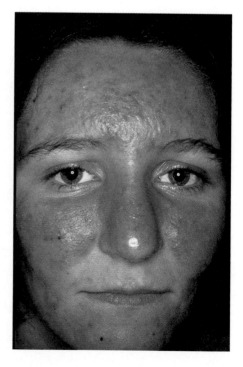

Lymphocyte Infiltrate of Skin
(Jessner-Kanof)

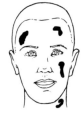

■ Morphology
Smooth, pink to reddish-brown papules and plaques that extend peripherally and clear centrally. Persistent, nonscarring, and recurrent.

■ Distribution
Face, neck most common sites.

■ Patient Profile
Most common in older men. Nonpruritic lesions. Usually unresponsive to therapy.

■ Diagnosis
Biopsy shows lymphocytes and histiocytes around vessels, and immunofluorescent studies for lupus erythematosus are negative.

■ Treatment
Class I or II topical corticosteroids; intralesional steroids.

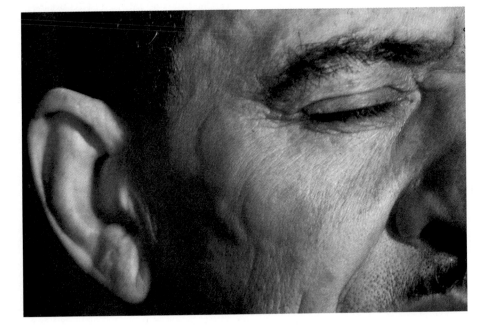

Lymphocytoma Cutis
(Spiegler-Fendt Sarcoid)

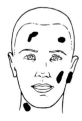

▪ **Morphology**
Smooth, red to yellow-brown papules up to 5 cm in diameter.

▪ **Distribution**
Most common on face and neck. Lesions are usually limited to one body area and rarely disseminate.

▪ **Patient Profile**
Adults of both sexes. Nonpruritic lesions. No photosensitivity or systemic disease.

▪ **Diagnosis**
Biopsy shows dense infiltrate of lymphocytes and histiocytes in follicular arrangement in the dermis. Nuclear dust, lack of invasion of normal structures, and slightly atypical cytology differentiate this disease from malignant lymphoma. Multiple papules around the ear and in scalp often have dense, lymphohistiocytic or eosinophilic infiltrate and have been called pseudopyogenic granuloma. Multiple lesions on the head and neck associated with a peripheral blood eosinophilia characterize angiolymphoid hyperplasia with eosinophilia.

▪ **Treatment**
Class I or II topical corticosteroids; intralesional corticosteroids.

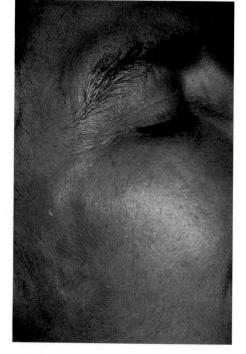

Polymorphous Light Eruption

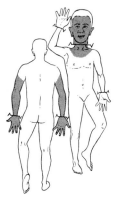

▪ Morphology
Sharply circumscribed red to purple papules and plaques that may become thickened, lichenified, and scaly. Some patients will develop papulovesicular lesions in a light-exposed distribution.

▪ Distribution
Light-exposed areas, especially face, back of neck, V of neckline, dorsum of hands, and extensor aspects of arms. Periorbital, submental, and underarms usually spared.

▪ Patient Profile
Adults of both sexes. Frequent in Native Americans. Lesions begin and flare up during periods of sun exposure. Lesions may itch.

▪ Diagnosis
Prominence of lesions in sun-exposed areas should suggest this diagnosis. Can be reproduced by repeated light exposure. Biopsy reveals dense, perivascular round-cell infiltrate and liquefactive degeneration of the basal cell layer. Lack of immunoglobulin deposition on immunofluorescent examination differentiates this syndrome from lupus erythematosus. A similar picture may be seen in photoallergic dermatitis; the latter is differentiated by positive photopatch test.

Other diseases with accentuation in light-exposed areas include actinic keratosis, porokeratosis, Darier's disease, drug photosensitivity and phototoxicity, lupus erythematosus, dermatomyositis, pellagra, porphyrias, solar urticarias, and rare hereditary syndromes (Bloom, Cockayne's, Hartnup, Rothmund-Thomson, xeroderma pigmentosum, photosensitive form of trichothiodystrophy).

▪ Treatment
Class I or II topical corticosteroids and sun protection with clothing. Sunscreens with UVA and UVB protection.

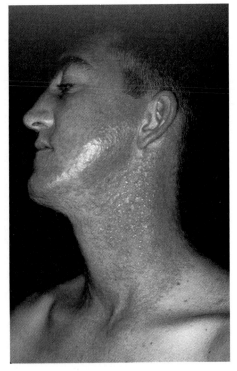

Relapsing Polychondritis

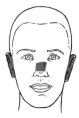

▪ Morphology
Macular erythema, tenderness, and swelling over the cartilaginous portions of the ear.

▪ Distribution
Ears and nose.

▪ Patient Profile
Adults, often with a history of arthritis. May have associated autoimmune disease.

▪ Diagnosis
The diagnosis is established by a biopsy of involved areas, which show loss of normal cartilage basophilia with perichondrial inflammation plus 3 out of 5 of the following: bilateral auricular chondritis; nonerosive, seronegative polyarthritis; nasal chondritis; ocular inflammation; respiratory chondritis; and audiovestibular damage.

▪ Treatment
Systemic corticosteroids.

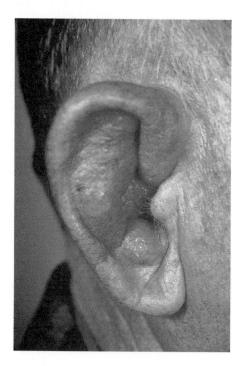

SCALY PAPULES

DIAGNOSTIC OBSERVATIONS

Surface irregularities and scaling characterize this group, which contains a large number of common and similar-appearing dermatologic diseases. All scaling lesions should be scraped and examined with potassium hydroxide (see p. 14) to exclude dermatophyte, *Candida* infection, and tinea versicolor. Certain lesions are more frequent on sun-exposed sites (e.g., actinic keratosis and cutaneous lupus erythematous). Several of the diseases often have from 1 to 10 lesions and are separated on that basis. Others frequently are generalized.

Limited Lesions (<10)

Actinic keratoses
Bowen's disease
Keratoacanthoma
Lichen simplex chronicus
Paget's disease
Warts, including condylomata

Multiple lesions

Atopic dermatitis (eczema)
Darier's disease
Dermatophyte infection
Drug eruptions
Exfoliative dermatitis
Kawasaki's disease
Keratosis pilaris
Lichen amyloidosis and lichen myxedematosus (see p. 178)
Lichen planus
Lupus erythematosus
Mycosis fungoides and parapsoriasis
Neurodermatitis (see p. 239)
Nummular eczema
Pityriasis rosea
Pityriasis rubra pilaris
Prurigo nodularis
Psoriasis
Seborrheic dermatitis
Seborrheic keratoses
Secondary syphilis
Squamous cell carcinoma
Tinea versicolor
Warts and condyloma acuminatum (see pp. 241–242)

Scaly Papules (Limited Lesions)

Actinic Keratoses

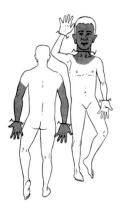

▪ Morphology
Poorly circumscribed, pink to red, slightly scaly lesions. Removal of scale often results in erosions or bleeding. Wrinkling, hyperpigmentation and hypopigmentation, telangiectasia, and evidence of sun damage is common. Palpation of lesions reveals a sandlike feel.

▪ Distribution
Sun-exposed areas such as face, head, neck, and dorsum of hands.

▪ Patient Profile
Adults in both sexes. Extremely common condition. Lesions increase in number with age. Patients often have fair skin and burn instead of tan. History of excessive sun exposure is common. Lesions may progress to squamous cell carcinoma.

▪ Diagnosis
The clinical picture is highly suggestive of the diagnosis. Biopsy should be performed on indurated lesions to rule out squamous cell carcinoma. Biopsy of actinic keratoses reveals hyperkeratosis, disordered maturation of keratinocytes, perivascular round-cell infiltrate, and basophilic degeneration of collagen.

▪ Treatment
Liquid nitrogen or electrodesiccation. Very hyperkeratotic lesions may have to be excised. Multiple lesions respond to topical 5-fluorouracil applied until lesions are inflamed (2 to 3 weeks).

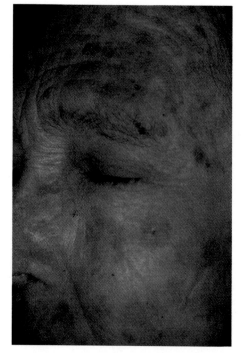

Bowen's Disease
(Squamous Cell Carcinoma in Situ)

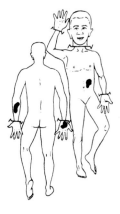

■ **Morphology**
Persistent, single, sharply circumscribed, pink scaly plaque that may crust.

■ **Distribution**
Anywhere, but often on sun-exposed areas.

■ **Patient Profile**
Adults of both sexes.

■ **Diagnosis**
Biopsy shows dyskeratosis and epithelial atypia extending through the full thickness of the epidermis. Superficial basal cell carcinoma resembles Bowen's disease. Disease on non–sun-exposed areas may suggest arsenic ingestion and internal malignancy.

■ **Treatment**
Surgical excision, curettage and electrodesiccation, topical 5-fluorouracil, cryotherapy.

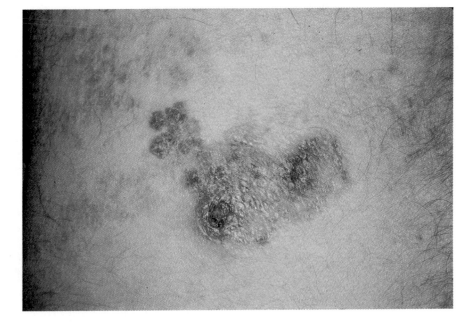

Keratoacanthoma

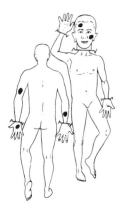

■ Morphology
Raised, red, firm, scaly lesion with a central volcano-like depression filled with scaly debris. Usually single, rarely multiple.

■ Distribution
Face or extremities, but can be anywhere.

■ Patient Profile
Late middle-aged adults in both sexes.

■ Diagnosis
Extremely rapid growth (weeks) and a volcano-like appearance suggest keratoacanthoma. Biopsy reveals atypical epithelial cells with a ground-glass appearance extending into dermis, a central area of keratotic debris, and inflammatory cells in the dermis.

■ Treatment
Excision, curettage and electrodesiccation, or intralesional 5-fluorouracil or methotrexate.

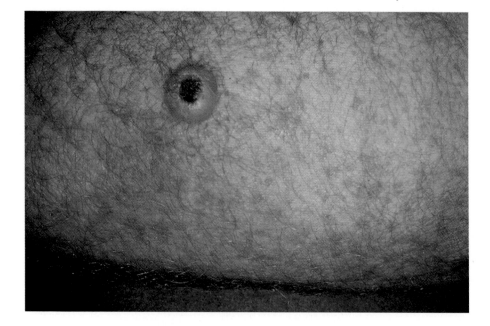

Lichen Simplex Chronicus
(Neurodermatitis)

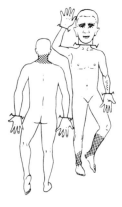

■ **Morphology**
Poorly circumscribed, raised, red, slightly scaly, large plaques with lichenification and excoriation. Heal with hyperpigmentation.

■ **Distribution**
Posterior neck, extremities, and over malleoli are common sites; may be anywhere but rare on face.

■ **Patient Profile**
Adults of both sexes. Extremely pruritic lesions, especially with stress.

■ **Diagnosis**
Biopsy reveals a nonspecific psoriasiform dermatitis. Lichen planus may simulate this disease but can be differentiated by biopsy.

■ **Treatment**
Class I or II topical corticosteroids, topical tars; Cordran tape or intralesional corticosteroids in selected cases.

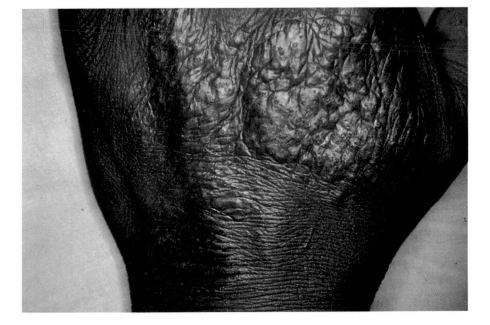

Paget's Disease

■ **Morphology**
A single red-brown, well-circumscribed plaque with scaling and loss of normal skin markings.

■ **Distribution**
Nipple and areola of breast are most common sites, but lesions also occur in genital area.

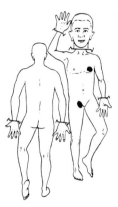

■ **Patient Profile**
Breast and extramammary Paget's diseases more commonly involve adult women. Extramammary disease most commonly involves the genital area but also is seen in the axillae, as well as presternal and periumbilical areas.

■ **Diagnosis**
Biopsy is diagnostic and shows large, pale cells with glycogen granules in the cytoplasm of the neoplastic cells. Paget's disease is frequently associated with intraductal carcinoma. Mammogram and surgical consultation.

■ **Treatment**
Surgical excision.

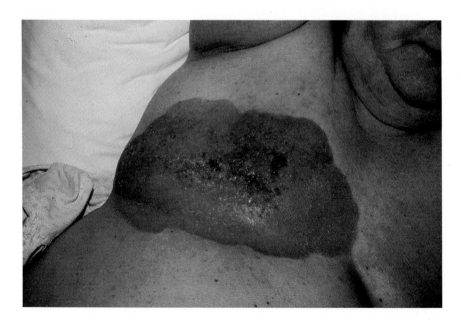

Warts (Common)
Verruca Vulgaris

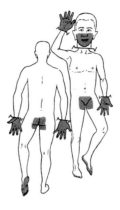

▪ Morphology
Discrete, raised, hypopigmented pink lesions with irregular, scaly-appearing "verrucous" surface. Paring of lesions produces multiple, fine bleeding points. Lesions may be linear or in groups. On the palms and soles, skin markings diverge around the wart.

▪ Distribution
Anywhere; common locations are hands, knees, palms and soles, nail beds, scalp, lips, and genitals. Immunosuppressed patients may have diffuse involvement, including the face.

▪ Patient Profile
Both sexes; more common in children, young adults, and immunosuppressed patients, including those who are HIV-positive. Refractory lesions in adults require ruling out HIV. Nonpruritic. Lesions on sole may be painful.

▪ Diagnosis
Lesions with an irregular surface that develop multiple, fine bleeding points when pared suggest the diagnosis of warts. Biopsy reveals hyperkeratosis, acanthosis, papillomatosis, and vacuolated cells in the upper stratum malpighii with intranuclear eosinophilic inclusions. Wartlike lesions due to inoculation of deep fungi or mycobacteria directly into the skin (prosector's wart) occur uncommonly.

▪ Treatment
Feet: 40% salicylic acid plasters under occlusion. General body: liquid nitrogen. Canthrone. Laser.

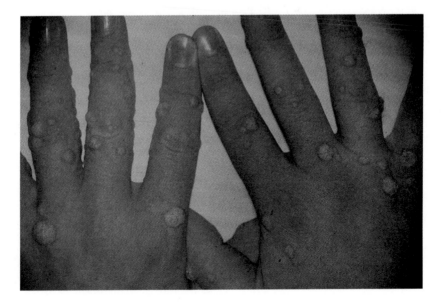

Warts
(Condylomata)

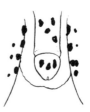

▪ Morphology
Single or multiple white, pink, or slightly hyperpigmented papules with a highly irregular verrucous surface that resembles cauliflower. Early lesions may be flat and pink. A probable variant of genital warts with multiple small brown lesions is bowenoid papules of the penis.

▪ Distribution
Anogenital region: penile, vaginal, or rectal mucosa, as well as lips and mouth may be involved. Other intertriginous areas such as axillae and groin may develop condylomata.

▪ Patient Profile
Sexually active adults of both sexes.

▪ Diagnosis
The verrucous, irregular surface of the lesion is highly suggestive of this diagnosis. The smaller papules may resemble lichen planus, syphilis, psoriasis, or Fabry's disease. Biopsy may be necessary to exclude the presence of squamous cell carcinoma. Biopsy is diagnostic and shows hyperkeratosis, acanthosis, papillomatosis, and vacuolated cells in the stratum malpighii. A serologic test for syphilis is indicated for atypical lesions and because of coexistence of other venereal diseases.

▪ Treatment
Podophyllin applied (contraindicated in pregnant patients), cantharone, or liquid nitrogen. With perirectal lesions, anoscopy and culdoscopy to detect intra-anal and vaginal involvement.

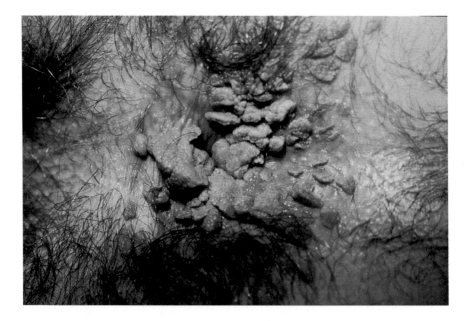

Scaly Papules (Multiple Lesions)

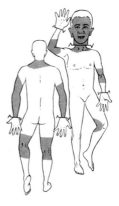

Atopic Dermatitis
(Eczema)

▪ Morphology
Red to red-brown, raised, scaly, poorly circumscribed lesions with accentuation of skin markings (lichenification) and excoriation. Lesions may become infected and crusted. Lesions heal with hyperpigmentation and hypopigmentation, especially in patients with very pigmented skin. Edema of the eyelids, conjunctivitis, and rhinitis are common.

▪ Distribution
Symmetric. Infants: cheeks, scalp, trunk, and lower leg. Children younger than 4 years and adults: antecubital and popliteal space, thighs, neck, and hands. At any age, eruption may be generalized.

▪ Patient Profile
This disease is extremely pruritic. It usually begins in infancy and early childhood, remits in late childhood, and flares in adolescence. The disease clears in 60% of patients in adulthood. Patients may have asthma, rhinitis, and autosomal dominant ichthyosis vulgaris (see p. 129).

▪ Diagnosis
Pruritic eruption in an atopic patient suggests the diagnosis of atopic dermatitis. Many patients have elevated IgE levels. Biopsy reveals nonspecific psoriasiform dermatitis. Atopic eczema frequently becomes infected with bacteria and less com-

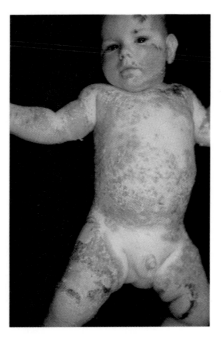

monly, with virus (eczema herpeticum), especially herpes simplex virus (p. 306).

■ Treatment

Household, especially patient's bedroom, should maintain a high relative humidity with a room humidifier. Avoidance of wool or other itch-provoking fabrics, dust, and animal dander. Use of mild, unscented soaps (e.g., Dove, Purpose). Soap should be removed completely after bathing. Retaining moisture in epidermis by applying moisturizers immediately after bathing (e.g., Eucerin, Aquaphor, Moisturel, Vaseline). Systemic antihistamines to control itching, especially at night. Application of topical corticosteroids class II or III to very pruritic lesions, topical tars, UVB or PUVA therapy in selected patients.

Darier's Disease

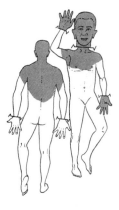

▪ Morphology
Raised, scaly red-brown papules (0.5 to 1 cm in diameter) occur around hair follicles. Smaller papules (1 to 2 mm) without scale may also be present. Crusting may occur. Some families have acral hemorrhagic lesions. The nails are thin and have chips and cracks at the free edge; nails also demonstrate parallel red and white stripes in the nail bed.

▪ Distribution
Symmetric. Scalp, posterior head, neck, chest, and back are the most common sites. Smaller papules may be seen on distal extremities, including palms and soles. Oral papules with a cobblestone appearance may be present.

▪ Patient Profile
Both sexes, beginning in childhood or adolescence. Autosomal dominant inheritance. Worse in summer, exacerbated by ultraviolet light. Herpes simplex infection may occur in the skin lesions.

▪ Diagnosis
The scaly, brown, perifollicular papules in the characteristic distribution are diagnostic. The biopsy demonstrates clefts above the basal layer and individual cell keratinization. Adults may develop a self-limited, highly pruritic disease with a similar appearance, distribution, and pathology (transient acantholytic disease). Systemic IL-4 lesions produce similar lesions.

▪ Treatment
Systemic retinoids for severe lesions. Treatment may be necessary only in spring and summer. Moisturizers and mild keratolytics (lachydrin 12%) may be useful.

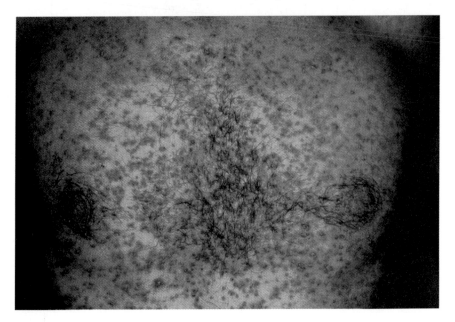

Dermatophyte Infection

▪ **Morphology**

One or more red, polycyclic, arciform, and annular lesions with scaling. Lesions tend to spread peripherally with central clearing. Candidiasis is associated with satellite pustules.

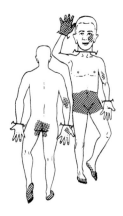

▪ **Distribution**

Anywhere, but commonly on thighs and trunk.

▪ **Patient Profile**

Any age, both sexes. Slowly enlarging, slightly pruritic lesions.

▪ **Diagnosis**

Lesions tested with potassium hydroxide preparations reveal hyphae. Fungal cultures grow pathogenic dermatophytes or *Candida albicans*.

▪ **Treatment**

Limited infections: topical antifungals and dry powders for 3 to 4 weeks or until clear. Widespread or resistant infection: systemic antifungal agents.

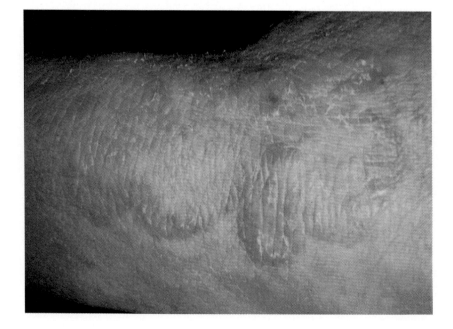

Drug Eruption

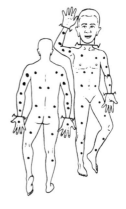

▪ Morphology
Multiple, symmetric, minimally raised, pink to red scaly papules.

▪ Distribution
Symmetric. Lesions usually spread over days. In bedridden patients, often in dependent areas. Oral lesions may be found.

▪ Patient Profile
Any age, both sexes. Lesions may itch. Patient has just begun drug or is taking drug chronically. Eosinophilia may be present. May take 4 to 6 weeks to clear after drug use is stopped.

▪ Diagnosis
Clearing of eruption after discontinuing drug, followed by recurrence of eruption with readministration of drug is diagnostic. Biopsy is not diagnostic.

▪ Treatment
Elimination of the offending agent is curative. Systemic antihistamines for symptomatic relief. A course of systemic steroids beginning with 60 mg prednisone over 2 to 3 weeks may be necessary with severely symptomatic patients. Topical steroids (class II or III) can be helpful.

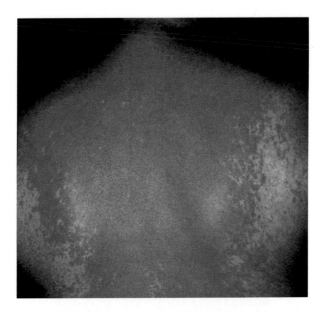

Exfoliative Dermatitis

▪ Morphology
Generalized redness, warmth, and scaling characterize this syndrome. The scales vary in size. Alopecia (complete or partial), ectropion, subungual debris, and malformations of the nail plate may be present.

▪ Distribution
Generalized, including palms and soles. Mucous membranes uninvolved.

▪ Patient Profile
Usually adults of both sexes. Lesions often very pruritic. Patients may have adenopathy, chills, fever, poor temperature control, tachycardia, peripheral edema, gynecomastia, and high-output heart failure.

▪ Diagnosis
Generalized redness and scaling suggest this diagnosis. Presence of exfoliative dermatitis from birth suggests the diagnosis of lamellar ichthyosis, epidermolytic hyperkeratosis, or congenital psoriasis. The causes of exfoliative dermatitis include:

Drug reaction: Gold, penicillin, or barbiturates are common causes, but any drug may cause this syndrome.

Eczematous dermatitis: Atopic or chronic contact dermatitis (see pp. 190, 243).

Idiopathic cause: Many patients with erythroderma may be followed up for many years without specific etiology being established.

Lymphoma (see p. 220).

Mycosis fungoides (see p. 253).

Pityriasis rubra pilaris (see p. 256).

Psoriasis (see pp. 258–259).

Seborrheic dermatitis (see p. 260).

Patients with the diagnosis of exfoliative dermatitis need a complete medical evaluation, including investigations for malignancy. Biopsy shows thickened epidermis with parakeratotic stratum corneum. The biopsy is not diagnostic of the etiology, except when the patient has mycosis fungoides.

▪ Treatment
Class I or II topical steroids under occlusion usually required, in addition to good supportive measures to maintain temperature and fluid balance. Systemic corticosteroids less often. Etretinate useful if psoriatic erythroderma is suspected.

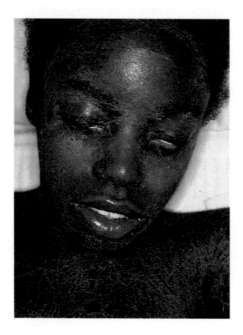

Kawasaki's Disease

▪ **Morphology**
Erythematous papules and macules.

▪ **Distribution**
Trunk and proximal extremities but can be
more generalized.

▪ **Patient Profile**
Child with a fever, lymphadenopathy, oral
involvement, and an exanthem. May have
complicating cardiac involvement, arthralgia or arthritis, urethritis, aseptic meningitis, and GI complaints.

▪ **Diagnosis**
Child with fever for 5 or more days with 4
or 5 of the following: bilateral conjunctival
injection, oropharynx involvement (injected or fissured lips, injected pharynx,
strawberry tongue), erythema of palms or
soles, edema of hands or feet, periungual
desquamation, polymorphous exanthem,
and acute cervical lymphadenopathy. Must
be differentiated from toxic shock syndrome, which is seen primarily in adults
and associated with fever, generalized
erythroderma, and hypotension.

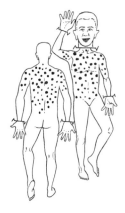

▪ **Treatment**
Aspirin, IV immunoglobulin, symptomatic support.

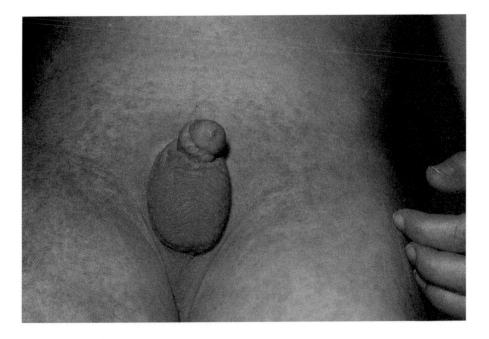

Keratosis Pilaris

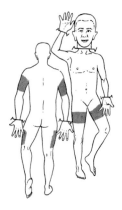

▪ **Morphology**
Perifollicular, pink, grouped, minimally raised, scaly lesions pierced by a small, curled hair.

▪ **Distribution**
Most common on extensor aspects of upper arms and thighs but can occur anywhere.

▪ **Patient Profile**
Both sexes; all ages, beginning in childhood; worse in winter. Lesions often associated with ichthyosis vulgaris (see p. 129) and atopic dermatitis (see p. 243).

▪ **Diagnosis**
A small, scaling, perifollicular papule with a central hair is characteristic. Biopsy is nondiagnostic. Rare causes of follicular hyperkeratosis are vitamin A and vitamin C deficiency.

▪ **Treatment**
Moisturization, mild keratolytics, Retin-A.

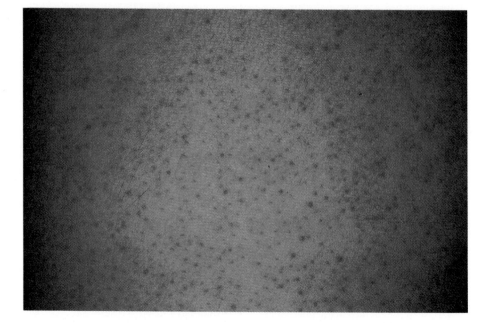

Lichen Planus

■ Morphology
Purple to blue-purple papules that are discrete or confluent and have reticulate white areas (Wickham's striae). There may be diffuse hyperkeratosis on palms and soles. Hyperpigmentation, hypopigmentation, and atrophy also occur. Rarely, vesicles are present. There may be ulcers on palms and soles.

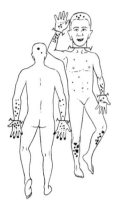

■ Distribution
Lesions are symmetric, on flexural surfaces, and are frequently linear or annular. Mucosal lesions (erosions or hyperkeratosis) are frequent in mouth and less common on genitalia. Nails may have pits or grooves. Scalp may have scarring alopecia.

■ Patient Profile
Usually adults of both sexes. Duration of several months to several years. Pruritus (often severe) is common.

■ Diagnosis
Biopsy is diagnostic and shows hyperkeratosis, thickening of the granular layer, basal cell liquefaction, basement-membrane thinning, and a bandlike lymphocytic and histiocytic upper dermal filtrate. Leg lesions have to be distinguished from lichen simplex chronicus and lichen amyloidosis.

■ Treatment
Class I or II topical corticosteroid can be used on skin and mucosal lesions. Severe generalized disease may require 3 to 6 weeks of oral corticosteroids until lesions are arrested, and then tapering steroids. UVB can control pruritus. PUVA therapy. Isotretinoin useful for severe disease.

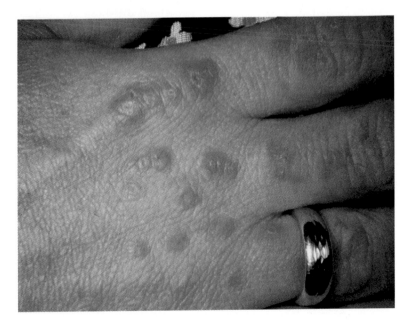

Lupus Erythematosus
(Discoid and Subacute)

■ **Morphology**

Multiple, sharply marginated, slightly raised red areas, several millimeters to many centimeters in size, that have irregular adherent scale and loss of skin markings. Lesions may demonstrate hyperpigmentation, hypopigmentation, atrophy, and telangiectasia.

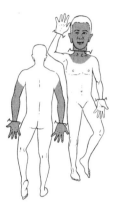

■ **Distribution**

Face; ears; scalp; sun-exposed areas of extremities, neck, upper chest, and palms and soles are most frequently involved.

■ **Patient Profile**

Systemic lupus is more common in young females. Patients often have systemic complaints with arthritis, serositis, and renal disease.

■ **Diagnosis**

Biopsy demonstrates an atrophic epidermis, basal cell vacuolization, thickening of the basement membrane, and perivascular and periadnexal round-cell infiltrate in the dermis. Immunofluorescent examination reveals deposition of immunoglobulin and complement at the dermal-epidermal basement membrane. Serologic tests for lupus erythematosus are listed in Table 5-4. Polymorphous light eruption (see p. 233) must be considered in this differential diagnosis.

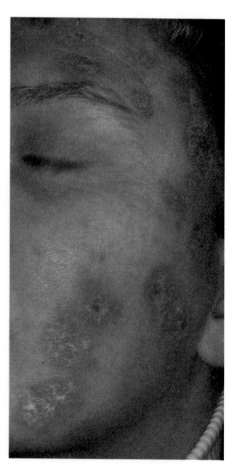

■ **Treatment**

Class I or II topical corticosteroids or intralesional corticosteroids may be necessary to control lesions. Broad spectrum UVB and UVA sunscreens and clothing for photoprotection.

Mycosis Fungoides and Parapsoriasis

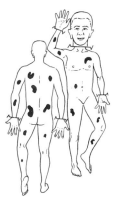

▪ Morphology
Pink, red, or brown minimally scaly papules and plaques. Lesions may be circular, ring-shaped, or polycyclic and have telangiectasia and mottled hyperpigmentation and hypopigmentation. Lesions may be very indurated on palpation and have associated hair loss. Tumors and ulcerations are found in mycosis fungoides.

▪ Distribution
Asymmetric. Anywhere; most common on trunk. Oral lesions uncommon.

▪ Patient Profile
Older adults, more common in men than in women. Lesions may be pruritic.

▪ Diagnosis
The clinical picture suggests either parapsoriasis or early mycosis fungoides. Parapsoriasis is a benign, chronic disease. Mycosis fungoides is a malignant T-cell lymphoma that may arise in a parapsoriasis-like eruption, especially with large plaques. Adenopathy and organomegaly favor the diagnosis of mycosis fungoides, in which biopsy reveals characteristic large, atypical lymphocytes in the epidermis and a polymorphous cellular infiltrate in the papillary dermis. T-cell receptor gene rearrangement from skin biopsy supports the diagnosis.

▪ Treatment
Parapsoriasis: class I or II corticosteroids, UVB, PUVA therapy. Large plaques of parapsoriasis may eventuate in systemic T-cell lymphoma and should be managed by those familiar with the disease and treatment modalities confined to skin: UVB, UVA; psoralens; interferon alfa-2; or topical nitrogen mustard.

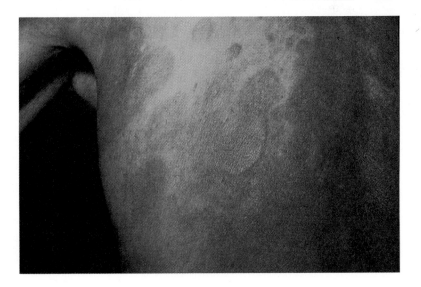

Nummular Eczema

▪ **Morphology**
Group of pinpoint vesicles and papules on a coin-shaped erythematous base.

▪ **Distribution**
Dorsum of hands, extensor aspect of arms, but may appear anywhere.

▪ **Patient Profile**
Younger women and older men. Very pruritic lesions. Lesions tend to be chronic and often worse in the winter.

▪ **Diagnosis**
Biopsy reveals eczematous dermatitis without presence of fungal elements.

▪ **Treatment**
Class I or II topical corticosteroids, emollients. Two to 4 weeks of systemic antibiotics may be helpful. Combined UVA and UVB light.

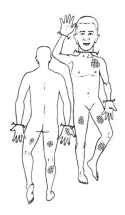

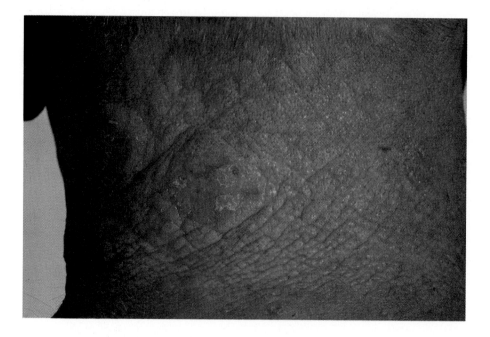

Pityriasis Rosea

■ Morphology
Oval and ring-shaped, pink to fawn-colored, raised, slightly scaly papules, 0.5 to 4 cm in diameter. Oval lesions are longest in horizontal dimension.

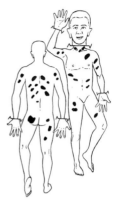

■ Distribution
Symmetric. Trunk and proximal extremities. Lesions are distributed along skin lines, giving a fir tree distribution. Face and lower extremities usually spared. Oral lesions rare.

■ Patient Profile
Young adults of both sexes. Disease frequently begins with a single oval herald patch on the trunk. Within a week, the truncal eruption begins. Often pruritic. Upper respiratory tract infections and mild adenopathy may occur. Eruptions may last up to 3 months before clearing spontaneously.

■ Diagnosis
Diagnosis is based on clinical observations. Biopsy is nondiagnostic and reveals spongiosis and perivascular round-cell in-filtrate. Serology for syphilis should be performed to rule out secondary syphilis.

■ Treatment
Pruritus may be extreme and require systemic histamines, UVB, or class II topical corticosteroids. Does not respond to oral corticosteroids.

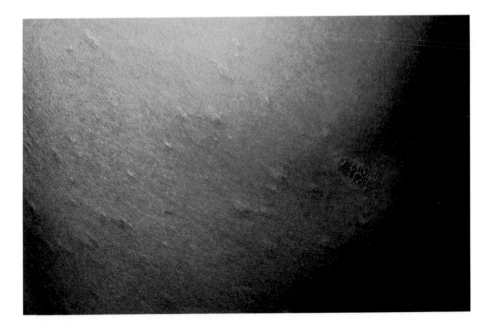

Pityriasis Rubra Pilaris

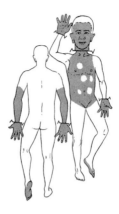

▪ Morphology
Scaly, pink to red, elevated perifollicular lesions that range in size from millimeters to centimeters. Pinpoint lesions begin around hair follicles and may enlarge to form large plaques; may involve total body. Islands of normal skin may occur between lesions. Diffuse red-yellow hyperkeratosis on palms and soles.

▪ Distribution
Anywhere; pinpoint perifollicular lesions are easily recognized over proximal phalanges of hands. Lesions may be accentuated in light-exposed areas.

▪ Patient Profile
Both sexes. In hereditary forms, may begin in childhood. In adults, lesions often begin on scalp and face. Chronic, usually lasts several years but may be life-long. May worsen with light exposure.

▪ Diagnosis
Perifollicular papules and islands of normal skin in a patient with a generalized, red scaling skin disease is highly suggestive. Biopsy shows hyperkeratosis with focal parakeratosis around hair follicles.

▪ Treatment
Topical class I or II corticosteroids for localized lesions. Systemic retinoids, isotretinoin or etretinate, or systemic methotrexate may be necessary. Phototherapy useful in nonphotosensitive patients.

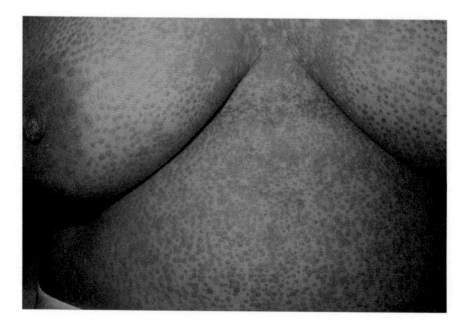

Prurigo Nodularis

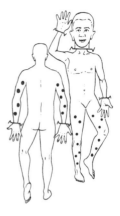

■ Morphology
Single or multiple flesh-colored to red-brown, dome-shaped lesions (up to 1 cm in diameter) with a central excoriation. Scaling and erythema are frequent.

■ Distribution
Lower legs, extensor aspect of arms are most common sites. Rarely involves the face.

■ Patient Profile
Most frequent in middle-aged women. Very pruritic lesions. Lesions may persist for years.

■ Diagnosis
Persistent, pruritic papules with excoriations in middle-aged women suggest this disease. Biopsy shows irregular epidermal hyperplasia and nerve fiber proliferation.

■ Treatment
Class I or II topical steroids with Cordran tape; intralesional corticosteroids (up to 1 month). Cryotherapy. More potent antihistamine-like drugs, such as doxepin, are often necessary. Thalidomide has been used for its antipruritic effects. If related to delusions of parasitosis, pimozide often effective.

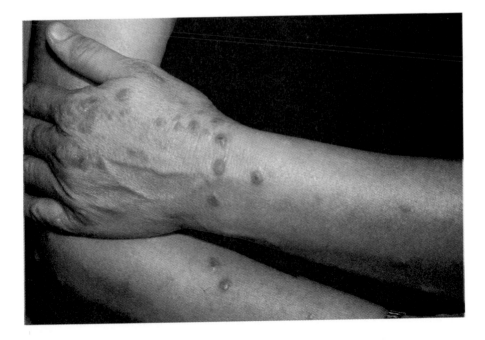

Psoriasis

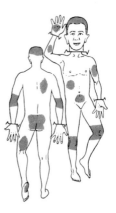

▪ Morphology
Sharply circumscribed red papules and plaques with a powdery white scale. Scale can be induced by rubbing the plaque with a tongue blade. Tiny bleeding points may appear after removal of scale (Auspitz sign). Lesions may vary in size from pinpoint to large plaques. Total body erythema and scaling, erythroderma, may occur. Pustules occur especially around the periphery of plaques and on the palms and soles. Pitting and dystrophy of nails is common. Oral lesions occur rarely.

▪ Distribution
Extensor aspect of elbows and knees, presacral area, and scalp are most common sites, but lesions can occur anywhere. Pustular lesions are found most commonly on palms and soles. Lesions can cover entire body.

▪ Patient Profile
Both sexes. Usually begins in childhood but may begin in infancy or in old age. Psoriasis is familial. Uncommon in West African blacks. Lesions may itch. Explosive onset of lesions may follow streptococcal infection. Arthritis of axial skeleton and distal phalanges is common. A rapid onset of refractory psoriasis occurs in HIV-positive patients.

▪ Diagnosis
Presence of sharply circumscribed plaques with fine white powdery scale on extensor aspect of extremities is highly suggestive of this diagnosis. Positive family history and arthritis further support this diagnosis. Biopsy reveals hyperkeratosis, para-

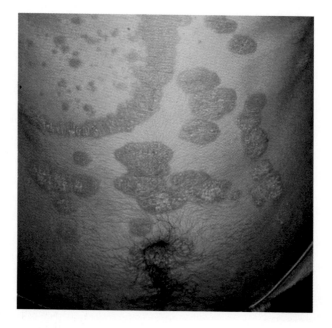

keratosis, papillomatosis, and accumulation of polymorphonuclear leukocytes in the stratum corneum (Munro microabscesses).

▪ Treatment

Class I to III topical steroids; IV or V in intertriginous lesions, which are common. Topical tars. Cordran tape or intralesional steroids in resistant plaques. Scalp often requires keratolytic agents before tar shampoos and steroids with occlusion will be effective. Topical vitamin D analogues (calcipotriol) effective. Systemic antistreptococcal antibiotics for 2 to 4 weeks in pharyngitis-associated flares and early episodes of guttate psoriasis. Systemic antihistamines are useful for pruritus, which may be severe. UVB or UVA with systemic psoralens for more extensive disease. Systemic retinoids (etretinate) or antimetabolites (e.g., methotrexate) or immunosuppressives (cyclosporine) for more advanced and refractory disease.

Seborrheic Dermatitis

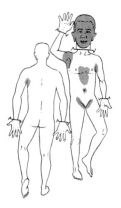

■ Morphology
Raised, scaly, red, greasy papules and plaques that may be sharply or poorly circumscribed. Discrete papules, pustules, and hypopigmentation often present. Secondary infection with crusting occurs.

■ Distribution
Symmetric. Scalp, eyebrows, eyelids, retro-auricular areas, cheeks, beard, anterior chest, axilla, and groin most commonly involved. Seborrheic dermatitis may be generalized.

■ Patient Profile
Usually adults, both sexes. In early childhood, involves scalp (cradle cap), diaper area. Severe in patients with Parkinson's disease or HIV infection.

■ Diagnosis
Red lesions in symmetric locations with a loosely attached, greasy scale characterize this disease. The scale in psoriasis is whiter and more compact. Persistent, severe seborrheic dermatitis in infancy associated with diarrhea and deficiency of the fifth component of complement is called *Lein-*

er's disease. Petechiae in severe seborrheic dermatitis in a young child should suggest the possibility of histiocytosis X (see p. 150). Biopsy shows a psoriasiform dermatitis and is not diagnostic.

■ Treatment
High-potency (class II or III) corticosteroids, with low-potency (class IV or V) corticosteroids on intertriginous sites and the face. Topical ketoconazole alone or with corticosteroids can be effective. Shampoos containing tar or ketoconazole.

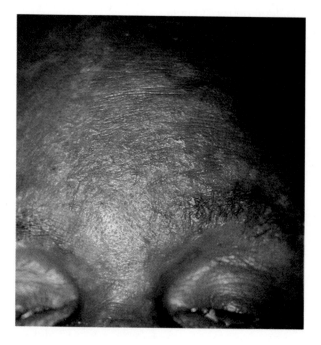

Seborrheic Keratoses

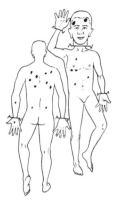

■ **Morphology**
Sharply circumscribed, elevated, pasted-on–appearing, brown to black papules (a few millimeters to several centimeters). The surface is irregular, slightly scaly, and rough. The lesions are often multiple, sometimes pedunculated, and, if irritated, they have a red base and associated tenderness.

■ **Distribution**
Trunk, but may be anywhere, including the face.

■ **Patient Profile**
Both sexes. Usually begin during the fourth decade and increase in prevalence with age. Usually asymptomatic. Rarely familial.

■ **Diagnosis**
This very common lesion persists. The color of an individual lesion is uniform. The pasted-on appearance of the lesion is characteristic. Scraping the surface produces brownish debris. The onset of multiple seborrheic keratoses may follow an inflammatory dermatosis or on rare occasions may be a sign of internal malignancy. Multiple, usually small seborrheic keratoses may be seen on the faces of blacks in their second and third decades (dermatosis papulosa nigra). Biopsy of seborrheic keratoses shows hyperkeratosis, papillomatosis, and acanthosis of benign cells.

■ **Treatment**
Light liquid nitrogen, electrodesiccation, removal of excess scale with lactic-acid–containing medications.

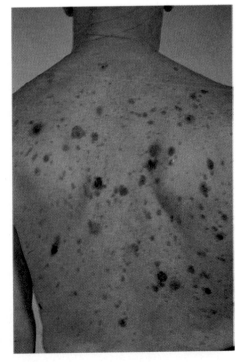

Secondary Syphilis

▪ **Morphology**
Red to raw ham-colored, sharply circum-scribed, circular or ring-shaped noncoales-cent papules with sparse scaling. In inter-triginous areas, papules may have a moist, wartlike surface (condylomata lata). Patchy alopecia may occur.

▪ **Distribution**
Symmetric lesions over the entire body, including palms and soles. Papules may split on two adjacent surfaces around nose and mouth. White plaques may be found on oral and genital mucosa.

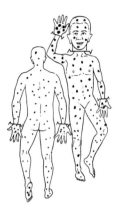

▪ **Patient Profile**
Any sexually active individual. Patient may have a history of chancre (see p. 464) occurring 3 weeks to 3 months before the eruption develops. Lesions may be associ-ated with adenopathy, hepatospleno-megaly, fever, coryza, neuropathy, or head-ache. Patients with HIV infection may have secondary syphilis with negative se-rologies and require careful histologic ex-aminations, including silver stains for spi-rochetes and dark-field examinations.

▪ **Diagnosis**
Sharply circumscribed, exanthematous, scaly eruption involving the palms and soles should suggest secondary syphilis. Serologic tests are positive for syphilis; serum must be diluted to exclude a pro-zone phenomenon. Biopsy reveals endo-thelial swelling and perivascular round-cell infiltrate that is rich in plasma cells. Dark-field examination of a lesion, espe-cially condyloma, reveals spirochetes.

▪ **Treatment**
Systemic antibiotics. See Table 14-12.

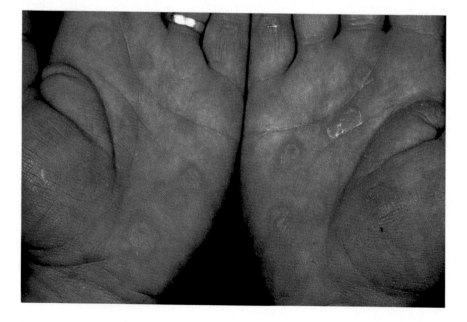

Squamous Cell Carcinoma

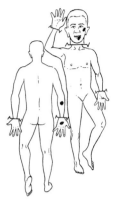

▪ Morphology
Firm, indurated, infiltrating lesion, sometimes circumscribed, with scaling and a central, scaly plug or ulceration.

▪ Distribution
Lesions are most common on sun-exposed areas, such as the lower lip, ears, face, dorsum of hands, but may occur anywhere.

▪ Patient Profile
Both sexes, usually older age group. Squamous cell carcinoma usually occurs in areas of sun exposure, x-ray therapy, chronic ulceration, lupus erythematosus, or lupus vulgaris.

▪ Diagnosis
Biopsy shows infiltration of dermis with neoplastic squamous cells. Chronic inflammatory cells are frequently seen.

▪ Treatment
Mohs' surgery, surgical excision; radiation therapy in selected cases.

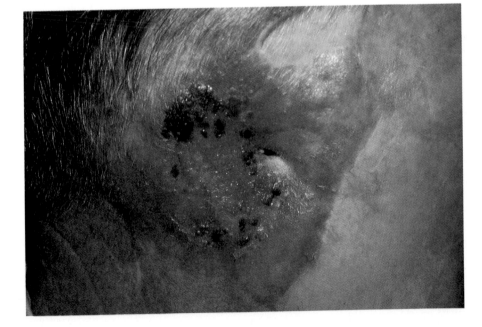

Tinea Versicolor

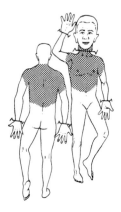

▪ **Morphology**
Minimally elevated brown or hypopigmented papules and plaques that scale when rubbed. Hypopigmentation may be seen.

▪ **Distribution**
Upper trunk, shoulders, neck, proximal arms; occasionally face; rarely below waist.

▪ **Patient Profile**
Usually adolescents or young adults of both sexes. Lesions may be slightly pruritic.

▪ **Diagnosis**
Lesion scrapings treated with potassium hydroxide preparation reveal large spores and thick hyphae.

▪ **Treatment**
Topical ketoconazole or 2% selenium sulfide. Ketoconazole, 200 to 400 mg for a 5-day course, and then once monthly as needed. Patient should be advised that normal pigmentation returns slowly.

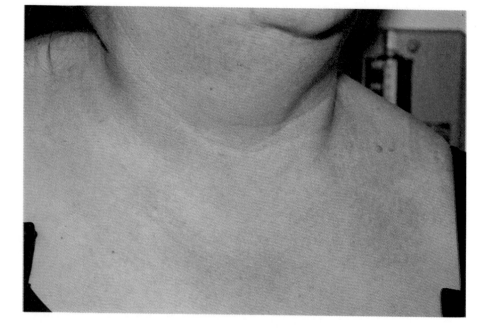

Rare Causes of Scattered, Scaly Papules

Acquired perforating dermatoses: Hyperkeratotic, pruritic papules are most common on extremities. Seen in patients with chronic renal failure, diabetes mellitus; oil-field workers.

Elastosis perforans serpiginosa: Papules are small, multiple, and grouped in ring or horseshoe arrangements on the neck, face, trunk, or upper extremities. The disease occurs in children or young adults and is associated with Down syndrome, Marfan syndrome, Ehlers-Danlos syndrome, osteogenesis imperfecta, or penicillamine therapy. Biopsy shows elastic tissue penetrating the epidermis.

Epidermal nevus: Groups of flesh-colored lesions, covered with thick scale, often patterned in lines or whorls. Present at birth or appear early in childhood.

Epidermodysplasia verruciformis: Papules and plaques develop on the extremities. Life-long disease with autosomal recessive and X-linked recessive inheritance. Multiple human papillomaviruses isolated from lesions, with HPV types 3 and 10 being common.

Kyrle's disease: Papules are large (1 to 2 cm), may occur anywhere, and are frequently found in middle-aged adults who may have diabetes. Biopsy shows a keratin plug penetrating into the dermis.

Lichen amyloidosis: Multiple, often symmetric, flesh-colored to red-brown papules develop on extensor aspect of extremities. Biopsy reveals amyloid but not associated with systemic amyloidosis.

Multiple keratoacanthoma: Multiple pink to red volcano-appearing lesions with a central area of keratinous debris.

Pemphigus foliaceus (see p. 333): This disease is rarely papular.

Perforating collagenosis: Small, frequently linear papules that may follow trauma. Biopsy shows collagen extending into the epidermis.

Perforating folliculitis: Papules are small, on the extremities, and caused by a hair perforating through the follicle.

Perforating granuloma annulare: Small papules with central umbilication or crust appear, most common on the hands. May be associated with diabetes mellitus.

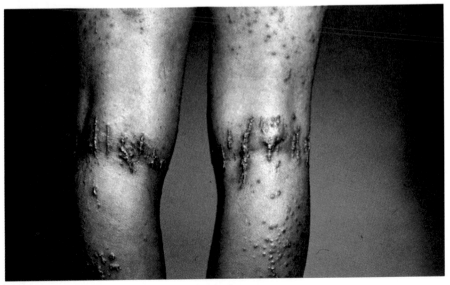

Kyrle's disease

YELLOW PAPULES

Actinic elastosis
Eruptive xanthomas
Necrobiosis lipoidica diabeticorum
Noneruptive xanthomas
Pseudoxanthoma elasticum
Sebaceous hyperplasia
Other yellow lesions: Goltz's syndrome, lupus vulgaris, nevus lipomatosus, nevus sebaceous, xanthogranuloma

Actinic Elastosis

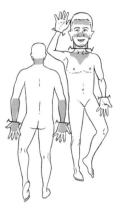

▪ Morphology
Coarse wrinkling of skin resulting in flesh-colored papules and nodules. Pigmented macules (lentigines) and telangiectases frequently seen.

▪ Distribution
Sun-exposed areas: face, neck, upper chest, extensor arms, and dorsum of hands.

▪ Patient Profile
Caucasian patients with history of extensive sun exposure. Most often observed in the southern United States. Similar changes on the face have been reported in heavy smokers.

▪ Diagnosis
Clinical lesions and distribution are diagnostic. Biopsy shows nodular aggregations of amorphous material in the papillary dermis, ectatic vessels, and altered pigmentation.

▪ Treatment
Sunscreens and topical Retin-A.

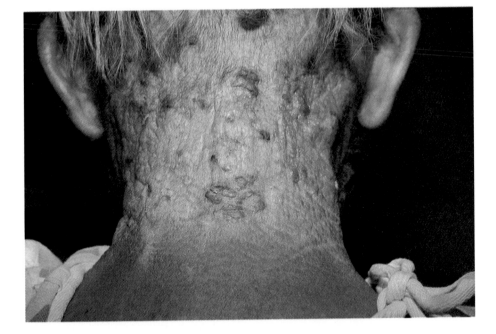

Eruptive Xanthomas

▪ **Morphology**
Multiple small (0.3 to 1 cm), uniform yellow papules with a red halo.

▪ **Distribution**
Symmetric; trunk, proximal extremities, extensors.

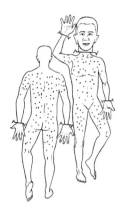

▪ **Patient Profile**
Both sexes; any age but usually adulthood. Frequently pruritic lesions. Frequently sudden onset of multiple lesions.

▪ **Diagnosis**
Plasma is lipemic owing to high triglycerides. Abnormalities of the liver, pancreas (diabetes), and other endocrine organs may cause eruptive xanthoma.

▪ **Treatment**
For dietary therapy, control of underlying disease, and systemic treatments, see an internal medicine text.

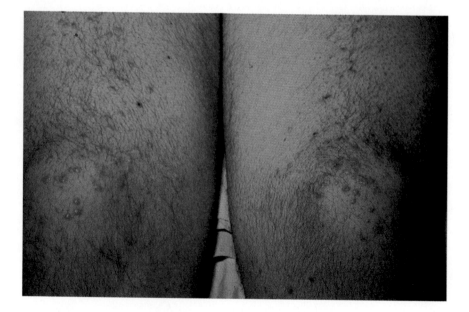

Necrobiosis Lipoidica Diabeticorum

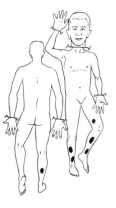

▪ Morphology
Yellow-tan plaques with dilated blood vessels and depressed atrophic areas showing loss of skin markings. Lesions may ulcerate. Borders are often scalloped.

▪ Distribution
Often symmetric; on shins but can occur anywhere.

▪ Patient Profile
Both sexes; any age. More common in adults. More than 50% of patients have or will have diabetes mellitus. Painful when ulcerated.

▪ Diagnosis
Yellow color with prominent superficial vessels in an atrophic plaque is very suggestive. Biopsy shows necrobiosis, inflammatory cells including giant cells, fibrosis, and increased mucin. Studies to exclude diabetes are necessary. Rarely, lupus vulgaris (see p. 385), granuloma annulare (see p. 161), and rheumatoid nodules may appear similar histologically to necrobiosis.

▪ Treatment
Class I topical corticosteroids, Cordran tape, and intralesional steroids helpful for inflammatory or ulcerative lesions.

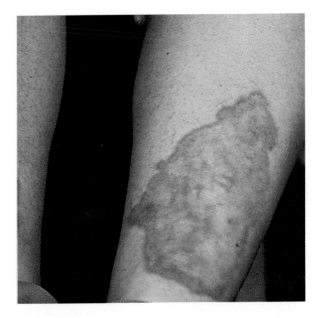

Noneruptive Xanthomas

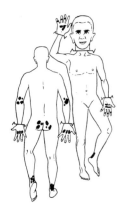

■ **Morphology**
Multiple yellow to yellow-orange, symmetric papulonodules.

■ **Distribution**
Eyelids (xanthelasma), extensors (elbows, knees, knuckles), axillae, Achilles tendon, and palmar creases. Lesions persist months to years. Nonpruritic.

■ **Patient Profile**
Both sexes, any age. Cardiovascular disease, liver disease, thyroid disease, nephrotic syndrome, or dysproteinemia may be associated with noneruptive xanthomas.

■ **Diagnosis**
Xanthomas are a sign of possible serious internal disease. A thorough evaluation is necessary. Biopsy shows lipid-laden cells.

■ **Treatment**
Dietary therapy and use of cholesterol-reducing agents. See an internal medicine text.

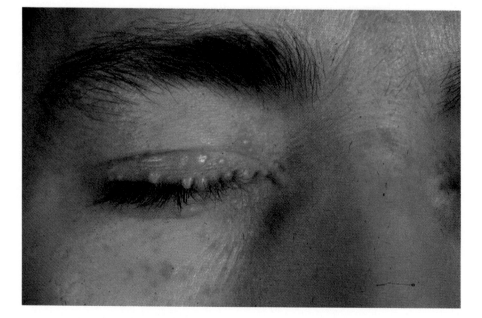

Pseudoxanthoma Elasticum

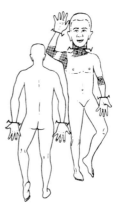

■ Morphology
Soft, small, grouped, pale-yellow papules separated by areas of normal skin; resembles skin of plucked chicken.

■ Distribution
Flexural areas, especially neck, antecubital fossae, and axillae. Labial mucosa involved.

■ Patient Profile
Both sexes; onset in late childhood or early adulthood. Associated with angioid retinal streaks, arterial insufficiency, and GI hemorrhage. Autosomal recessive and autosomal dominant forms.

■ Diagnosis
Biopsy is diagnostic and shows fragmented, calcified elastic tissue.

■ Treatment
Low-calcium diet; observation for signs or symptoms of coronary artery disease.

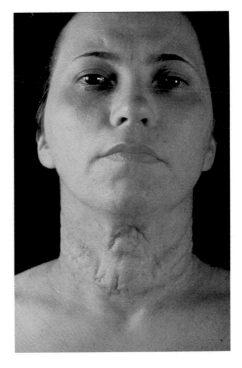

Sebaceous Hyperplasia

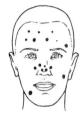

▪ Morphology
Yellowish papules (3 to 10 mm in diameter) have a central depression or are multilobulated; there may be telangiectases over the lesions. Lesions are usually multiple.

▪ Distribution
Face, especially forehead and nose.

▪ Patient Profile
Older adults of both sexes.

▪ Diagnosis
These lesions are more yellow than a basal cell carcinoma but closely mimic that tumor. Biopsy is diagnostic and shows large, mature sebaceous glands.

▪ Treatment
Liquid nitrogen, electrodesiccation, chemical peel.

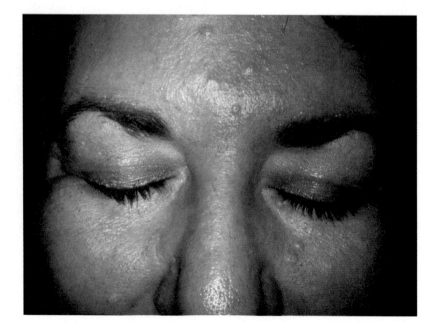

Other Yellow Lesions

Focal dermal hypoplasia (Goltz's syndrome): This syndrome is characterized by yellow papules, and often by red papules and atrophic skin lesions.

Lupus vulgaris: This plaque begins in children or young adults and is characterized by atrophy and a yellow-brown color (see p. 385).

Nevus lipomatosus: Group of yellow, soft papules, usually on the buttock, presents at birth. Biopsy shows fat cells in the dermis.

Nevus sebaceous: Raised yellow-red plaques that have an irregular surface usually appear on the scalp and have less hair over them than on remainder of scalp. Lesions are present at birth or appear early in childhood and increase in size with age. Lesions may develop appendageal tumors and can be associated with bone defects, epilepsy, and mental retardation.

Some of the lesions in Tables 5-1 and 5-2 (pp. 174–175, 178–179) may appear yellow, especially xanthogranuloma, amyloid, sarcoid, gout, and calcinosis cutis.

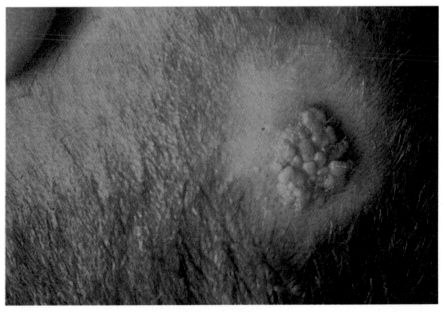

Nevus sebaceous

PALM AND SOLE PAPULES WITH SCALING

DIAGNOSTIC OBSERVATIONS
Many general body diseases affect the palms and soles. Several disorders show a propensity for involving these sites. The general body surface should be carefully examined, because the disorders in this section often have involvement elsewhere.

Arsenical keratoses
Diffuse palm and sole scaling
Digital fibromas
Hereditary keratodermas
Hyperhidrosis
Tyrosinemia II

Arsenical Keratoses

■ **Morphology**
Discrete, multiple, irregular, hyperkeratotic lesions, often surrounded by a shallow depression.

■ **Distribution**
Palms and soles.

■ **Patient Profile**
Adults past middle age. More common in men.

■ **Diagnosis**
History of arsenic exposure, often through farming activities or ingestion of inorganic arsenic-containing medication. Hyperpigmentation may be present. Biopsy shows vacuolization of epidermal cells but is not diagnostic. Acute arsenic poisoning has associated desquamative palmar lesions.

■ **Treatment**
Surgical removal of lesions suspicious for malignancy. Propylene glycol, salicylic acid, or alpha-hydroxy-acid–containing preparations.

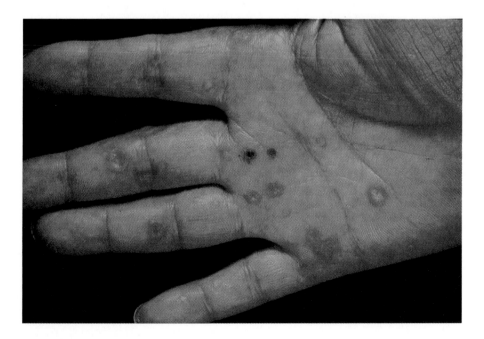

Diffuse Palm and Sole Scaling

The following diseases have diffuse scaling of the palms and soles, often without discrete papules:
Acanthosis nigricans
Arsenic ingestion
Chronic eczematous dermatitis
Dermatophyte infection
Drug-related eruption
Hidrotic ectodermal dysplasia
Ichthyosis secondary to other diseases
    HIV
    Carcinoma
    Lymphoma
Ichthyosis vulgaris
Lamellar ichthyosis
Lupus erythematosus
Psoriasis

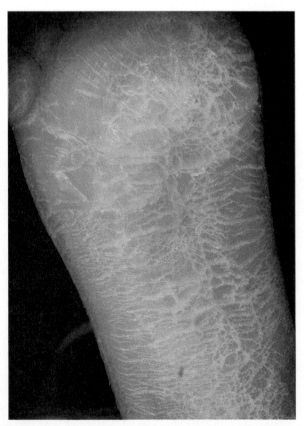

Ichthyosis secondary to lymphoma

Digital Fibromas

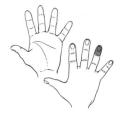

■ **Morphology**
Erythematous, dome-shaped papules developing on the fingers of an infant or child.

■ **Distribution**
Most common on the dorsum of the fingers and toes.

■ **Patient Profile**
Infant or child who experiences the sudden growth of a papule distally on a digit.

■ **Diagnosis**
Dome-shaped digital papule on an infant is characteristic for the diagnosis. Biopsy shows interdigitating sheets of fibroblasts and collagen.

■ **Treatment**
Spontaneous regression has been reported. Surgical excision.

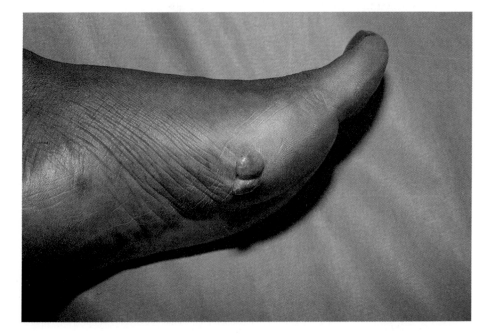

Hereditary Keratodermas
(Keratosis Palmaris et Plantaris)

▪ Morphology
Discrete or confluent hyperkeratotic lesions. Hyperhidrosis and fissures may occur, especially in the diffuse forms.

▪ Distribution
Palms and soles, with rare involvement of knees or Achilles tendon.

▪ Patient Profile
Onset in first two decades of life, often early childhood. Dominant and recessive disorders are in this group of diseases.

▪ Diagnosis
Family studies and pedigree analysis are necessary to establish the form of keratoderma present in a family (Table 5-5).

▪ Treatment
Treatment may include propylene glycol, salicylic-acid–containing preparations, and

TABLE 5–5. **Major Types of Hereditary Keratodermas**

Type	Genetics	Association
Howel-Evans' syndrome	Dominant	Carcinoma of esophagus
Mal de Meleda	Recessive	Mental and physical retardation
Papillon-Lefèvre syndrome	Recessive	Periodontal disease
Mutilating keratoderma	Dominant	Ainhum and loss of digits
Unna-Thost syndrome	Dominant	None

lactic-acid– or alpha-hydroxy-acid–containing preparations. These are most effective when used after hydration of the epidermis and when applied under plastic occlusion.

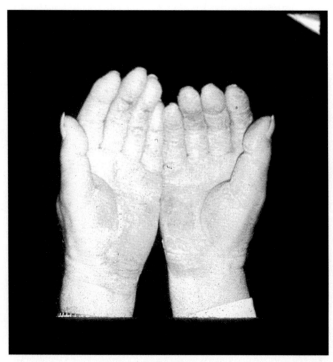

Keratosis palmaris et plantaris

Hyperhidrosis

▪ Morphology
Increased moisture on the palms and soles. Some vesicles may be seen on distal digits.

▪ Distribution
Palms and soles. Axilla and perineal areas also may be involved.

▪ Patient Profile
Patients may note excessive perspiration with emotional stress. Hyperhidrosis often accompanies disorders with palms or plantar hyperkeratosis.

▪ Diagnosis
Clinical evidence of perspiration.

▪ Treatment
Aluminum chlorohydrate solution, systemic anticholinergics, injections of botulism toxin.

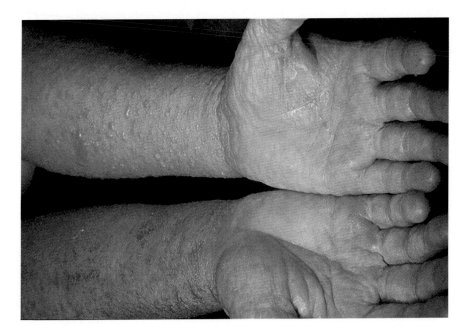

Tyrosinemia II

▪ **Morphology**
Discrete, crusted, erosive or hyperkeratotic lesions, often linear. Subungual hyperkeratosis may be present.

▪ **Distribution**
Palms and soles.

▪ **Patient Profile**
Infancy or early childhood, both sexes. Autosomal recessive. Keratitis. Painful.

▪ **Diagnosis**
Plasma and urinary tyrosine levels are markedly elevated; liver and renal function is normal. The disease responds to a low-tyrosine and low-phenylalanine diet. This response is diagnostic.

▪ **Treatment**
Low-tyrosine, low-phenylalanine diet.

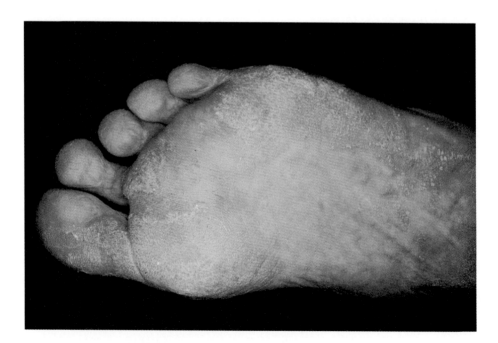

Chapter 6

■ ■

Blisters, Erosions, and Excoriations

BLISTERS

DIAGNOSTIC OBSERVATIONS

Vesicles are sharply marginated, elevated lesions that contain clear fluid. Blisters >1 cm in diameter are known as bullae. The freshest blister should always be examined, because blisters break and become eroded, pustular, hemorrhagic, and crusted with time. The blister should be examined carefully for a central dell or umbilication. Associated papules should be observed and their color noted.

MAJOR CATEGORIES

Blisters with red papules
Blisters with nonred papules
Umbilicated blisters
Blisters without other lesions

Blisters with Red Papules

DIAGNOSTIC OBSERVATIONS
These diseases have red papules that are distinct and separate from the blisters. There are usually tense, rounded vesicles and bullae. Hemorrhage into the blister can occur in any disease in this group. Some blistering diseases have prominent hemorrhage early in their course. Determine whether lesions are distributed symmetrically over the body.

Multiple Symmetric Blisters
Autoeczematization
Bullous pemphigoid (see p. 291)
Contact dermatitis
Dermatitis herpetiformis
Erythema multiforme
Vasculitis

Asymmetric Blisters
Bullous pemphigoid
Contact dermatitis (see p. 284)
Dermatophyte infection
Insect bites
Nummular eczema
Scabies

Rare Causes of Blisters with Red Papules
Congenital syphilis (see p. 296)
Erysipelas
Fixed drug reaction
Gas gangrene
Herpes gestationis
Lichen planus (see p. 251)
Lupus erythematosus (LE) (see p. 252)
Pemphigus vegetans
Pityriasis lichenoides et varioliformis acuta (see p. 221)
Rickettsialpox
Tumor

Multiple Symmetric Blisters with Red Papules

Autoeczematization

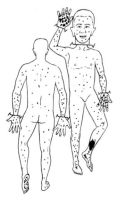

■ Morphology
Vesicles are small, on a red base, multiple, and can be scattered or grouped. Papules are multiple, small, red, and can scale.

■ Distribution
Symmetric, frequently generalized; especially prominent on palms and soles. The limbs are usually involved more often than the trunk.

■ Patient Profile
Any age but usually adults of both sexes. The generalized eruption is usually pruritic, evolves over a few days, and may persist for 2 to 4 weeks. Frequently begins with a focal area of dermatitis or infection.

■ Diagnosis
The generalized eruption is secondary to a preexisting active inflammatory dermatitis. Localized inflammatory fungal infections, contact dermatitis, or stasis dermatitis are common antecedent conditions. In the absence of a local site of skin inflammation, this diagnosis is unlikely.

■ Treatment
Potent (class II or III) topical steroids; frequently systemic corticosteroids (0.75 to 1.0 mg/kg prednisone) tapered over 2 to 3 weeks are necessary. Systemic antihistamines. Cool soaks to relieve pruritus. Antibiotics if local skin infection exists.

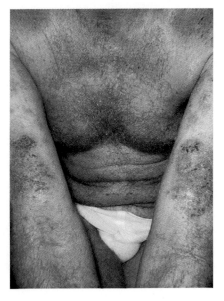

Contact Dermatitis

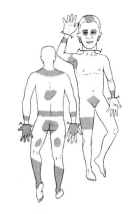

▪ Morphology
Papules and plaques are red, hivelike, and sharply circumscribed. Vesicles are tense and on a red base. They may be excoriated and frequently become pustular or crusted.

▪ Distribution
Anywhere, but more frequent in exposed areas. Lesions correspond to the area of contact and frequently have linear edges. Because of the mode of exposure, linear lesions are frequently seen. Palms and soles may be spared because of thickness of keratin.

▪ Patient Profile
Any age, both sexes. Lesions appear 12 to 48 hours after contact with allergen and last 11 to 14 days without therapy. Lesions usually pruritic.

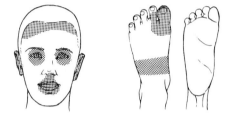

▪ Diagnosis
The configuration and location of the dermatitis are the most important clues to diagnosis (Table 6–1). Diagnosis is established by performing a patch test with the offending agent after the dermatitis has subsided. A small amount of the substance, preferably in liquid form, is obtained and placed on a small bandage,

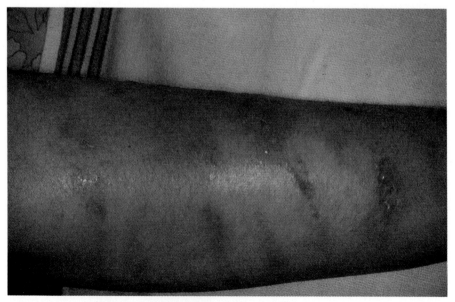

Contact dermatitis due to poison ivy

which is then placed in contact with the skin. The entire bandage is covered with impermeable tape and left on the skin for 48 hours. After removing the patch, the tester should wait 30 minutes and then observe the skin for erythema and vesicles. In contact dermatitis due to delayed hypersensitivity to an allergen, there is prominent perivascular round-cell infiltration in the dermis. In irritant contact dermatitis, there is necrosis of the epidermis and infiltration with polymorphonuclear leukocytes.

■ **Treatment**

Topical (class II or III) corticosteroids for mild to moderate cases. Oral corticosteroids (0.75 to 1 mg/kg prednisone, tapering doses over 2 weeks) for severe cases. Antihistamines for pruritus.

Table 6–1.**Characteristic Bodily Locations of Contact Dermatitis and the More Common Contact Allergens Involved**

Location	Cause
Ears	Metal earrings, plastics, perfumes.
Eyelids, neck, face	Nail polishes, perfumes, face creams, cosmetics.
Lips	Lipstick, foods, lip licking.
Feet	Shoe materials (rubber, dyes, polishes), sock and stocking dyes and finishes, professional dust (e.g., cement).
Hands and forearms	Household cleaning agents, waxes, soaps, rubber gloves. Chemicals used in professional work, cement, plants, poison ivy (gardeners).
Scalp	Hair tonics and dyes, setting lotions, permanent wave solutions.
Trunk	Clothing, brassieres, girdles, underwear, bathing materials, ointments, soaps, lotions.
Thighs and legs	Materials carried in trousers, clothing material, garters (rubber, metals, dyes), plants.
Any site	Ointments, lotions, pastes, plasters, tapes.
Airborne contact: face, neck, and dorsum of hands	Exposed areas without sparing of eyelids, areas under nose and under chin: chemical sprays.
Photocontact: face and dorsum of hands	Light-exposed areas, usually sparing eyelids, areas under nose and under chin: lime, cosmetics, soaps.

From deWick AL: Contact Eczematous Dermatitis. In Fitzpatrick TB et al (eds). *Dermatology in General Medicine.* McGraw-Hill, New York, 1993. Reproduced with permission of The McGraw-Hill Companies.

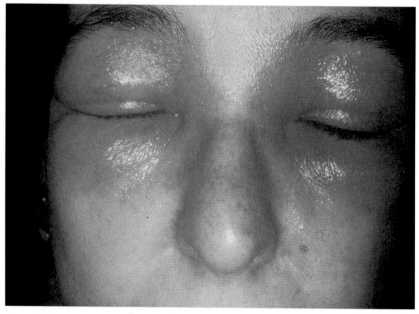

Contact dermatitis due to nail polish

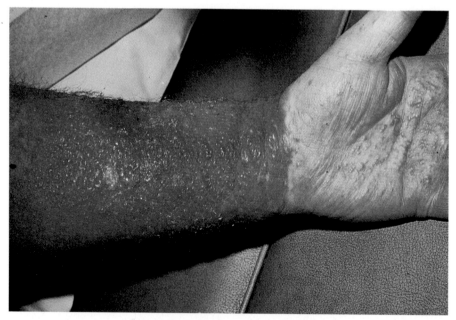

Contact dermatitis due to topical anesthetic

Dermatitis Herpetiformis

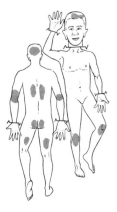

▪ Morphology
Vesicles are usually small, tense, and grouped on an erythematous base. Crusting is frequent. Papules are usually small, red, and are frequently excoriated. Scarring, mottled hyperpigmentation, and hypopigmentation are frequently seen.

▪ Distribution
Groups of lesions are striking in their bilateral symmetry. Lesions are prominent over the elbows, knees, buttocks, scalp, posterior neck, and thigh. Oral erythema and erosions may be present.

▪ Patient Profile
Primarily adults. More frequent in men. Disease lasts months to years. Lesions extremely pruritic. The absence of pruritus practically excludes the diagnosis.

▪ Diagnosis
Biopsy of an early papulovesicle reveals an accumulation of neutrophils and eosinophils at the tip of the dermal papillae. Later lesions demonstrate subepidermal bullae with a predominance of neutrophils. Immunofluorescent study of skin biopsy reveals IgA accumulations immediately below the dermal-epidermal basement membrane in a clumped pattern. A dramatic remission with the use of sulfones supports the diagnosis of dermatitis herpetiformis. Many patients have an associated spruelike syndrome with minimal malabsorption or hypothyroidism. Increased risk of intestinal lymphoma.

▪ Treatment
Dapsone (50–200 mg qd) after G6PD testing, follow-up hematologic studies. Strict low-gluten diet can control the disease.

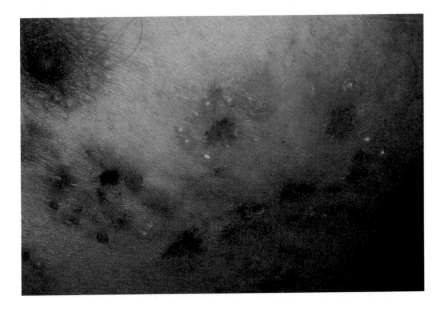

Erythema Multiforme

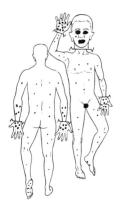

▪ Morphology
Vesicles are initially tense, on an erythematous base, and may be hemorrhagic. Blisters frequently erode and crust. Papules and plaques are erythematous and hivelike. Unlike common hives, these lesions last longer than 24 hours. Target lesions, very suggestive of erythema multiforme, have a central dark red area, a rim of pallor, and an outermost rim of erythema.

▪ Distribution
Generalized, symmetric with accentuation over extensor aspect of distal limbs, including palms and soles. Mucosal blisters and erosions are frequent.

▪ Patient Profile
Usually children and adults, uncommon in infants and patients older than 50. Disease evolves over several days and usually lasts 2 to 3 weeks. May be recurrent. Lesions may itch and burn.

▪ Diagnosis
This disease has numerous causes. The most common are drugs, herpes simplex, other viral infections, bacterial infections, deep fungal infections, systemic lupus erythematosus, neoplasms, and x-ray treatment of internal malignancies. Biopsy demonstrates subepidermal blisters and no deposition of IgG or complement at the dermal-epidermal basement membrane. The latter finding helps to differentiate this disease from bullous pemphigoid.

▪ Treatment
The cause should be identified and eliminated. Systemic antihistamines for pruritus. Oral acyclovir to prevent recurrent herpes simplex is useful when that infection precipitates erythema multiforme. Oral or topical corticosteroids have not been proven efficacious.

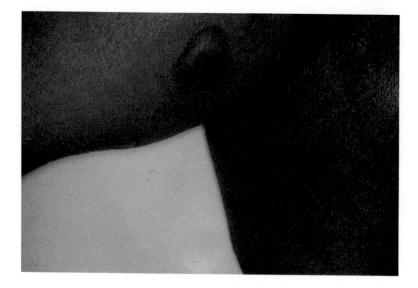

Vasculitis
(Allergic Vasculitis)

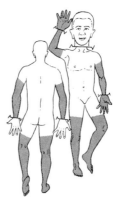

▪ Morphology
Vesicles are hemorrhagic and arise from papular lesions. Red, hivelike papules have flecks of purpura (palpable purpura). The purpura is demonstrated by pressing the lesion with a slide to blanch out the erythema (diascopy) and observing the residual hemorrhage, which does not blanch. Flat areas of purpura, 1 to 2 mm in diameter, are also frequently seen.

▪ Distribution
Symmetric, predominantly distal; frequently more lesions on lower extremities. Hundreds of lesions may be present, often with accentuation of lesions under areas of pressure (e.g., beneath belts or tight clothing).

▪ Patient Profile
All ages, both sexes. Usually sudden onset with acute forms lasting days to weeks. Chronic forms last months to years. Burning may precede eruption of lesions; usually nonpruritic. Disease may be associated with arthritis, abdominal pain, and renal disease.

▪ Diagnosis
Multiple etiologies. Some classic groupings have been given special names:

Schönlein-Henoch purpura (anaphylactoid purpura): A disease of children and young adults characterized by arthritis, abdominal pain, and skin and renal lesions.

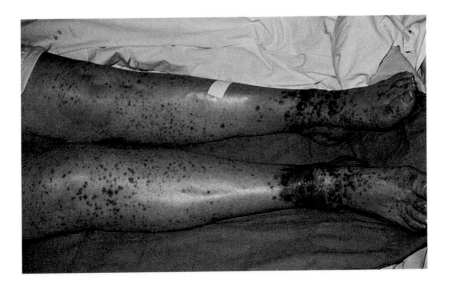

Allergic cutaneous vasculitis: A form of vasculitis seen at any age and frequently caused by drugs. Lupus erythematosus, cryoglobulinemia, macroglobulinemia, infectious hepatitis are among the underlying causes of this cutaneous syndrome, and appropriate tests for these diseases should be done. When a limited number of lesions are present, septic vasculitis (see p. 348) must be ruled out. The existence of multiple, definitely palpable, symmetric purpuric lesions is the clinical clue to allergic vasculitis. Biopsy reveals leukocytoclastic angiitis, representing immune complex disease.

▪ Treatment

Identification and treatment of primary disease, especially stopping drugs if they are suspected etiology. Systemic steroids efficacious for connective tissue diseases; severe disease may require immunomodulating agents such as azathioprine or cyclophosphamide.

Asymmetric Blisters with Red Papules

Bullous Pemphigoid

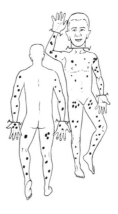

▪ Morphology
Vesicles are initially tense. Most blisters are on an erythematous base, but a blister on normal-appearing skin is highly suggestive of bullous pemphigoid. Erosions and crusting are frequent. Early lesions appear as papules and plaques that are erythematous and nonscaly.

▪ Distribution
Generalized without grouping or symmetry. Flexors, limbs, and abdomen are frequently involved. Occasionally oral lesions and desquamative gingivitis are seen.

▪ Patient Profile
All ages but more frequent in older age group. Both sexes. Disease lasts months to years. Lesions may be mildly pruritic.

▪ Diagnosis
Biopsy reveals subepidermal blister with eosinophils. Immunofluorescent examination demonstrates linear deposition of IgG and complement at dermal-epidermal basement membrane in approximately 90% of patients. Serum contains circulating antibodies to human dermal-epidermal basement membrane components bp-230 or bp-180 in 70% of patients.

▪ Treatment
Oral corticosteroids, starting at 0.75 to 1 mg/kg prednisone, usually effective. Some patients require higher doses of corticosteroids; addition of immunosuppressive agents, especially azathioprine, is common. Tetracycline and nicotinamide have been reported to be effective.

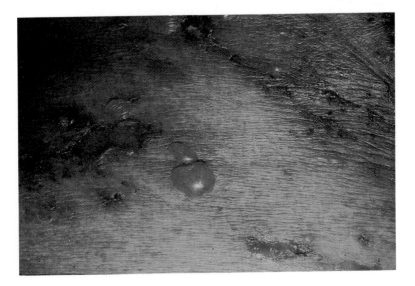

Dermatophyte Infection

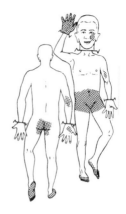

▪ Morphology
Vesicles and pustules may be in a ring. Red, scaly papules and erosions are common. Bullous lesions on feet may occur.

▪ Distribution
Symmetric. Anywhere, but vesicular lesions are most common on palms and soles.

▪ Patient Profile
Very common. Both sexes, all ages. Most common in adolescent and adult males; can occur in childhood. This is a chronic dermatosis with acute exacerbations.

▪ Diagnosis
Scraping the roof of the vesicle or pustule demonstrates septate hyphae on potassium hydroxide preparations. Lesions often become secondarily infected.

▪ Treatment
Topical antifungal creams or powders for 3 to 4 weeks or until clear for widespread or resistant infection; oral griseofulvin, ketoconazole, itraconazole, or fluconazole.

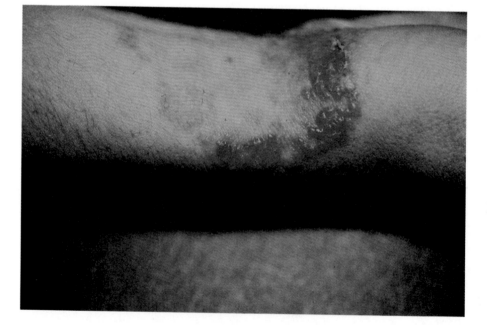

Insect Bites

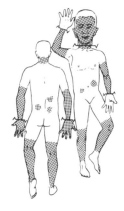

▪ Morphology
Vesicles appear on a red base and may become hemorrhagic. Papules are red, hivelike, often excoriated, and may have a central punctum.

▪ Distribution
Anywhere, but more frequently occur on exposed areas. Lesions often erupt simultaneously and appear in a group. No oral lesions.

▪ Patient Profile
Any age, both sexes. Insect bites appear acutely, but patients may be bitten recurrently over a period of months. Usually pruritic.

▪ Diagnosis
Biopsy shows neutrophils, eosinophils, and a dense lymphohistiocytic infiltrate.

▪ Treatment
Topical corticosteroids (class I or II). Systemic antihistamines. For severe multiple lesions (e.g., from fire ants), a course of corticosteroids is indicated. Systemic antibiotics if infected.

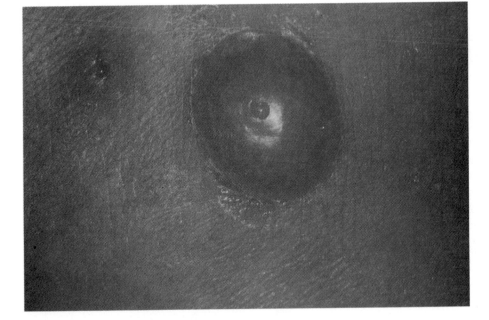

Nummular Eczema

▪ Morphology
Group of pinpoint vesicles and papules on a coin-shaped erythematous base.

▪ Distribution
Dorsum of hands, extensor aspect of arms, but may appear anywhere.

▪ Patient Profile
Younger women and older men. Very pruritic lesions. Lesions tend to be chronic and often worse in the winter.

▪ Diagnosis
Biopsy reveals eczematous dermatitis without presence of fungal elements.

▪ Treatment
Class I or II topical corticosteroids; emollients. Two to 4 weeks of systemic antibiotics may be helpful. Combined UVA and UVB light.

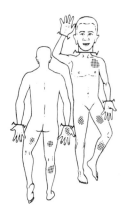

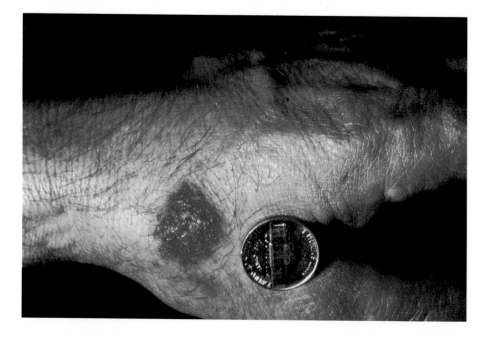

Scabies

▪ Morphology
Vesicles are small, arise on an erythematous base, and may be located at the end of a 1- to 3-cm curved, threadlike burrow. Papules are small, hivelike, and excoriated. Nodules may be seen on the genitalia. Multiple crusted lesions in older patients.

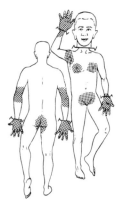

▪ Distribution
Flexor aspects of wrists, between fingers, ulnar border of hand, anterior axillary fold, around nipple, and penis. In older patients, lesions may be numerous.

▪ Patient Profile
All ages but more frequent in young adulthood. Disease may last for months. Very pruritic lesions. Perirectal lesions may occur in older patients.

▪ Diagnosis
Scraping lesion to demonstrate scabietic mite, eggs, or feces microscopically (see p. 17).

▪ Treatment
Permethrin (Elimite) applied over the body from the neck down overnight is preferred. Lindane (Kwell) often effective. Pruritus may persist for several weeks after treatment and should be treated with topical steroids and systemic antihistamines. Postscabietic nodules may require treatment with class I or II corticosteroids or intralesional corticosteroids.

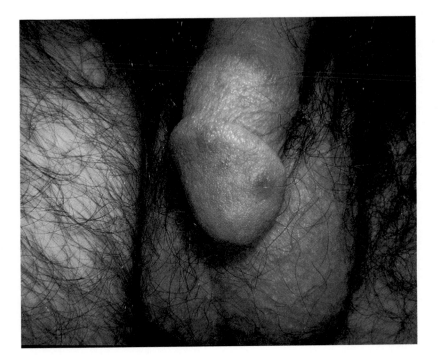

Rare Causes of Blisters with Red Papules

The following diseases manifest blisters and papules. However, they are so rare that they are grouped together here for completeness of differential diagnosis.

Congenital syphilis: Newborn infants may exhibit red-brown papules and flaccid bullae. Rhinorrhea, oral lesions, jaundice, generalized adenopathy, and bone pain are associated with congenital syphilis. Diagnosis is made by demonstrating an IgM antibody for syphilis in the infant.

Erysipelas: A rapidly spreading, red, hot, often purpuric, sharply circumscribed plaque, which may develop tense blisters at the periphery in a febrile patient, should suggest this diagnosis. Cultures are positive for *Streptococcus.*

Fixed drug reaction: Patients may develop one or several papules that become blistered after taking a drug. These lesions recur in exactly the same location each time the drug is ingested. Tetracycline, phenolphthalein, and quinine are common causes.

Gas gangrene: A red, deeply indurated plaque with blisters and crepitation of the surrounding subcutaneous tissue suggests *Clostridium perfringens* infection. Medical emergency.

Herpes gestationis: A rare bullous eruption found in pregnancy or in patients taking oral contraceptives. It is generalized and pruritic, with hivelike papules or blisters, or both. It resembles bullous pemphigoid (see p. 291) clinically, and anti–basement-membrane antibody (anti–bp-180) is present. This disease remits with parturition or discontinuation of oral contraceptives.

Lichen planus: In addition to the papules of lichen planus (see p. 251), erosions in the mouth resulting from dermal-epidermal separation and blisters on the palms and soles may be present.

Lupus erythematosus (LE) (see p. 252): The lesions of LE may blister. Blisters may appear without the classic lupus lesions. Blistering LE lesions may respond to dapsone treatment.

Pemphigus vegetans: Intertriginous and flexural hyperkeratotic plaques with vesicles at their borders. Blisters also

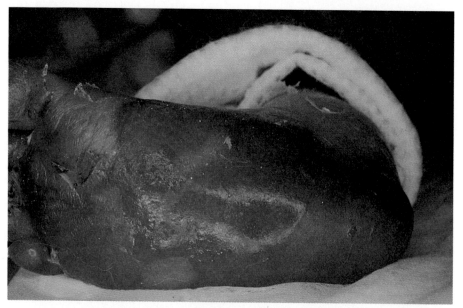

Congenital syphilis

occur on normal skin. Acantholysis is seen on smear and biopsy.

Pityriasis lichenoides et varioliformis acuta (see p. 221): Papules evolve through transient vesicles into hemorrhagic crusts and hypopigmented depressed ulcers. The multiplicity and polymorphic character of the lesions in a healthy young person suggest this diagnosis.

Rickettsialpox: At the site of a mite bite is a papule that progresses to a single vesicle and then to a hemorrhagic, adherent crust. Generalized papules and non-umbilicated vesicles, sparing the palms and soles, then develop.

Tumor: On rare occasions, tumor nodules may develop blisters. This phenomenon is most common with leukemia cutis and lymphoma.

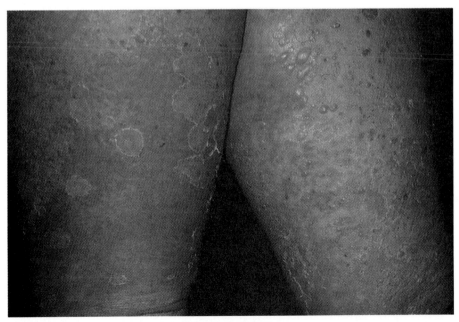

Herpes gestationis

Blisters with Nonred Papules

Dystrophic epidermolysis bullosa
Incontinentia pigmenti
Linear IgA disease
Lymphangioma circumscriptum
Porphyria cutanea tarda
Urticaria pigmentosa (infants)
Rare diseases with blistering and nonred
  papules

Dystrophic Epidermolysis Bullosa

■ **Morphology**
Vesicles and bullae occur in response to trauma. Erosions, crusts, and scars are common. Dystrophy or absence of nails, scarring alopecia, and hypopigmentation are frequent. Fusion of the digits of hands and feet are complicating sequelae. Milia (smooth white papules, 1 to 2 mm in diameter) represent intraepidermal inclusion cysts.

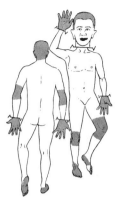

■ **Distribution**
Generalized, but especially common over the knees, elbows, and ankles. Oral lesions and oral scarring are common.

■ **Patient Profile**
Onset at birth or infancy in both sexes. Life-long. Autosomal dominant and recessive forms. Squamous cell carcinomas may develop in scarred lesions.

■ **Diagnosis**
Blisters, erosions, and scarring secondary to trauma beginning in infancy are highly suggestive of this diagnosis. Biopsy shows subepidermal blisters and absence of anchoring fibrils. Genetic defect in collagen VII.

■ **Treatment**
Minimizing trauma and treating infected lesions. Prenatal genetic analysis possible.

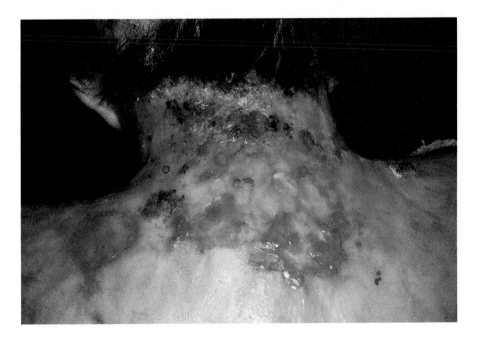

Incontinentia Pigmenti

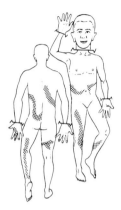

▪ Morphology
Vesicles are linear, tense, and arise on red skin. Papules are scaly. Hyperpigmentation (blue-gray to brown) is swirl-like.

▪ Distribution
Vesicles occur on the lateral aspect of trunk and flexor aspect of extremities.

▪ Patient Profile
Early infancy; affects females predominantly. Scarring alopecia, abnormal teeth, small nails, eye abnormalities, mental and motor retardation are sometimes present. Two genetic loci on X chromosome.

▪ Diagnosis
Biopsy shows intraepidermal bullae containing eosinophils. X-chromosome translocations in some patients.

▪ Treatment
Prenatal diagnosis possible in some cases by genetic testing.

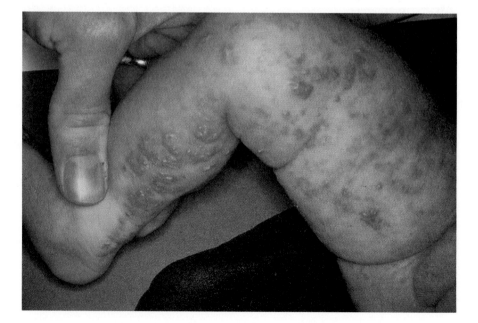

Linear IgA Disease

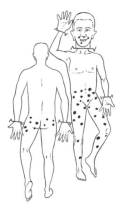

▪ **Morphology**
Tense blisters on an erythematous base. Often arranged in an annular or polycyclic distribution.

▪ **Distribution**
Perioral area, lower abdomen, perineum, and lower extremities. Can be generalized.

▪ **Patient Profile**
Children, often before age 10 years, and adults. Drugs may precipitate eruption.

▪ **Diagnosis**
Biopsy demonstrates a subepidermal blister with neutrophils and eosinophils. Immunofluorescence demonstrates linear deposition of IgA at the dermal-epidermal junction.

▪ **Treatment**
Dapsone, sulfapyridine.

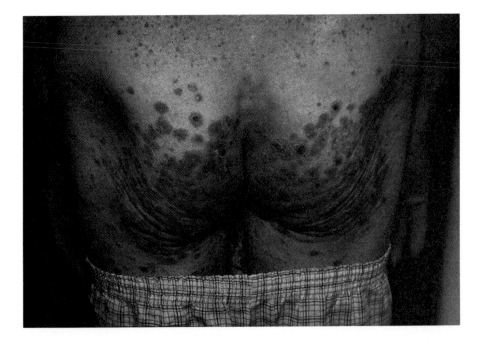

Lymphangioma Circumscriptum

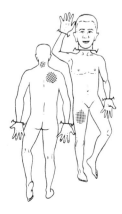

▪ Morphology
Vesicles are small, deep yellow-brown or filled with blood. Papules are scaly and wartlike.

▪ Distribution
Lesions are grouped, appearing like frog spawn with a few scattered peripheral vesicles. Anywhere, but trunk, shoulder, neck, and proximal limbs are most common sites.

▪ Patient Profile
Lesions present at birth or appear during early childhood in both sexes. Life-long. May be associated with large, deep lymphangiomas.

▪ Diagnosis
Biopsy reveals proliferation of dilated lymphatic vessels.

▪ Treatment
Destruction with laser or, for very superficial lesions, electrodesiccation. Recurrence is common if deeper portion not removed.

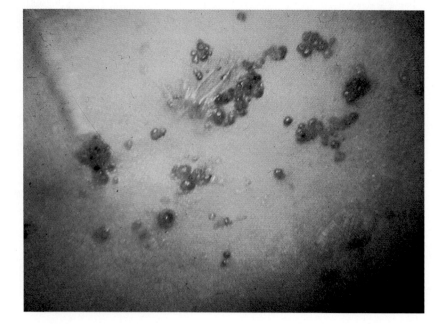

Porphyria Cutanea Tarda

■ **Morphology**
Vesicles usually number fewer than 5, may be hemorrhagic, and progress to crusting and scarring. Papules are milia—white, smooth, 2- to 4-mm epidermal inclusion cysts at the site of old blisters.

■ **Distribution**
The vesicles and milia are usually on sun-exposed or traumatized areas, especially the dorsum of the hands. Hyperpigmentation may be generalized. There may be purple coloration around the eyes and hypertrichosis of the face. Sclerodermatous changes and hyperpigmentation usually occur in sun-exposed areas. No oral lesions, but conjunctival injection.

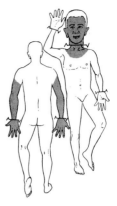

■ **Patient Profile**
Usually adults (30 to 60 years old) with a slight male preponderance. Sometimes familial. Insidious onset with duration of several months to a few years. Burning sensation in affected sites. Defect in uroporphyrinogen decarboxylase activity.

■ **Diagnosis**
Excess liver uroporphyrin production, the metabolic basis of this disease, is most commonly precipitated by chronic ethanol usage or drugs (estrogen, birth control pills, griseofulvin, and NSAIDs). Serum ferritin and transferrin markedly elevated. Screening test: Urine fluoresces pink with an ultraviolet A light if >1 mg/L of uroporphyrin is present. A 24-hour urine collection for uroporphyrin is more sensitive and should be obtained when this diagnosis is suspected. Skin biopsy reveals subepidermal bullae with a sparse lymphocytic infiltrate and deposition of PAS-positive amorphous material in the dermis.

■ **Treatment**
Removal of inciting agent. Phlebotomy or low-dose antimalarials usually effective.

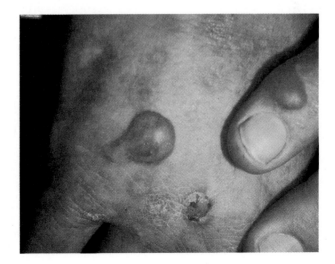

Rare Diseases with Blistering and Nonred Papules

Darier's disease (see p. 245): Vesicles are usually flaccid and associated with symmetric, greasy, keratotic brown papules that are located on scalp, neck, upper chest, and flexural areas. Blisters may be hemorrhagic.

Lichen sclerosus et atrophicus: Porcelain white papules and atrophic macules may develop blisters that may become hemorrhagic. Lesions are most common on genitalia in older adults.

Urticaria pigmentosa (childhood) (see p. 44): Papules are light brown, often single, and form hives when stroked. In newborns and young infants, they may vesiculate. Erythema and edema after stroking are diagnostic.

Urticaria pigmentosa (diffuse, cutaneous, severe mastocytosis): Papules are diffuse, and the skin is diffusely indurated. Large vesicles and denudation follow trauma. Erythema and edema after stroking is diagnostic.

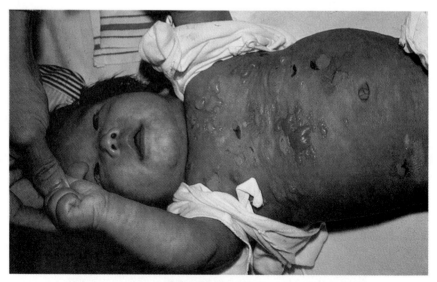

Bullous mastocytosis

Umbilicated Vesicles

Herpes simplex
Herpes zoster (shingles)
Kaposi's varicelliform eruption
Orf and milker's nodule
Smallpox
Vaccinia
Varicella (chickenpox)

TZANCK SMEAR

This test is very important in the diagnosis of patients with umbilicated vesicles. The demonstration of multinucleated giant cells indicates that the causative agent is either herpes simplex or zoster virus.

Method

1. Select a fresh umbilicated vesicle.
2. Unroof the vesicle with a scalpel blade.
3. Gently scrape the base of the vesicle with a scalpel blade and smear on a microscope slide.
4. Fix with 95% alcohol.
5. Stain with Giemsa stain using the technique for routine white cell differential counts.
6. Examine under the microscope using oil immersion for fine detail.

A positive smear demonstrates very large multinucleated giant cells with deep blue cytoplasm or very enlarged nuclei. Intranuclear inclusions (seen in tissue sections) usually are not seen.

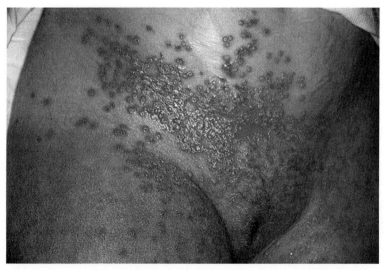

Giant cell from a Tzanck smear

Herpes Simplex

▪ Morphology
Grouped, umbilicated vesicles on an ery-thematous base. Lesions begin as ery-thematous papules and plaques that de-velop umbilicated vesicles that become pustular and crust.

▪ Distribution
Primarily perioral, labial, and genital areas but can be anywhere on skin; occasionally a zosteriform distribution. In newborns and immunosuppressed patients, disease may disseminate over entire body (see also Kaposi's varicelliform eruption, p. 000). Intraoral lesions are unusual in recur-rence. Keratitis occurs.

▪ Patient Profile
Any age, but most frequently in young adulthood. The initial exposure to herpes simplex may cause severe stomatitis with fever, balanitis, or vulvovaginitis. Recur-rent herpes frequently occurs at the same location. Lesions are frequently preceded by a burning sensation. Recurrent herpes simplex is a common cause of recurrent erythema multiforme. Chronic herpes sim-plex lesions are seen in HIV-positive and other immunosuppressed patients.

▪ Diagnosis
Grouped, umbilicated vesicles on an ery-thematous base strongly suggest this diag-nosis. Tzanck smear shows multinucle-ated giant cells. Viral cultures grow herpes simplex within 48 hours. Biopsy demon-strates reticular and ballooning degenera-tion of the epidermis, multinucleated gi-ant cells, and intranuclear inclusions.

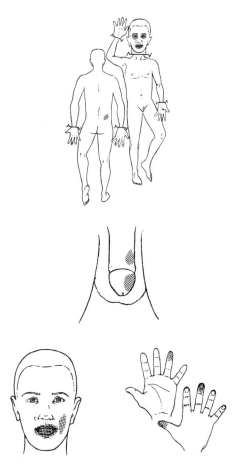

▪ Treatment
Acyclovir orally (400 mg five times a day) for 7 to 10 days for acute episode. In those with recurrent erythema multiforme, acy-clovir (200 mg twice a day) for many months usually can prevent recurrences.

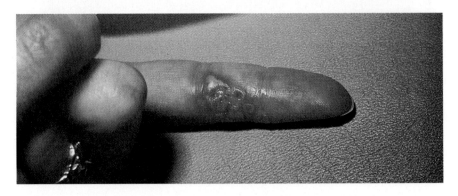

Herpes Zoster

▪ Morphology

Umbilicated vesicles arise on groups of erythematous papules or urticarial plaques after 2 to 3 days. The lesions may be hemorrhagic. Crusting occurs rapidly, and scarring is common.

▪ Distribution

Herpes zoster begins in a dermatomal distribution. Thoracic, cervical, trigeminal, and lumbosacral involvement are most common. Ophthalmic zoster may involve the ciliary body and appears clinically as vesicles on the tip of the nose. Vesicles in the mouth may be seen when the mandibular and maxillary branches of the trigeminal nerve are affected.

▪ Patient Profile

This disease is most common in patients older than 40 years and in HIV-positive and other immunosuppressed patients. Frequently begins with pain and burning in a dermatomal distribution. After 3 to 4 days, groups of erythematous papules erupt that develop into characteristic umbilicated vesicles. Lesions and surrounding skin frequently are hypoalgesic.

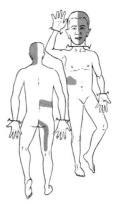

▪ Diagnosis

Groups of umbilicated vesicles in a dermatomal distribution are characteristic. Tzanck smear reveals multinucleated giant cells. Contact with herpes zoster in a previously uninfected patient can result in varicella. Biopsy shows reticular and ballooning degeneration of the epidermis, multinucleated giant cells, and intranuclear inclusion.

▪ Treatment

Acyclovir (800 mg five times a day), valacyclovir (1 g tid), or famciclovir (500 mg tid) until lesions crust, usually 7 to 10 days. Symptomatic pain relief.

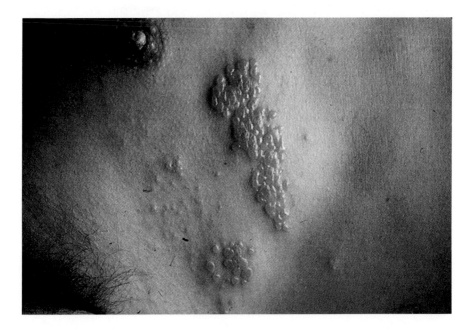

Kaposi's Varicelliform Eruption
(Eczema Herpeticum)

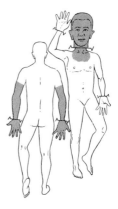

▪ Morphology
Umbilicated vesicles on erythematous bases in sites of preexisting dermatitis. Lesions rapidly become pustular and crusted. Lesions are not grouped.

▪ Distribution
Entire body, especially in areas with preexisting dermatitis. May affect mucous membranes of mouth, eyes, and genitalia.

▪ Patient Profile
Both sexes; all age groups, but most common in children. Patient always has a preexisting dermatologic disease or altered immune response. Atopic dermatitis, which may be quiescent, is the most common preexisting disease. Rarely, this disease occurs in patients with active pemphigus, Darier's disease, or ichthyosis. When the lesions of the preexisting atopic dermatitis are infected with herpes simplex, the condition is called *eczema herpeticum*.

▪ Diagnosis
Disseminated umbilicated vesicles in a patient with preexisting dermatologic disease or history of atopic dermatitis strongly suggest this diagnosis. Tzanck smear is positive in patients infected with herpes simplex. The biopsy in eczema vaccinatum reveals intracytoplasmic inclusions and an absence of giant cells. In eczema herpeticum it reveals nuclear inclusions and multinucleated giant cells.

▪ Treatment
Systemic antibiotics for secondary staphylococcal infection and acyclovir (400 mg five times a day) for 7 to 10 days.

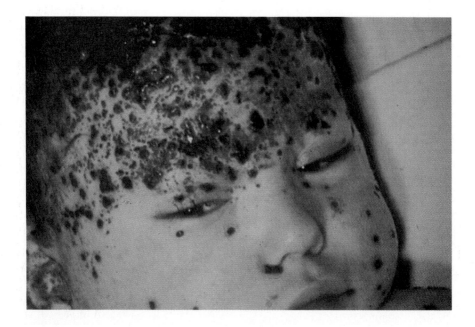

Orf and Milker's Nodule

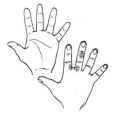

■ **Morphology**
One or several umbilicated vesicles are tense, large, and firm on a red or hemorrhagic base. Lesions resolve over weeks.

■ **Distribution**
Almost always on hands.

■ **Patient Profile**
Any age or sex in patient who has had contact with cows (milker's nodule) or sheep (orf). *Orf* (ecthyma contagiosum) begins with fever and lymphadenopathy, which resolves after 3 to 4 days. Papular lesions evolve into a weeping nodule that develops a surface crust. In *milker's nodule*, typically a single lesion on the finger begins as a red macule that becomes papular. A papulovesicle develops and evolves into a weeping, crusted nodule.

■ **Diagnosis**
Five days after contact with infected sheep or cows, sparse lesions develop on hands that go through the characteristic progression. Biopsy reveals edema and ballooning degeneration of the epidermis and a dense, lymphohistiocytic dermal infiltrate indicative of a poxvirus infection.

■ **Treatment**
Self-limited, treatment not necessary.

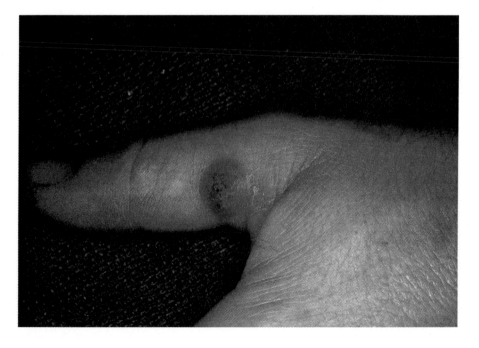

Smallpox
(For Historical Interest)

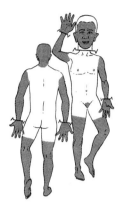

▪ Morphology
Umbilicated vesicles are tense, sharply demarcated, approximately 1 cm in diameter, and may be hemorrhagic. They are preceded by indurated red papules that may last 1 to 2 days. Umbilicated vesicles become pustules within several days and then progress to crusting and scarring. All lesions are in the same stage of development.

▪ Distribution
Eruption begins on the face, neck, and upper trunk and then spreads to distal arms and legs. Lesions have a regular, uniform distribution. Mucosal vesicles and erosions are seen.

▪ Patient Profile
Currently infection is possible only in laboratory personnel working with organisms, frozen tissue specimens, and other such contaminants.

▪ Diagnosis
Disease begins with fever, headache, and backache 8 to 14 days after exposure. Skin eruption has a characteristic progression and distribution. Biopsy reveals intracytoplasmic inclusions. Tzanck smear does not show giant cells. Electron microscopy of lesions demonstrates the poxvirus and is the most rapid method of diagnosis. The disease is highly contagious and, if the diagnosis is suspected, the patient should be isolated.

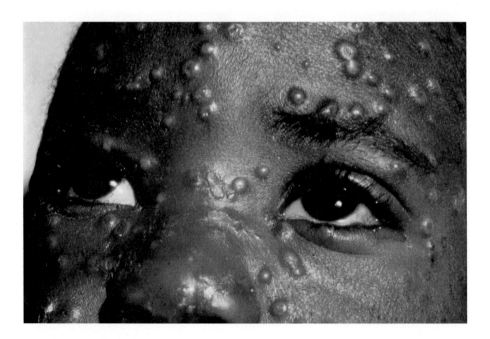

Vaccinia
(For Historical Interest)

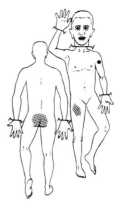

■ **Morphology**
Umbilicated vesicle on erythematous base
that is usually >1 cm at the site of inoculation.

■ **Distribution**
Lesions occur at the site of inoculation.
Multiple lesions can occur by self-inocula-
tion if the patient has scratched himself or
herself.

■ **Patient Profile**
Disease usually occurs in childhood, but it
can occur at any age. Patients have been
vaccinated for smallpox or have been in
contact with another person who has been
vaccinated. Because these vaccinations are
not part of normal childhood immuniza-
tions, this disease is presented mainly for
historical interest.

■ **Diagnosis**
History is essential for the diagnosis. Giant cell preparation is negative.

■ **Treatment**
Symptomatic treatment.

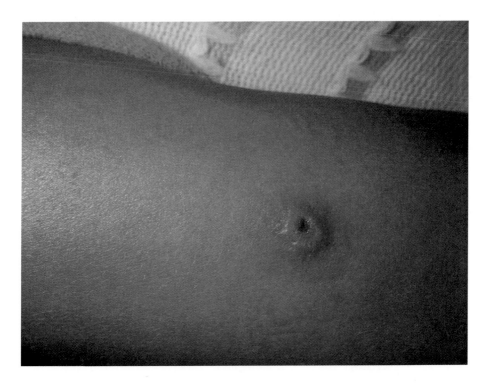

Varicella
(Chickenpox)

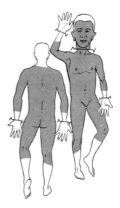

▪ Morphology
Two- to three-millimeter umbilicated vesicles arise from preexisting red papules within a matter of hours. The umbilicated vesicles rapidly become pustules on red bases and then crust. Characteristic of varicella is that lesions are in different stages of development. Rarely, lesions become hemorrhagic.

▪ Distribution
Lesions begin on the trunk, are usually scattered, and are sparse acrally. Lesions may be seen on mucosal surfaces and especially on the hard palate.

▪ Patient Profile
The usual patient is a child between the ages of 2 and 10 years who develops mild constitutional symptoms 2 to 3 weeks after exposure to varicella. After several days, the characteristic rash erupts. Pruritus is common. Encephalitis occurs rarely. Pneumonia may also occur. Secondary staphylococcal or streptococcal infection seen.

▪ Diagnosis
Umbilicated vesicles in different stages of development are characteristic, and demonstration of multinucleated giant cells on Tzanck smear confirms the diagnosis. Such cells are absent in smallpox. Biopsy is similar to that in herpes simplex.

▪ Treatment
Adults or immunosuppressed children with acyclovir (800 mg five times a day) until all lesions crust; intravenous acyclovir may be needed in debilitated patients.

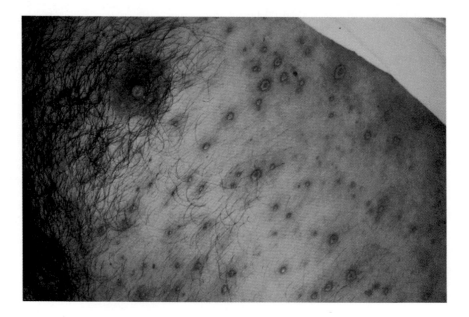

Blisters without Other Lesions

DIAGNOSTIC OBSERVATIONS
These diseases present with nonumbilicated blisters, and distinct, separate papules are not present. Sequelae of blisters include erosions, pustules, and crusts. Heat, sunlight, x-ray, or extreme cold may produce tense, sometimes hemorrhagic, blisters. The history of trauma and the shape and distribution of the blisters suggest this diagnosis.

Pinpoint, Tiny Vesicles

Dyshidrosis (hands, feet)
Miliaria

Vesicles and Bullae

Bites
Bullous impetigo
Bullous lupus erythematosus (p. 252)
Burns
Cicatricial pemphigoid (see p. 492)
Coma, drug-related, and neuropathic bullae
Dystrophic epidermolysis bullosa (see p. 299)
Epidermolysis bullosa acquisita
Epidermolysis bullosa letalis
Epidermolysis bullosa simplex
Familial benign pemphigus (see p. 333)
Hand-foot-and-mouth disease
Linear IgA bullous dermatoses (see p. 301)
Pemphigoid
Pemphigus foliaceus
Pemphigus vulgaris
Toxic epidermal necrolysis (staphylococcal or drug-related)

Pinpoint, Tiny Vesicles

Dyshidrosis
(Pompholyx)

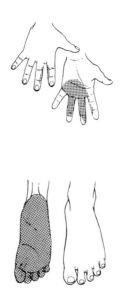

▪ Morphology
Groups of clear vesicles and pustules involve lateral aspects of fingers, palms, and soles. The lesions begin as small (2 to 3 mm) vesicles but can evolve into larger blisters and crusts.

▪ Distribution
Hands and feet. Initially, lateral portions of digits. Usually symmetric.

▪ Patient Profile
Both sexes; adults, rarely children. This is a chronic disease with recurrent episodes of vesicles on hands and feet. Individual episodes have a sudden onset; lesions are very pruritic. Pustulation may be secondary to bacterial superinfection. Hyperhidrosis is common, and emotional stress may precipitate vesiculation.

▪ Diagnosis
Vesicles and pustules that are pruritic on lateral aspects of fingers, palms, and soles suggest this diagnosis. If lesions are very localized, contact dermatitis (see p. 284) and fungus infection (see p. 292) should be considered. Biopsy reveals intraepidermal spongiotic vesicles.

▪ Treatment
Identification of potential contactant. Topical corticosteroids (class I or II), tar soaks, systemic antihistamines.

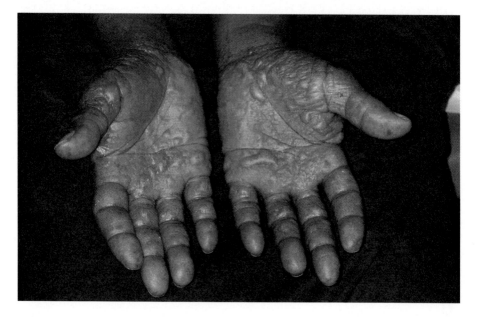

Miliaria
(Miliaria Crystallina)

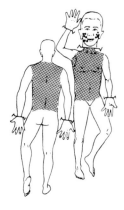

■ **Morphology**
Vesicles are 1 to 2 mm in diameter, have clear or opaque thin walls, rupture easily, and may have associated redness.

■ **Distribution**
Lesions are uniformly distributed at the orifice of sweat ducts. Clear vesicles are more frequent on the trunk, and inflammatory papules may be found on flexural surfaces.

■ **Patient Profile**
Any age but much more common in infancy; both sexes. Sudden onset; self-limited disease. Lesions prickle rather than itch, but patients may scratch.

■ **Diagnosis**
Fever, occlusive therapy, and hot, humid weather are common predisposing factors.

■ **Treatment**
Cool environment.

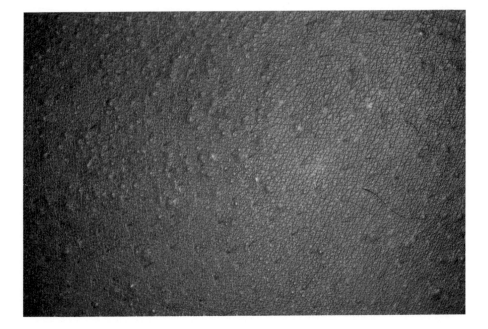

Vesicles and Bullae

Bites

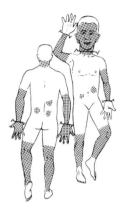

▪ **Morphology**
Tense blister, may be hemorrhagic, and is on an erythematous base. Several blisters may be grouped together.

▪ **Distribution**
Grouped lesions usually in exposed areas.

▪ **Patient Profile**
Patient notices sudden onset of pruritic blisters after appropriate exposure.

▪ **Diagnosis**
Clinical pattern is highly suggestive of diagnosis. Biopsy reveals subepidermal blister with eosinophilia and dense, perivascular mononuclear cell infiltrate.

▪ **Treatment**
Corticosteroids (I or II), antihistamines, antibiotics if secondarily infected.

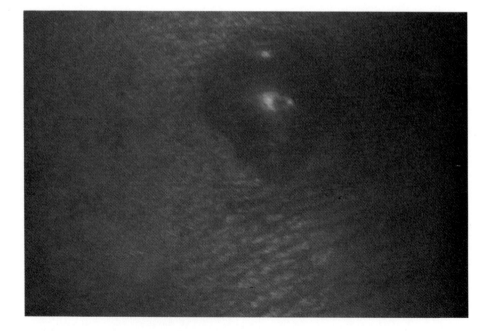

Bullous Impetigo

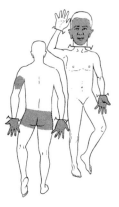

▪ Morphology
Bullae with thin, easily broken roofs evolve from red macules. Lesions rapidly become weeping erosions, or they develop a tightly adherent honey-colored crust. Satellite lesions occur close to the initial lesions; these lesions and the central healing of older lesions can lead to polycyclic and annular lesions.

▪ Distribution
Face, especially around mouth and nose, but can be anywhere.

▪ Patient Profile
More common in children; both sexes. Frequently found in epidemics during summer in patients with poor hygiene. Lesions may itch. Disease is very contagious.

▪ Diagnosis
Large, flaccid bullae with honey-colored crusts are characteristic of this diagnosis. Gram-positive cocci in chains and clumps and polymorphonuclear leukocytes are seen on Gram's stain of blister fluid. Culture yields *Staphylococcus aureus*, usually bacteriophage group I, and frequently streptococci as well.

▪ Treatment
Lesions usually require systemic antibiotics for 7 to 10 days (erythromycin, dicloxacillin, or a cephalosporin). Very localized lesions respond to topical mupirocin. Cleansing with soap and water is important.

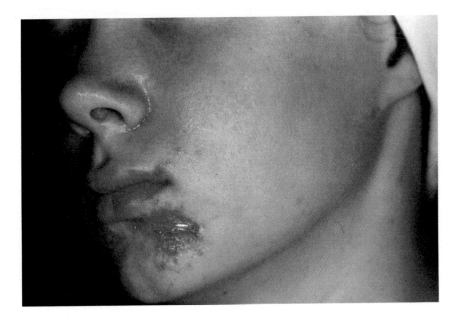

Burns

Heat, sunlight, x-ray, or extreme cold may produce tense, sometime hemorrhagic blisters. History of trauma and shape and distribution of the blister suggest this diagnosis.

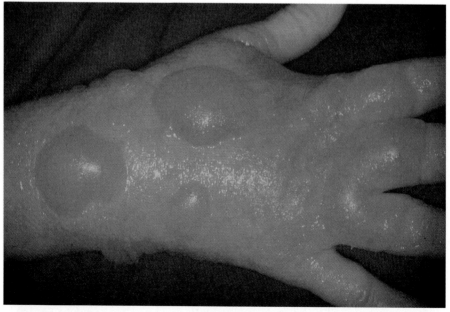

Thermal burn

Coma, Drug-Related, and Neuropathic Bullae

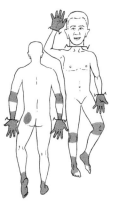

▪ Morphology
Vesicles or bullae are clear, tense, and located on a red, indurated plaque. Dusky erythematous plaques without vesicles may also occur.

▪ Distribution
Located on areas of pressure, such as fingers, wrists, ankles, heels, dorsa of feet, toes. Some blisters are in linear groups; distribution may depend on position of comatose patient.

▪ Patient Profile
Any age, both sexes. Blisters occur within 24 hours of drug ingestion. Lesions resolve over several days. Only one crop of lesions occurs.

▪ Diagnosis
History of unconsciousness or drug overdose. Biopsy shows intraepidermal and subepidermal bullae and sweat gland necrosis. Smear of blisters shows no cells or bacteria. Lesions are not specific for any one type of drug. Similar blisters are seen in patients with chronic renal disease and diseases of the nervous system with peripheral neuropathy, such as syringomyelia. Diabetics may have similar lesions, often associated with neuropathy. Blisters rarely occur with granulocyte-macrophage colony-stimulating factor and pyridoxine.

▪ Treatment
Supportive care; removal of pressure.

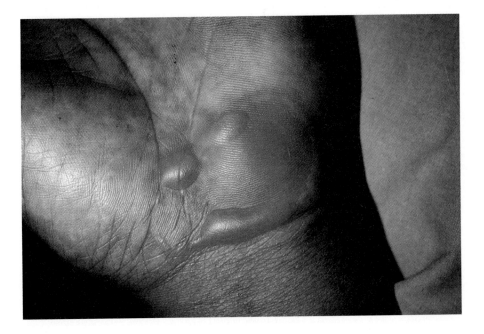

Epidermolysis Bullosa Acquisita

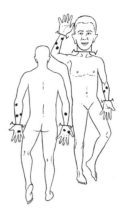

▪ Morphology
Blister on a nonerythematous base. Erosions, scars, and milia frequently present. A second variant shows widespread blisters on an erythematous or even urticarial base. Some blisters may become hemorrhagic.

▪ Distribution
Usually acral for noninflammatory blister, but widespread for inflammatory blisters.

▪ Patient Profile
Patient presents with blistering eruption with scarring. Clinically is similar to porphyria cutanea tarda but lacks associated hyperpigmentation, hirsutism, photodistribution, or scleroderma-like changes. Has been described in patients with systemic lupus erythematosus and inflammatory bowel disease.

▪ Diagnosis
Biopsy shows a subepidermal blister with few inflammatory cells. Direct immunofluorescence of the specimen treated with 1 mol NaCl shows deposition of IgG on the blister floor. This is differentiated from bullous pemphigoid, which has its antigen located on the blister roof of a salt split skin section.

▪ Treatment
Systemic corticosteroids, immunosuppressants, dapsone.

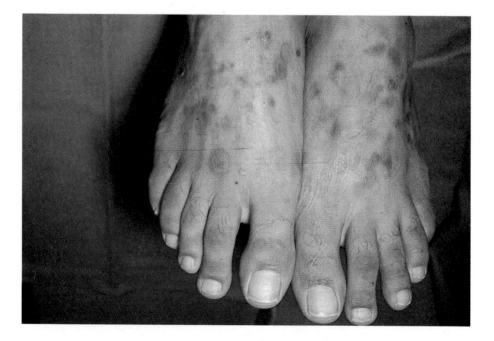

Epidermolysis Bullosa Letalis
(Junctional Disease)

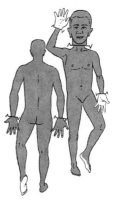

▪ Morphology
Bullae and erosions in areas of trauma. Blisters may be hemorrhagic. Nails may shed. Lesions heal with thin, abnormally pigmented skin, but scarring and milia are uncommon. Hypertrophic granulation tissue in erosions is common. Teeth are abnormal.

▪ Distribution
Any area of trauma but usually spares palms and soles. Mucosal lesions and especially oral erosions are common.

▪ Patient Profile
Disease begins at birth or soon after. Autosomal recessive inheritance. Disease may be fatal.

▪ Diagnosis
Biopsy reveals sharp dermal-epidermal separation. Cleavage plane bisects the basement membrane when electron microscopy is performed. Deficiency of laminin 5. Prenatal genetic analysis on DNA possible.

▪ Treatment
Symptomatic, including prevention of pressure and overhydration of epidermis; treatment of secondary infections; maintenance of good nutrition.

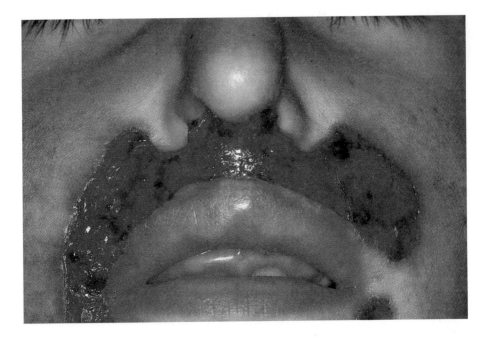

Epidermolysis Bullosa Simplex

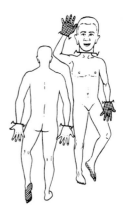

▪ Morphology
Blisters arise at sites of trauma and rapidly erode. May be hemorrhagic. No scarring or milia.

▪ Distribution
Palms, soles, areas of tight clothing. Oral lesions may occur.

▪ Patient Profile
Infants, children, young adults. Worse in summer. Often autosomal dominant inheritance. Blisters may be painful.

▪ Diagnosis
Biopsy of very fresh blisters reveals dissolution of the basal cells. Most cases due to a point mutation in keratin 5 or keratin 14.

▪ Treatment
Prevention of trauma; treatment of secondary infection.

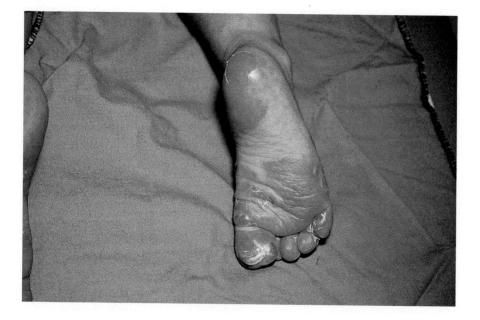

Hand-Foot-and-Mouth Disease

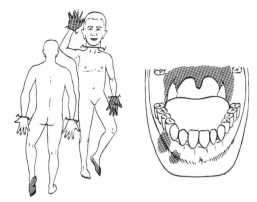

▪ Morphology
Vesicles progress to form opaque, discrete, oblong blisters with red rims. Nonblistered papules occur.

▪ Distribution
Palms, soles, and dorsal portions of hands and feet (especially periungually). Oral bullae rapidly evolve into erosions.

▪ Patient Profile
Any age but most common in young children; both sexes. Skin and mucosal lesions are painful.

▪ Distribution
Culture reveals coxsackievirus A16 (and rarely A10 and A5) to be the etiologic agent.

▪ Treatment
Analgesics may be necessary for painful mouth lesions.

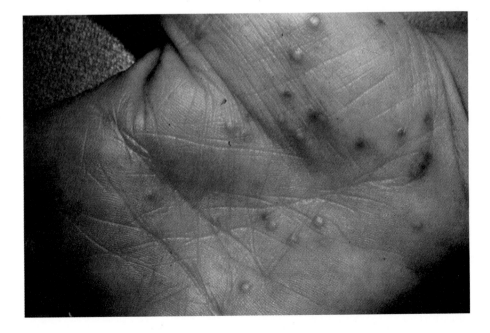

Pemphigus Foliaceus

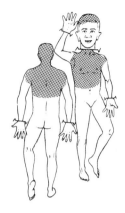

■ **Morphology**
Superficial vesicles, erosions with scaling and crusts are characteristic.

■ **Distribution**
Primarily scalp, face, neck, and upper trunk, but can occur anywhere; oral lesions very uncommon.

■ **Patient Profile**
Middle-aged adults. Disease may persist for years.

■ **Diagnosis**
Biopsy and immunofluorescence. Antibodies against desmoglein I bind to upper spinous and granular layers.

■ **Treatment**
Disease may respond to lower doses of corticosteroids but can be quite resistant to therapy and require the full course of drugs used to treat pemphigus vulgaris (see p. 325).

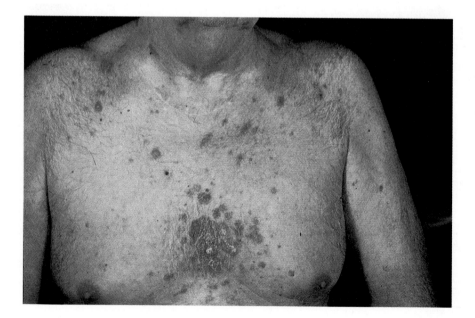

Pemphigus Vulgaris

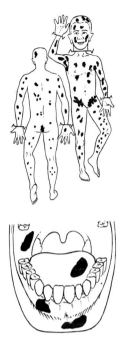

▪ Morphology
Flaccid vesicles and bullae on normal or red skin. Pressure on normal skin induces lesions (Nikolsky's sign), and pressure on lesions extends them laterally (Asboe-Hansen sign). Fresh lesions are not hemorrhagic. Erosions and crusts are common sequelae of blisters.

▪ Distribution
Generalized, nongrouped. Mucosal erosions, especially of the mouth, are common. Intertriginous areas are often severely involved.

▪ Patient Profile
Any age, but middle-aged adults most frequently involved; both sexes. More frequent in Jews. Usually nonpruritic blisters. May present as persistent oral erosions without skin lesions. Lethal without therapy.

▪ Diagnosis
Flaccid blisters that can be induced by pressure on normal skin and are associated with mucosal lesions strongly suggest pemphigus. Smear of blister fluid with Wright's or Giemsa stain demonstrates acantholytic cells. Biopsy shows intraepidermal blisters and acantholysis. Direct immunofluorescence shows IgG in the intercellular spaces; serum contains an antibody against a component of the epidermal cell surface, a desmosomal protein, desmoglein III.

▪ Treatment
High-dose oral corticosteroids necessary for treatment. If patient is unresponsive, immunosuppressives may be necessary. Secondary infection should be treated with systemic antibiotics.

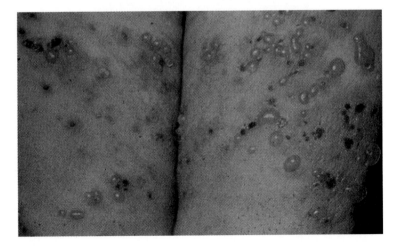

Toxic Epidermal Necrolysis

▪ **Morphology**
Intact bullae and vesicles are rarely seen; moist, red erosions and crusts are the most prominent features of this clinical syndrome. Mechanical pressure extends the blister (Asboe-Hansen sign). Pressure on normal-appearing skin may induce lesions (Nikolsky's sign).

▪ **Distribution**
Generalized; frequently begins in axillae and groin. Perioral and perigenital involvement and conjunctivitis are common. Oral lesions are seen in drug-induced disease.

▪ **Patient Profile**
Usually adults. Skin is tender, and high fever and malaise are common.

▪ **Diagnosis**
Sudden onset of painful blisters at the periphery of a tender, red, scalded-appearing plaque is highly suggestive of this diagnosis. In adults, drugs (phenobarbital, phenylbutazone commonly) and lymphoma may cause this syndrome; blister-

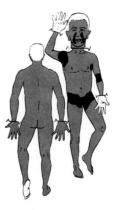

ing is frequently subepidermal and the prognosis is much worse. Gasoline or kerosene soaking of the skin causes similar lesions. May be confused with staphylococcal scalded skin syndrome, which is usually limited to children and lacks oral lesions. Immunocompromised adults and adults with renal failure are susceptible to staphylococcal scalded skin syndrome.

▪ **Treatment**
Intensive supportive care with intravenous fluid, topical dressings, treatment of secondary infection.

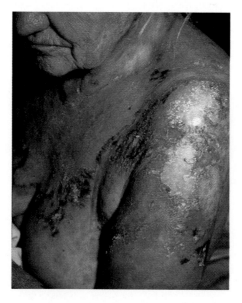

EROSIONS AND CRUSTING

DIAGNOSTIC OBSERVATIONS

Erosions are moist, red, shiny, circumscribed lesions that lack the upper layers of skin. The skin around an erosion may be raised and red. These lesions are frequently secondary to the rupture of a blister. Some diseases cause the skin to be unusually fragile, leading to erosions. To diagnose a disease causing erosions, the nature of the antecedent lesion must be established.

Crusts are yellow-brown to black, circumscribed, moist collections of serum and inflammatory cells on the surface of the skin. Crusting is a secondary lesion. Ruptured blisters, erosions, and excoriations may have fine crusts. Vasculitic infarctions, dry gangrene, *Pseudomonas* sepsis, and factitial ulcerations may have thick, adherent black hemorrhagic crusts (eschars).

Candidiasis
Dermatophyte infection
Fragile skin: Ehlers-Danlos syndrome, epidermolysis bullosa, epidermolytic hyperkeratosis, porphyria cutanea tarda, sundamaged skin, and corticosteroid ingestion or topical application
Impetigo
Intertrigo
Pemphigus: foliaceus, vulgaris, and Hailey-Hailey disease
Perlèche
Toxic epidermal necrolysis

Candidiasis
(Moniliasis)

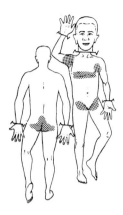

▪ **Morphology**
Eroded plaque with scaling, crusting, and satellite pustules.

▪ **Distribution**
On groin, axillae; under breasts; in skin folds; and between fingers.

▪ **Patient Profile**
Any age, both sexes. Lesions may itch. Lesions are moist and macerated. More common in diabetics.

▪ **Diagnosis**
Fungal scraping is positive for budding yeast and pseudohyphae 50% of the time. Culture positive within 48 to 72 hours.

▪ **Treatment**
Topical imidazoles; systemic ketoconazole often necessary because of intraoral, perirectal, and vaginal lesions.

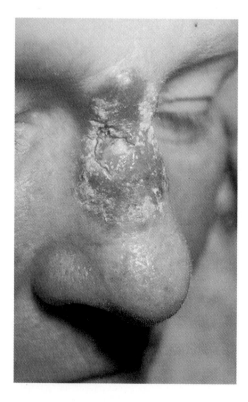

Dermatophyte Infection

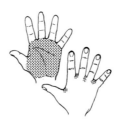
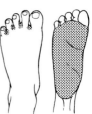

■ **Morphology**
Red erosion covered with gray-white scale and crust.

■ **Distribution**
Between palms and soles and between fingers and toes.

■ **Patient Profile**
Adults, more common in men.

■ **Diagnosis**
Fungal scraping reveals septate hyphae.

■ **Treatment**
For limited infections: use of topical antifungals and dry powders for 3 to 4 weeks or until clear. For widespread or resistant infection: systemic antifungal agents.

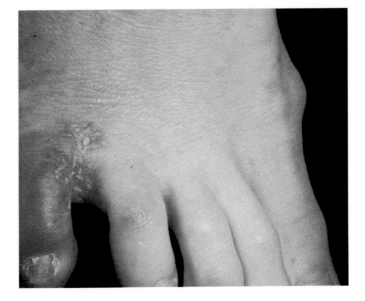

Fragile Skin

Actinically damaged skin and corticosteroid ingestion or topical application: This type of skin damage is characterized by transparent paper-thin skin that tears and erodes easily. Purpura is commonly seen.

Ehlers-Danlos syndrome: Patients with specific subtypes of this genetic syndrome have thin, fragile skin that tears easily. They also have hyperelastic, stretchable skin and skeletal abnormalities.

Epidermolysis bullosa: This uncommon genetic disease is present at birth or in neonatal period. Patient develops blisters and erosions with trauma (see pp. 299, 321, 322).

Epidermolytic hyperkeratosis: This scaly disease is present at birth, and patient develops erosions. Erosions are especially prominent in flexural areas (see p. 126).

Porphyria cutanea tarda: Erosions on the dorsa of the hands are secondary to trauma and light exposure. They are associated with milia, hyperpigmentation, and hirsutism (see p. 303).

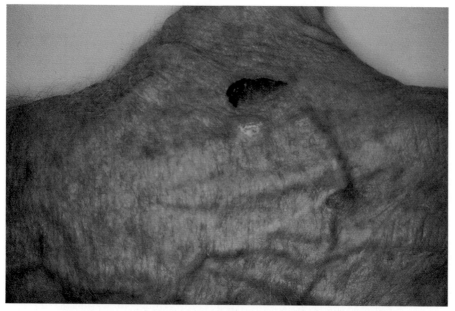

Erosion in actinically damaged skin

Impetigo

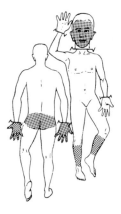

▪ Morphology
Fine, yellow-brown, honey-colored crusts surrounded by erythema.

▪ Distribution
Face, upper chest, extremities, groin.

▪ Patient Profile
Young children, often with a history of trauma. Older patients often have poor personal hygiene. Glomerulonephritis may follow streptococcal impetigo. Very contagious.

▪ Diagnosis
Gram's stain and culture reveal streptococci or staphylococci, or both.

▪ Treatment
Treatment usually requires systemic antibiotics for 7 to10 days (erythromycin, dicloxacillin, or a cephalosporin). Very localized lesions respond to topical mupirocin. Aggressive cleansing with soap and water important.

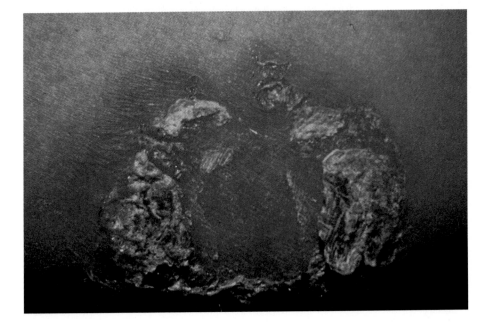

Intertrigo

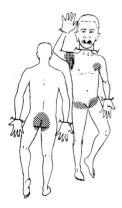

▪ **Morphology**
Pink to red erosions and slight scaling.

▪ **Distribution**
Skin folds; under pendulous breasts, on obese abdomen, groin, buttocks, axillae; under diapers.

▪ **Patient Profile**
Obese patients with deep skin folds and poor hygiene. Young babies, especially in diaper area.

▪ **Diagnosis**
Potassium hydroxide preparations are negative for fungus. Diagnosis is confirmed by rapid response to local drying therapy.

▪ **Treatment**
Drying powders.

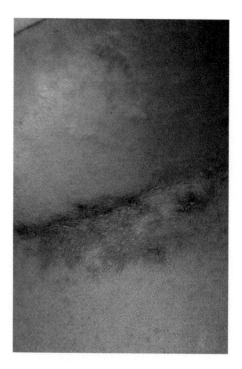

Pemphigus Foliaceus and Vulgaris and Hailey-Hailey Disease

▪ Morphology
Multiple red erosions with crusting and scaling. Flaccid blisters may be present in pemphigus vulgaris.

▪ Distribution
Hailey-Hailey disease: neck, axillae, groin
Pemphigus foliaceus: scalp, upper trunk, axillae
Pemphigus vulgaris: generalized

▪ Patient Profile
Usually adults of both sexes.

▪ Diagnosis
Rubbing lesions produces erosions and extension of lesion. Biopsy is diagnostic and results depend on disease.

▪ Treatment
See individual disease: pemphigus foliaceus (see p. 324); pemphigus vulgaris (see p. 325); familial benign pemphigus (Hailey-Hailey disease) (see p. 333).

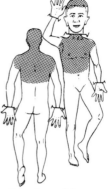

Pemphigus foliaceus

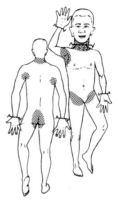

Familial benign pemphigus

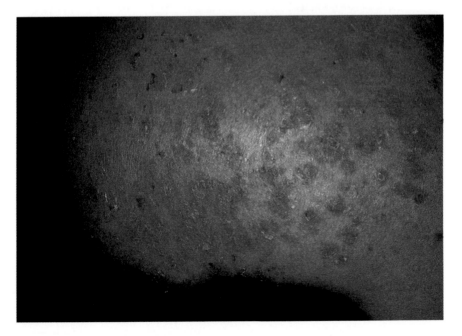

Perlèche

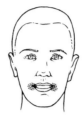

▪ **Morphology**
Red erosions, crusts, fissures, and occasional bleeding.

▪ **Distribution**
Corners of mouth, usually bilateral.

▪ **Patient Profile**
Older patients with loss of vertical height of mouth, resulting in pooling of saliva at corners of mouth. Oral candidiasis, especially under poorly fitting dental plates, and riboflavin deficiency are also associated.

▪ **Diagnosis**
Fungal scraping shows *Candida*. Riboflavin deficiency is associated with malnutrition and glossitis.

▪ **Treatment**
Systemic imidazoles may be necessary in some cases.

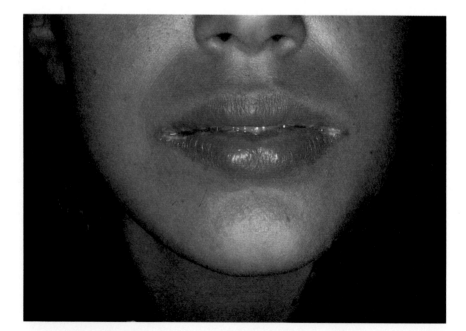

Toxic Epidermal Necrolysis

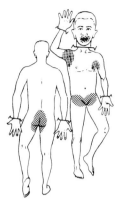

▪ Morphology
Bright red lesions that become eroded when touched. There may be blisters at the periphery of the lesion.

▪ Distribution
Generalized; perioral, perigenital areas, groin, axillae.

▪ Patient Profile
Usually adults. Lesions are tender. High fever and malaise common. Leukopenia is a bad prognostic indicator.

▪ Diagnosis
Disease is related to drug ingestion (phenobarbital, phenylbutazone common), lymphoma, or is idiopathic. Cleft is deep in lower epidermis or is subepidermal.

▪ Treatment
Supportive management and inpatient treatment as for a severe burn. Use of systemic steroids is controversial.

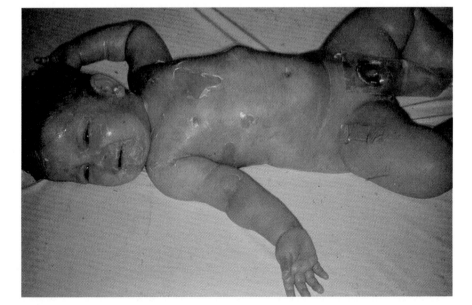

EXCORIATIONS

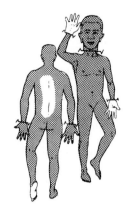

> ### DIAGNOSTIC OBSERVATIONS
> Excoriations are erosions produced by scratching. Excoriations are often linear and may crust, scale, scar, and have surrounding redness. Excoriations are associated with very pruritic skin diseases or generalized pruritus without primary skin diseases. It must be determined whether there was an itchy lesion that became excoriated or whether the patient had an intense itching before a skin lesion appeared. Patients with chronic pruritus will have evidence of linear hypopigmented or hyperpigmented macules.

MAJOR CATEGORIES

Skin Diseases That May Be Extremely Pruritic and Result in Excoriations
Atopic dermatitis (see p. 80)
Drug eruptions (see p. 196)
Insect bites and infestations (see p. 293)
Lichen planus (see p. 251)
Mycosis fungoides (see p. 253)
Neurodermatitis (see p. 239)
Prurigo nodularis (see p. 410)
Scabies (see p. 224)
Stasis dermatitis (see p. 48)
Swimmers' itch (see p. 350)

Pruritus and Excoriations without Skin Disease
Central nervous system disease
Delusions of parasitism
Diabetes
Drug reactions: codeine, amphetamines
Hyperparathyroidism
Hyperthyroidism
Infestations: pubic or body lice, worms
Leukemia
Liver disease
Lymphoma
Neuropathy
Polycythemia rubra vera
Pregnancy
Psychosis
Renal disease: often with uremia
Sarcoidosis

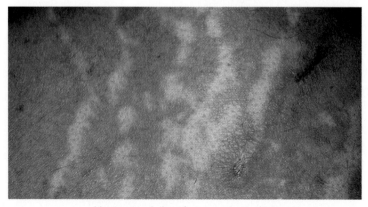

Linear excoriations from uremic pruritus

Chapter 7

■ ■

Pustules, Abscesses, and Sinuses

DIAGNOSTIC OBSERVATIONS

Pustules are focal accumulations of polymorphonuclear cells and serum in the skin. Nicking a pustule with a scalpel blade releases yellow-white purulent material. Abscesses are purulent lesions that involve the deep dermal and subcutaneous tissues. Blistering diseases may become pustular. Sinuses often are associated with inflammatory reactions and are included in this chapter.

The patient should be examined carefully for vesicles and bullae. Umbilicated viral vesicles (see p. 305), scabies (see p. 295), miliaria (see p. 315), and dermatitis herpetiformis (see p. 287) often become pustular. Pustules often crust. All pustules should be examined for bacteria by Gram's stain and for fungi by potassium hydroxide preparation. The number and distribution of pustular lesions should be observed. Sparse acral pustules (often with purpura) frequently are cutaneous manifestations of septic vasculitis. *Gonococcus* is a common cause, but *Meningococcus, Staphylococcus, Pseudomonas,* and deep fungi may cause similar lesions. Gram's stain and culture of the lesion and blood culture are essential.

PUSTULES

Pustules in Generalized or Nonspecific Locations
Acrodermatitis enteropathica
Acute generalized exanthematous pustulosis (AGEP)
Blastomycosis
Candidiasis (moniliasis)
Dermatophyte infection
Drug-related eruptions
Folliculitis
Impetigo
Pustular psoriasis
Septic vasculitis
Subcorneal pustular dermatoses
Rare pustular eruptions: impetigo herpetiformis, myiasis, pyoderma gangrenosum, secondary syphilis, swimmers' itch

Pustules or Abscesses on the Face
Acne
Rosacea

Sycosis barbae, folliculitis
Tinea barbae

Pustules or Abscesses on the Scalp
Dermatophyte infection
Dissecting cellulitis
Folliculitis decalvans

Pustules or Abscesses on the Palms and Soles
Acropustulosis
Dermatophyte infection
Dyshidrosis
Epidermolysis bullosa simplex (see p. 322)
Pustular psoriasis
Septic vasculitis (see p. 348)

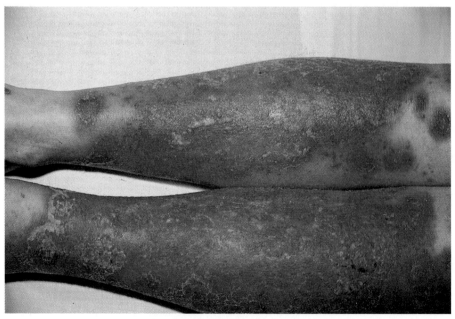

Pustular psoriasis

Pustules in Generalized or Nonspecific Locations

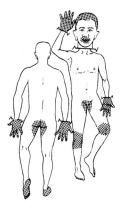

Acrodermatitis Enteropathica

▪ Morphology
Vesicles appear in crops around orifices and rapidly progress to pustules and to crusting. Red, scaly plaques are also present. In many cases, candidal infection with pustules occurs. Loss of hair is common.

▪ Distribution
Lesions are common acrally, on face, and around orifices.

▪ Patient Profile
Disease begins in infancy. Babies fail to thrive and develop diarrhea. Physical growth and sexual maturation are slowed; superimposed candidal infection is common. Autosomal recessive inheritance. Patients receiving hyperalimentation without supplemental zinc may develop an acrodermatitis enteropathica–like eruption.

▪ Diagnosis
The clinical picture associated with decreased serum zinc suggests the diagnosis. Serum alkaline phosphatase often low.

▪ Treatment
Supplemental dietary zinc induces remission.

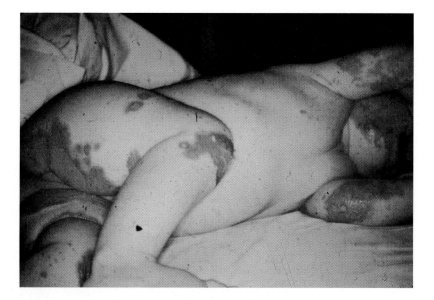

Acute Generalized Exanthematous Pustulosis (AGEP)

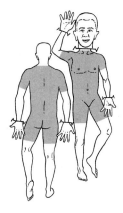

▪ Morphology
Superficial, 2- to 4-mm pustules that may coalesce. May have excoriated papules.

▪ Distribution
Often generalized.

▪ Patient Profile
Most common in adults. Rapid onset of pustules that resolve within 7 to 10 days. Usually associated with drug or viral infection. No fever or arthritis. Allopurinol and antibiotics (e.g., amoxicillin, ampicillin) are a frequent cause.

▪ Diagnosis
This disease must be differentiated from pustular psoriasis and bacterial infection. Skin biopsy shows epidermal neutrophils.

▪ Treatment
Discontinuing drug use.

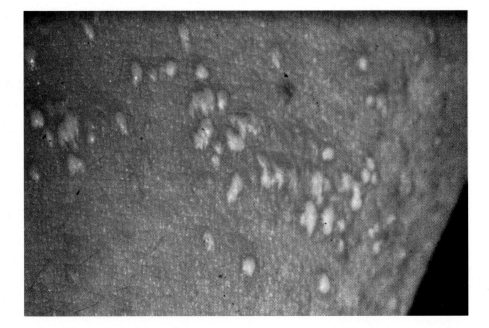

Blastomycosis

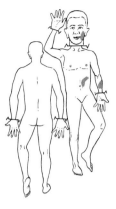

■ **Morphology**
Lesion begins as an erythematous papule
that becomes an indurated, boggy, erythematous plaque studded with pustules.
The lesion frequently ulcerates and heals
with scarring. There is a tendency for
central healing with peripheral spread.

■ **Distribution**
Usually single. It can appear anywhere but
most frequently is on face, wrists, hands,
and feet. Nasal and oral mucosae may be
involved.

■ **Patient Profile**
Much more common in males than in
females. Usually adults older than 40 years
from rural southeastern United States or
other endemic areas. Portal of entry is
usually lung; pulmonary lesions are frequently found. Accidental skin inoculation may occur. Urogenital, bone, and
central nervous system involvement may
occur.

■ **Diagnosis**
Pus mixed with 10% potassium hydroxide
may reveal the budding organism on
smear. Biopsy shows pseudoepithelioma-
tous hyperplasia, acute and chronic inflammatory cells, and organisms. Culture of
the organisms confirms diagnosis. Similar
lesions may be seen in patients ingesting
iodides and bromides.

■ **Treatment**
Systemic itraconazole or amphotericin.

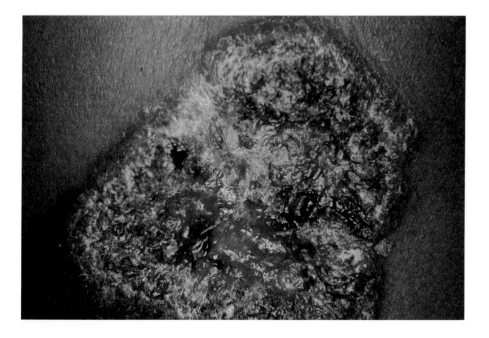

Candidiasis
(Moniliasis)

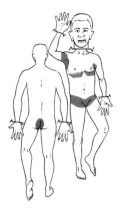

▪ Morphology
Scaly, erythematous plaque with satellite pustules. Discrete vesicopustules also occur. Plaque may progress to erosions and scaling. Usually multiple lesions are present.

▪ Distribution
Warm, moist areas such as groin, axilla, under breasts, but lesions can be anywhere. *Candida* may affect mouth (thrush), penis (balanitis), or vagina (vaginitis). Paronychia and subungual involvement are common.

▪ Patient Profile
Any age, both sexes. Lesions may be moderately pruritic. Disease is more common in patients with diabetes or altered delayed hypersensitivity, including HIV infection.

▪ Diagnosis
Potassium hydroxide preparation of pustules reveals pseudohyphae and spores. Fungal cultures demonstrate *Candida*.

▪ Treatment
Topical imidazoles or systemic ketoconazole or fluconazole.

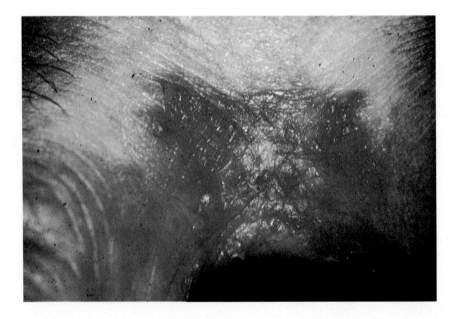

Dermatophyte Infection
(Tinea)

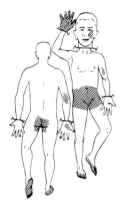

■ Morphology
Erythematous plaques studded with pustules. Pustular component is most marked at the periphery. Scaling is common.

■ Distribution
Anywhere. May be single or up to 20 to 30 discrete lesions.

■ Patient Profile
Any age, both sexes. Fungi causing pustular reactions are frequently contracted from animals. Eruption may itch.

■ Diagnosis
Potassium hydroxide preparations from lesions reveal septate hyphae. Culture on Sabouraud's agar demonstrates the pathogenic fungi.

■ Treatment
Limited infections: topical antifungals and dry powders for 3 to 4 weeks or until clear. Widespread or resistant infection: systemic antifungal agents.

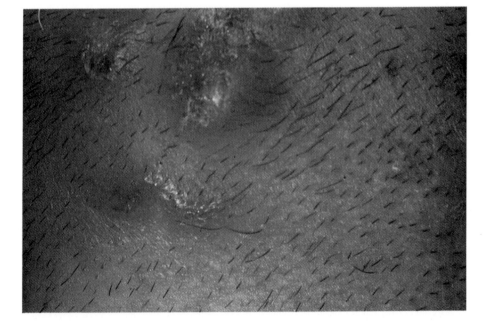

Drug-Related Eruptions

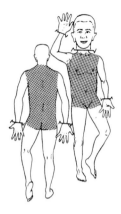

▪ Morphology
Small, acnelike pustules and papules without open comedones (whiteheads) or closed comedones (blackheads).

▪ Distribution
Symmetric; trunk.

▪ Patient Profile
Any age, both sexes. Drugs most commonly causing this reaction are corticosteroids, adrenocorticotropic hormone, iodides, bromides, lithium, phenytoin (Dilantin), and isoniazid. Sudden onset of generalized, superficial pustules has been associated with the use of systemic antibiotics and has been termed acute generalized exanthematous pustulosis (AGEP). This must be differentiated from pustular psoriasis, which is often accompanied by fever and joint complaints that are not part of AGEP.

▪ Diagnosis
Remission of eruption with discontinuation of therapy is suggestive of drug-related eruption. Miliaria (see p. 315) that becomes pustular may be confused with a drug eruption.

▪ Treatment
Discontinuation of drugs leads to clearing of eruption.

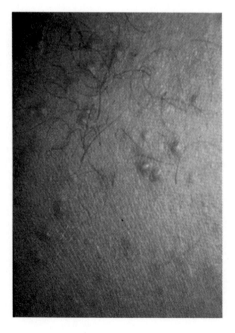

Folliculitis

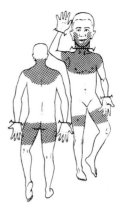

▪ Morphology
Pustules are located in hair follicles, which are surrounded by erythema. Pustules are frequently in groups.

▪ Distribution
Hairy areas of skin, especially face, chest, thighs, buttocks, and groin.

▪ Patient Profile
Both sexes; more frequent in adults. Abrupt onset of lesions, most commonly in areas of irritation. Bacterial and *Pityrosporum* folliculitis frequently occur in HIV-positive patients. Eosinophilic folliculitis is a nonbacterial folliculitis characterized by numerous eosinophils and usually occurs in AIDS patients.

▪ Diagnosis
Follicular pustules demonstrate pyogenic organisms, especially staphylococci on Gram's stain and culture. *Pseudomonas* from hot tubs with inadequate chlorine has lesions with wide rims of erythema.

▪ Treatment
Systemic antistaphylococcal and antistreptococcal agents (oral erythromycin, dicloxacillin, or cephalosporin). Oral ciprofloxacin for *Pseudomonas* folliculitis. Eosinophilic folliculitis is treated with UVB, topical corticosteroids, and antihistamines.

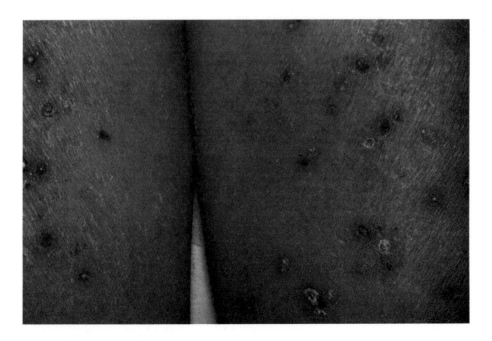

Impetigo

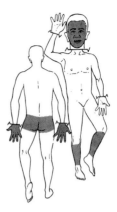

▪ Morphology
Small, flaccid, superficial pustules with a rim of erythema; pustules spread peripherally and rapidly develop crusts and scales. Large bullae may be seen. Lesions heal with slight discoloration.

▪ Distribution
Anywhere, but more frequently on face. Impetigo can complicate preexisting dermatitis, especially atopic dermatitis. Under these circumstances, the lesions follow the distribution of the underlying dermatitis. No oral lesions.

▪ Patient Profile
Usually children, in warm weather and with poor hygiene. Frequently precipitated by arthropod bites. Lesions may itch. Impetigo with a nephrogenic strain of *Streptococcus* may cause glomerulonephritis.

▪ Diagnosis
Culture reveals β-hemolytic streptococci or *Staphylococcus aureus*. Gram's stain reveals streptococci and staphylococci. Ecthyma indicates that lesions of impetigo have eroded through the epidermis to produce adherent crusts and superficial ulcers. Ecthyma is usually due to β-hemolytic streptococci.

▪ Treatment
Usually systemic antibiotics for 7 to 10 days (erythromycin, dicloxacillin, or a cephalosporin). Localized lesions respond to topical mupirocin.

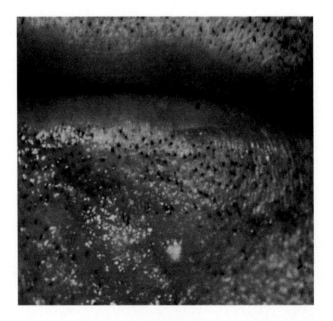

Pustular Psoriasis

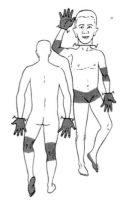

▪ Morphology
Pustules may appear around the rim of plaque of psoriasis and spread peripherally. Pustular von Zumbusch's psoriasis begins with pustules that coalesce into lakes of pus.

▪ Distribution
Anywhere; lesions are most common in acral, flexural, and genitocrural areas. Geographic tongue and erosions of buccal mucosa occur.

▪ Patient Profile
Usually adults of both sexes; chronic disease. Lesions may be painful. This disease may occur in a patient with routine psoriasis after streptococcal infection or after treatment with corticosteroids or chloroquine. High fever, leukocytosis, malaise, arthralgia, arthritis, hypocalcemia, and hypoalbuminemia may be associated with this disease. These cutaneous findings may also occur in Reiter's disease.

▪ Diagnosis
Pustules are sterile, and biopsy reveals spongiform pustules in the epidermis.

▪ Treatment
Potent (class I) topical corticosteroids, often with occlusion, can give rapid relief of erythema. Acitretin will improve lesions over 5 to 10 days. Systemic corticosteroids may be necessary.

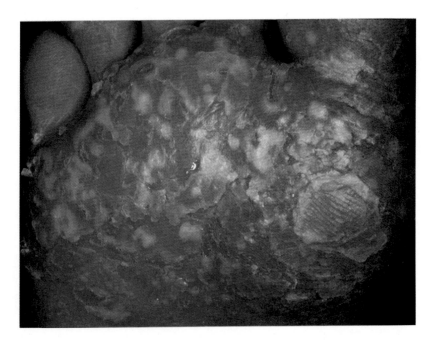

Septic Vasculitis

▪ Morphology
Sparse, acral, elevated, purpuric lesions that become pustular in hours to days. Cutaneous infarcts and splinter hemorrhages in the nails may be seen.

▪ Distribution
Acral, tips of fingers and toes, extensor aspect of elbows and knees. Usually asymmetric.

▪ Patient Profile
All ages. Gonococcemia usually seen in young adults. Arthralgias, periarthritis, fever, and leukocytosis common. Often present in the immunosuppressed host.

▪ Diagnosis
Biopsy reveals leukocytoclastic vasculitis. Gram's stain of pustule demonstrates organisms consistent with staphylococcal, pseudomonal, or meningococcal infection; organisms difficult to demonstrate in gonococcemia. Cervical, pharyngeal, and rectal cultures in Thayer-Martin agar demonstrate gonococcus. Blood culture and lesion culture demonstrate organisms in other infectious processes.

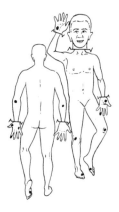

▪ Treatment
Appropriate antimicrobial treatment of the underlying infection. Systemic steroids efficacious for connective tissue diseases.

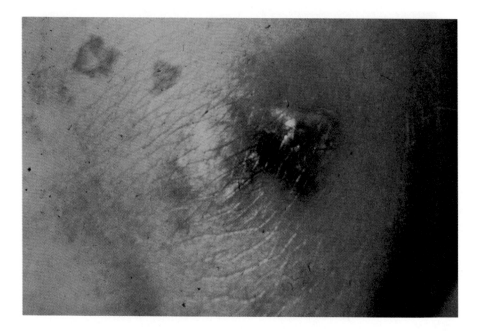

Subcorneal Pustular Dermatoses
(Sneddon-Wilkinson Disease)

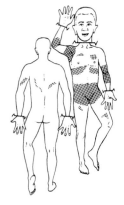

▪ Morphology
Flaccid, very superficial pustules that are on a red base and show a fluid level of pus. Lesions are in groups, rings, and arcs.

▪ Distribution
Groin, axilla, upper back, submammary trunk, and flexors of arms. No oral lesions.

▪ Patient Profile
More frequent in women than in men. Forty- to 60-year-old age group. Condition lasts years; mildly pruritic.

▪ Diagnosis
Histologic examination reveals a subcorneal pustule. Pustules are sterile, differentiating this disease from impetigo. Immunofluorescent studies of skin biopsy usually do not reveal deposits of immunoglobulin.

▪ Treatment
Dapsone (50 to 200 mg per day) is the treatment of choice.

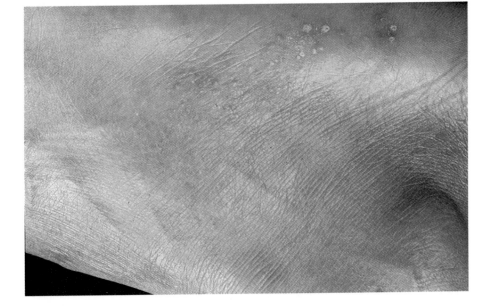

Rare Pustular Eruptions

Impetigo herpetiformis: This is a very rare pustular disease of pregnancy.

Myiasis: Fly larvae (maggots) can be deposited in skin with formation of pustules. Treatment: Occlusion with Vaseline or Aquaphor.

Pyoderma gangrenosum: Diffuse pustular eruptions may be associated with this condition.

Secondary syphilis: Pustules are rarely seen in secondary syphilis.

Swimmers' itch: This is a sensitization reaction to penetration of skin by cercariae of schistosomes.

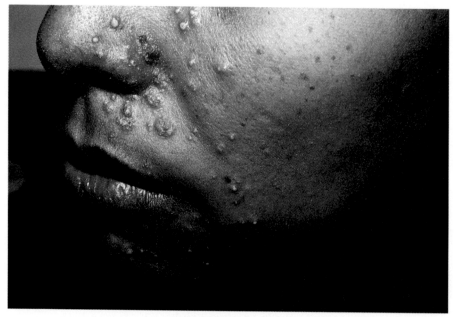

Secondary syphilis

Pustules or Abscesses on the Face

Acne

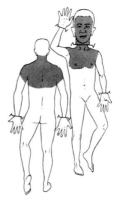

▪ Morphology
Pustules, papules, open comedones (blackheads), closed comedones (whiteheads), occasional cysts, and scarring.

▪ Distribution
Entire face, especially forehead, nose, and cheeks. Lesions may be scattered on chest, neck, and back.

▪ Patient Profile
Both sexes. Teenagers and young adults. Family history of acne and premenstrual flare-ups is common. Corticosteroids, anabolic steroids, halogens, and anticonvulsives may induce or exacerbate acne. Industrial cutting oils, pomades, and oily cosmetics also can aggravate acne.

▪ Diagnosis
This extraordinarily common disease is diagnosed by its characteristic clinical picture; numerous variants include acne necrotica, acne cosmetica, cystic acne, and so forth.

▪ Treatment
Topical desquamating agents, antibiotics, tretinoin. Systemic tetracycline or erythromycin. Rarely does this form of acne require systemic isotretinoin. Perioral dermatitis responds to oral tetracycline and low-potency topical corticosteroid.

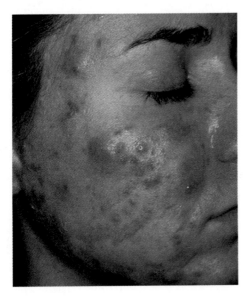

Rosacea

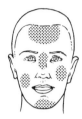

▪ Morphology
Pustules, papules, thickening of nasal skin (rhinophyma), telangiectasia, and flushing. Open and closed comedones (whiteheads and blackheads) are uncommon.

▪ Distribution
Central portion of face, especially bridge of nose, cheeks, and chin. Lesions uncommon on chest and back. May be associated with conjunctivitis, blepharitis, and keratitis.

▪ Patient Profile
Both sexes. Chronic disease found in patients between 30 and 50 years of age. Flushing may be aggravated by alcohol, coffee, tea, chocolate, highly spiced foods, and heat.

▪ Diagnosis
Papules, pustules, telangiectasia, and flushing in central area of face in adults suggest this diagnosis. Biopsy usually reveals lymphohistiocytic infiltrate but, on occasion, granulomas and giant cells are seen.

▪ Treatment
Topical erythromycin or clindamycin; topical metronidazole. Systemic tetracycline or minocycline.

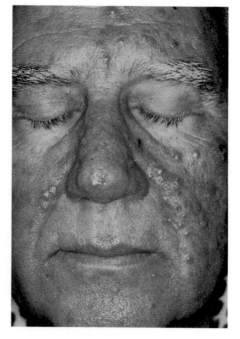

Sycosis Barbae
(Barber's Itch, Folliculitis)

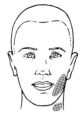

▪ Morphology
Pustules in hair follicles of beard, often associated with red papules. Crusting very common. Beard hair does not usually fall out; scarring may occur.

▪ Distribution
Limited to bearded areas of face and neck.

▪ Patient Profile
Males with poor hygiene who shave irregularly and have disease for weeks to months.

▪ Diagnosis
Pustules in beard area not associated with broken hairs suggest this diagnosis. This disease is more common in unshaven males, whereas pseudofolliculitis occurs more frequently in African-Americans with tightly curled hairs who shave frequently. Gram's stain demonstrates bacteria; fungal scrapings are negative. Culture yields staphylococci.

▪ Treatment
Systemic antistaphylococcal antibiotics (dicloxacillin, cephalosporin).

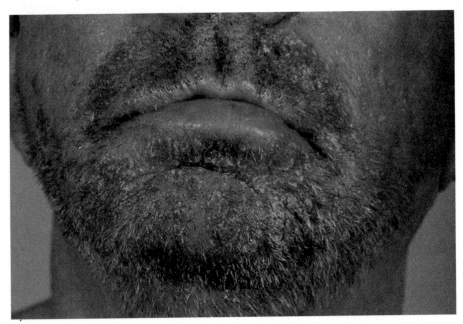

Tinea Barbae
(Fungal Infection of Face)

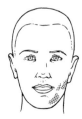

▪ **Morphology**
Boggy, nodular, cystic lesions studded with pustules. Crusting, foul odor, and scarring common. Hair in infected areas is broken.

▪ **Distribution**
Beard.

▪ **Patient Profile**
Males with beards. Secondary infection with bacteria is common.

▪ **Diagnosis**
Inflammation, pustules, and broken-off hairs suggest this diagnosis. Fungal scraping is positive, and fungal culture usually reveals *Trichophyton verrucosum* or *Trichophyton mentagrophytes*. Superficial forms of this disease may be vesicular.

▪ **Treatment**
Topical imidazoles; systemic itraconazole, ketoconazole, or griseofulvin.

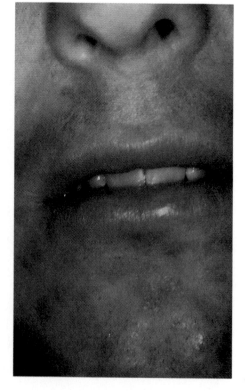

Pustules or Abscesses on the Scalp

Dermatophyte Infection

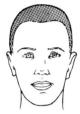

▪ Morphology
Pustules, vesicles, scales, and crusting. Focal reaction is a kerion. Hair may break off at scalp level or it can come through the crust. Scarring alopecia may occur. Black dots on scalp represent broken hairs with endothrix infection, most commonly *Trichophyton tonsurans* in United States.

▪ Distribution
Scalp.

▪ Patient Profile
Usually young children. Disease may last weeks to months. It is often self-limited but can continue for years. In African-Americans, *T. tonsurans* most common cause. Frequent asymptomatic carriers among family members.

▪ Diagnosis
Potassium hydroxide preparation reveals hyphae and spores. Fungal cultures demonstrate *Trichophyton schoenleinii, Trichophyton violaceum, Trichophyton mentagrophytes, Trichophyton verrucosum, Microsporum gypseum,* and *Microsporum canis.*

▪ Treatment
Systemic griseofulvin or ketoconazole. Selenium sulfide shampoo is often a useful adjuvant.

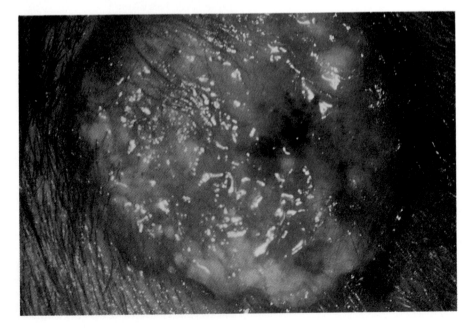

Dissecting Cellulitis
(Perifolliculitis Capitis Abscedens et Suffodiens)

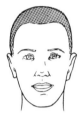

▪ **Morphology**
Superficial and deep abscesses that do not originate in hair follicles. Process leads to severe cordlike scarring and alopecia.

▪ **Distribution**
Scalp.

▪ **Patient Profile**
Most common among young black males. This chronic disease is frequently associated with hidradenitis suppurativa and cystic acne.

▪ **Diagnosis**
Perifollicular abscesses with scarring and alopecia in a black male suggests the diagnosis of dissecting cellulitis. May be mimicked by *Trichophyton tonsurans,* so a fungal culture is part of evaluation.

▪ **Treatment**
Long-term broad-spectrum antibiotics (e.g., tetracycline or minocycline).

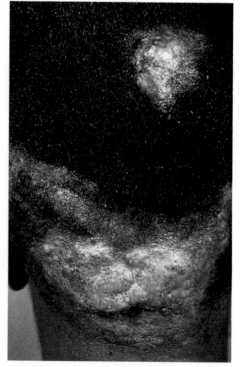

Folliculitis Decalvans

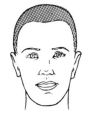

▪ Morphology
Clusters of pustules in hair follicles. Eruption spreads peripherally and results in crusting and scarring alopecia.

▪ Distribution
Scalp.

▪ Patient Profile
Younger adults. Lesions are chronic.

▪ Diagnosis
Chronic disease with clusters of follicular pustules, which results in scarring alopecia. Cultures reveal pyogenic organisms.

▪ Treatment
Topical corticosteroids (class I or II). Antibiotics, including rifampicin, should be tried but are often ineffective.

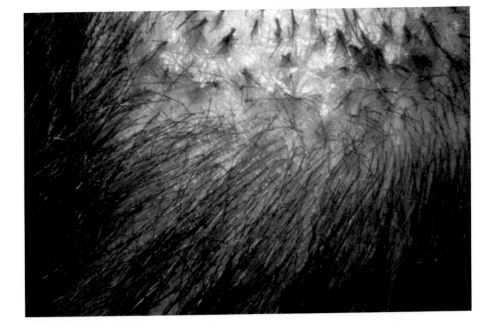

Pustules or Abscesses on the Palms and Soles

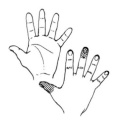

Acropustulosis
(Pustular Acrodermatitis, Acrodermatitis Perstans, Acrodermatitis Continua of Hallopeau, or Dermatitis Repens)

▪ **Morphology**
A plaque of deep-seated vesicles and yellow pustules. The lesions usually begin on one digit and then spread to other fingers. Destruction of nails and digits may occur.

▪ **Distribution**
Lesions confined almost entirely to hands and feet.

▪ **Patient Profile**
Both sexes, usually adults. Chronic disease. Lesions may be painful.

▪ **Diagnosis**
Pustules are sterile. Biopsy demonstrates psoriasiform changes with spongiform pustules.

▪ **Treatment**
Class I corticosteroids, etretinate, topical PUVA therapy.

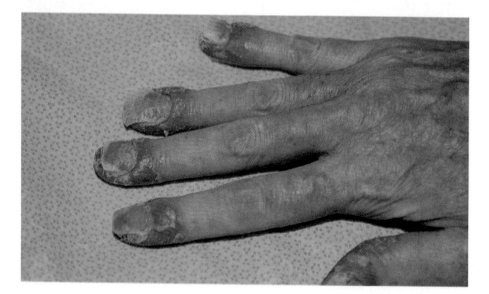

Dermatophyte Infection of Hands and Feet

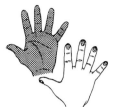 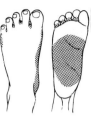

■ **Morphology**
Pustules and vesicles are asymmetric and may be in a ring. Toe web erosions and scaling are common.

■ **Distribution**
Pustules and vesicles usually occur on soles or between toes. Scaling is frequent on the lateral portion of the feet.

■ **Patient Profile**
Very common, particularly in adolescent and adult males. This is a chronic dermatosis with acute episodes.

■ **Diagnosis**
Potassium hydroxide preparations reveal branching hyphae. Fungal cultures are positive.

■ **Treatment**
Limited infections: topical antifungals and dry powders for 3 to 4 weeks or until clear. Systemic antifungal agents for widespread or resistant infection.

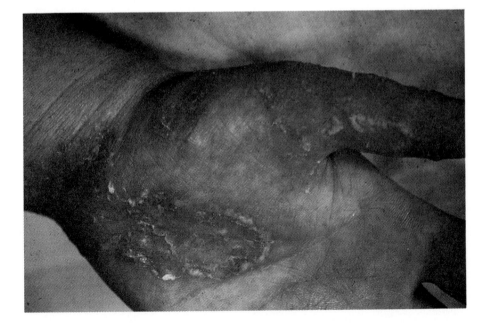

Dyshidrosis
(Pompholyx)

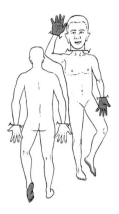

▪ Morphology
Groups of clear vesicles and pustules involve lateral aspects of fingers, palms, and soles. The lesions are small (2 to 3 mm), frequently light brown, and often evolve into crusts.

▪ Distribution
Hands and feet. Initially lateral portions of digits. Usually symmetric.

▪ Patient Profile
Both sexes; adults, rarely children. This is a chronic disease with recurrent episodes of vesicles on hands and feet. Individual episodes have a sudden onset; lesions are very pruritic. Pustulation may be secondary to bacterial superinfection. Hyperhidrosis is common, and emotional stress may precipitate vesiculation.

▪ Diagnosis
Vesicles and pustules that are pruritic on lateral aspects of fingers, palms, and soles suggest this diagnosis. If lesions are localized, contact dermatitis (see p. 284) and fungal infection (see p. 359) should be considered. Biopsy reveals intraepidermal spongiotic vesicles.

▪ Treatment
Identification of potential contactant. Topical corticosteroids (class I or II); systemic antihistamines.

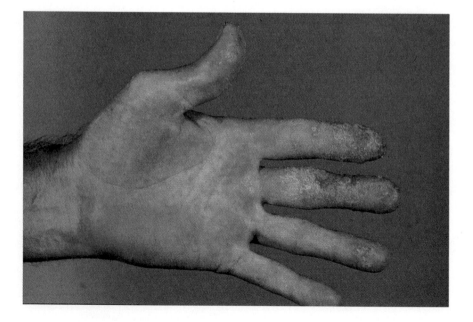

Pustular Psoriasis

■ Morphology
Symmetric sheets of pustules and single pustules are common.

■ Distribution
Pustules are primarily on thenar and hypothenar eminences of palms, soles of feet; along lateral aspect of heel; and around nails. Lesions of psoriasis may be found on other areas of the body.

■ Patient Profile
Chronic disease occurring in adults of both sexes. Lesions may be painful. This disease may occur de novo or in a patient with routine psoriasis after streptococcal infection or after treatment with corticosteroids or chloroquine. These cutaneous findings may also occur in Reiter's disease.

■ Diagnosis
Sterile, symmetric pustules in a patient with psoriatic lesions elsewhere on the body suggest this diagnosis. A very similar condition without psoriasis elsewhere has been called *palmoplantar pustulosis* (pus-

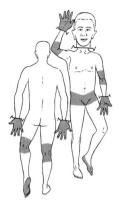

tular bacterid). Biopsy reveals spongiform pustule.

■ Treatment
Potent (class I) topical corticosteroids, often with plastic occlusion, can give rapid relief of erythema. Acitretin improves lesions after 1 to 3 weeks.

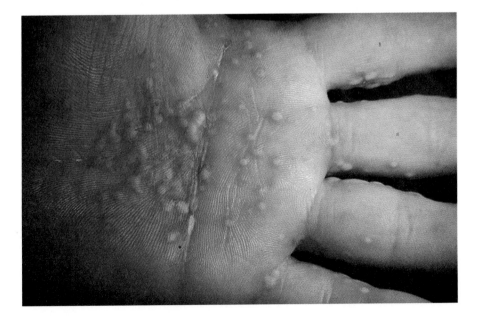

ABSCESSES

DIAGNOSTIC OBSERVATIONS

Abscesses are fluctuant, red, warm, indurated, and often tender. These lesions are accumulations of inflammatory cells that involve the skin and subcutaneous tissue. A number of infectious ulcerating processes may begin with abscesslike lesions; the differential diagnosis of those conditions is listed in Chapter 15. Most abscesses are due to bacteria. All abscesses should be incised and their contents cultured for bacteria and fungi, including *Actinomyces* and mycobacteria.

Distinctive Abscesses

Anthrax
Furuncle-carbuncle
Hidradenitis suppurativa

Anthrax

■ Morphology
The lesion begins as an inflammatory papule that develops within several days into a painless, hemorrhagic, and necrotic abscess. There is characteristic brawny, gelatinous, nonpitting edema around the lesions. Satellite vesicles and pustules may be seen on the edematous area. A dense, black, necrotic eschar gradually forms over the initial lesion.

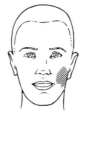

■ Distribution
Single lesion on exposed area of body, most frequently the hands, neck, or face.

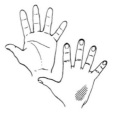

■ Patient Profile
Patient invariably has had contact with raw wool, rawhides, or bone meal. Butchers and wool sorters are frequently affected.

■ Diagnosis
Gram's stain of lesion reveals large, square-ended gram-positive rods that grow easily on blood agar.

■ Treatment
Systemic antibiotics (e.g., penicillin intravenously).

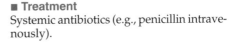

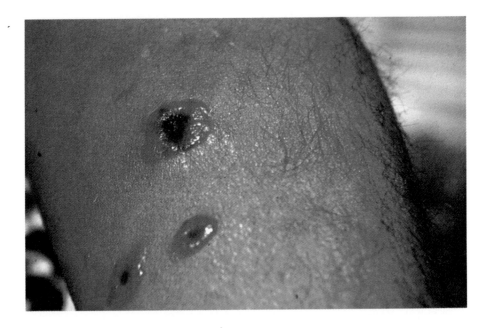

Furuncle-Carbuncle

■ **Morphology**

Erythematous, tender, deeply indurated, 1-cm or larger lesion that surrounds one or several pustular hair follicles. Lesions drain creamy pus when incised and may heal with scarring.

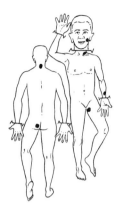

■ **Distribution**

Usually single but may appear in crops. Lesions occur on any hairy area of the body but most commonly on the neck, wrist, gluteal cleft, and perianal areas.

■ **Patient Profile**

Any age, both sexes. Multiple, recurrent furuncles are seen in patients with diabetes, hypogammaglobulinemia, and defects of granulocyte function.

■ **Diagnosis**

Gram's stain of the purulent contents generally demonstrates staphylococci. A furuncle involves one hair follicle; a carbuncle involves multiple contiguous follicles.

■ **Treatment**

Systemic antibiotics (dicloxacillin or a cephalosporin). Incision and drainage often necessary.

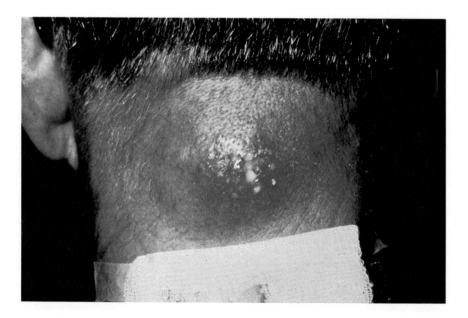

Hidradenitis Suppurativa

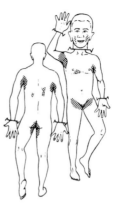

▪ Morphology
Abscesses, cysts, pustules, papules, double comedones, nodules, and draining sinuses result in scarring and fibrotic bands.

▪ Distribution
Bilateral in axillae, perineum, perianal areas, and occasionally around breast.

▪ Patient Profile
Both sexes. Onset at puberty. Disease sometimes associated with cystic acne and dissecting cellulitis of scalp.

▪ Diagnosis
This disease should be suspected in adolescents or adults with abscesses and sinus tract formation in apocrine areas. Biopsy is not specific in later stages.

▪ Treatment
Systemic antibiotics (tetracycline or minocyline). Systemic metronidazole sometimes effective. Isotretinoin (Accutane) 1 mg/kg daily has been effective in inducing remissions in some patients. Surgical excision of quiescent lesions is the only long-term definitive form of therapy.

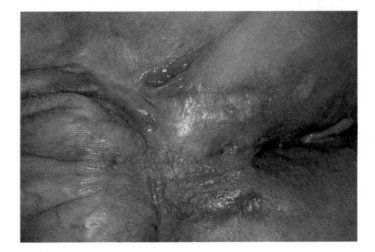

SINUSES

DIAGNOSTIC OBSERVATIONS

A sinus is a connection between the skin and an underlying structure (Table 7–1). Congenital sinuses are present at birth but may go unnoticed until they become infected. They appear as small depressions that may drain material. They are frequently hereditary and more than one family member may be affected. Acquired sinuses are due to specific diseases not present at birth. Diseases that cause suppurative adenitis (tularemia, cat scratch fever, lymphopathia venereum, sporotrichosis, coccidioidomycosis, and histoplasmosis) or abscesses may mimic sinus formation. A rare cause of sinuslike formation is deep fungal infection. Purulent sinus drainage should be cultured for bacteria, mycobacteria, and fungi.

Actinomycosis and nocardiosis
Dental sinus
Hidradenitis suppurativa
Mycetoma
Scrofuloderma

TABLE 7–1. **Characteristic Locations of Sinuses**

Face
Actinomycosis and nocardiosis
Dental sinus, cheek, chin
Lip sinus: congenital
Midline of nose: congenital, dorsum of nose
Preauricular clefts: congenital, anterior to ear

Intraoral
Dental sinus

Neck
Scrofuloderma
Thyroglossal sinus: congenital, often bilateral
    and multiple

Axillary
Hidradenitis suppurativa

Genitocrural and Perineal
Amebic colitis
Carcinoma of colon
Deep fungal infection
Granulomatous ileitis
Hidradenitis suppurativa
Lymphogranuloma venereum
Pilonidal cyst: congenital, presacral
Sigmoid diverticulitis
Ulcerative colitis

Feet
Maduromycosis, mycetoma

Finger or Toe Webs
Hair sinuses: arise from penetration of hairs
    into finger webs; barbers, dog groomers,
    and cow milkers are predisposed

Overlying Bones
Osteomyelitis

Actinomycosis and Nocardiosis

▪ Morphology
Lesions begin as firm, nontender, indurated erythematous nodules or plaques that gradually develop multiple sinuses draining yellowish material.

▪ Distribution
Angle of jaw, below jaw, anterior neck, thoracic wall, and abdominal wall.

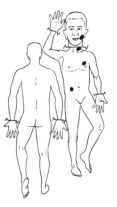

▪ Patient Profile
More common in males than in females, usually older than 40 years. Patients with cervicofacial actinomycosis frequently have a history of trauma to the jaw or a tooth extraction.

▪ Diagnosis
Pus contains characteristic sulfur granules, which are yellow and about 0.5 to 1 mm in size. Gram's stain shows branching gram-positive mycelial segments at the periphery of the granule. Anaerobic cultures grow *Actinomyces israelii*. *Nocardia asteroides* is aerobic, gram-positive, and slightly acid-fast. Thoracic and abdominal actinomycoses are extensions of pulmonary or intra-abdominal disease.

▪ Treatment
Penicillin or tetracycline for actinomycosis. Sulfisoxazole or trimethoprim-sulfamethoxazole for nocardiosis.

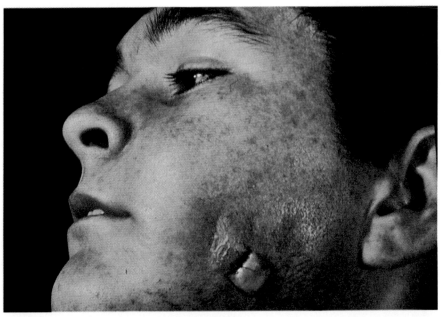

Actinomycosis

Dental Sinus

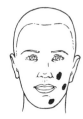

▪ Morphology
Red, indurated papule that progresses to drain purulent material. Skin around sinus may become scaly or warty.

▪ Distribution
Cheek over the maxilla, lower jaw over the mandible, or under the chin.

▪ Patient Profile
Patient with abscessed tooth who develops skin lesions.

▪ Diagnosis
This diagnosis should be suspected in all sinuses of upper and lower jaw. Examination of mouth and teeth demonstrate an apical abscess and dental x-ray confirms the diagnosis.

▪ Treatment
Removal of affected tooth and drainage of abscess.

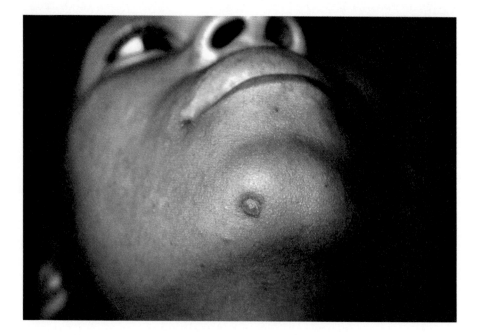

Hidradenitis Suppurativa

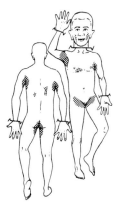

■ Morphology
Abscesses, cysts, pustules, papules, double comedones, nodules, and draining sinuses result in scarring and fibrotic bands.

■ Distribution
Bilateral in axillae, perineum, perianal areas, and occasionally around breast.

■ Patient Profile
Both sexes. Onset at puberty. Disease sometimes associated with cystic acne and dissecting cellulitis of scalp. Subareolar abscesses should be considered if lesions are limited to the breasts.

■ Diagnosis
This disease should be suspected in adolescents or adults with abscesses and sinus tract formation in apocrine areas. Biopsy is not specific in later stages.

■ Treatment
Systemic antibiotics (tetracycline or minocycline). Systemic metronidazole sometimes effective. Isotretinoin has been reported to be of value. Surgical excision of quiescent lesion is the only definitive cure.

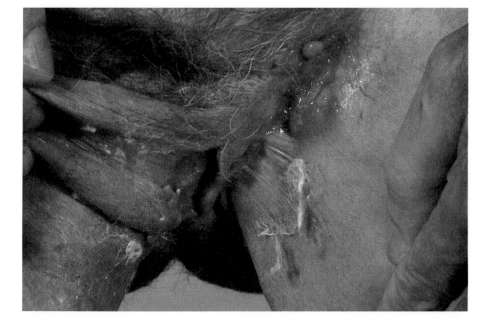

Mycetoma
(Madura Foot)

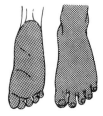

■ **Morphology**
Nodules enlarge, coalesce, and develop numerous draining sinuses and abscesses. Lesions may involve subcutaneous tissue and bone.

■ **Distribution**
Almost always foot but can occur anywhere.

■ **Patient Profile**
Males in tropical or subtropical climates who go barefoot. Disease evolves over years and pain is minimal.

■ **Diagnosis**
Granules of varying colors composed of fungal colonies are found in the pus. Cultures of pus and biopsy material reveal the causative agent, which is either a variety of actinomycetes or a fungus.

■ **Treatment**
Systemic antifungal agents such as itraconazole or amphotericin may be used.

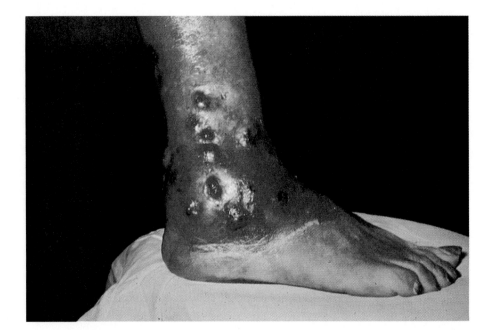

Scrofuloderma
(Tuberculosis)

■ **Morphology**
Firm, subcutaneous nodules become red-purple and develop sinuses. Lesions are undermined and heal with cordlike bridging scars.

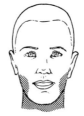

■ **Distribution**
Parotid, submandibular, and supraclavicular areas are common but can occur anywhere. Lesions may be bilateral.

■ **Patient Profile**
Most commonly lesions begin in childhood and are painless. Seen in patients with HIV infection.

■ **Diagnosis**
Histologic examination reveals caseation necrosis and acid-fast bacilli. Atypical mycobacteria as well as *Mycobacterium tuberculosis* cause this disease. Chest x-ray.

■ **Treatment**
Systemic antituberculosis agents.

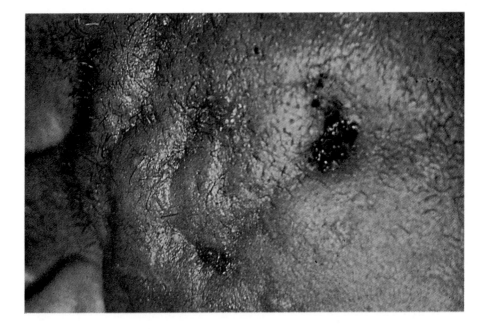

Chapter 8

■ ■

Induration, Sclerosis, and Atrophy

INDURATION AND SCLEROSIS

DIAGNOSTIC OBSERVATIONS
These lesions are flat and are discovered because palpation of the skin reveals hardness and thickening. The surface of the skin may have prominent follicular orifices *(peau d'orange)*. Diseases may be diffuse or circumscribed. Previous trauma, including injection of drugs such as pentazocine (Talwin) and insulin, may produce localized areas of sclerosis.

Edema
Lymphedema
Mastocytosis
Pachydermoperiostosis
Scleredema
Scleroderma
Rare scleroderma-like diseases

Edema

■ **Morphology**
Poorly circumscribed areas of tissue swelling that pit with moderate pressure.

■ **Distribution**
Dependent areas, especially legs, genitals, and feet. May be generalized.

■ **Patient Profile**
Dependent on cause; may last hours to years.

■ **Diagnosis**
The causes include a variety of systemic diseases, including cardiovascular, renal, and hepatic. A complete history and physical examination are mandatory for the patient presenting with pitting edema.

■ **Treatment**
Dependent on underlying disorder.

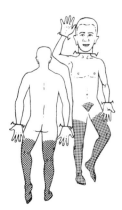

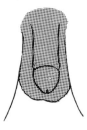

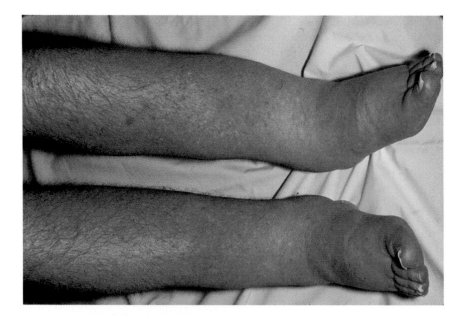

Lymphedema
(Elephantiasis)

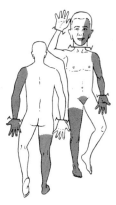

■ Morphology
Persistent, poorly circumscribed, flesh-colored to red areas of induration. Initially the swelling may pit. Skin becomes thick, hyperpigmented, and takes on a cobblestone appearance. Occasionally, patients also have yellow nails.

■ Distribution
Legs, genitals, arms, and face.

■ Patient Profile
Dependent on etiology. Primary lymphedema (Milroy's disease) is most common in women and begins at around age 35 years; it may be familial (autosomal dominant). Patients may develop lymphosarcoma in areas of chronic lymphedema (Stewart-Treves syndrome).

■ Diagnosis
Chronicity, progression, nonpitting quality, and epidermal change in this disease distinguish it from edema. Biopsy is usually not helpful. Etiologies of lymphedema include:

Inflammatory Diseases
Acne and recurrent streptococcal infections: These may cause persistent areas of lymphedema of the face.
Filariasis: This is a common cause of lymphedema in the tropics.
Lymphogranuloma venereum: This diagnosis should be considered with chronic genital edema.
Melkersson-Rosenthal syndrome: This syndrome is characterized by persistent edema of the lips and face, scrotal tongue, and facial nerve paralysis.
Tuberculosis.

Fibrosis
Malignancy: Including lymphoma.
Milroy's disease: Primary (congenital lymphatic defect).
Radiation fibrosis.
Surgical destruction: Possible consequence of radical breast surgery.
Destruction of venous system: Condition associated with cellulitis.

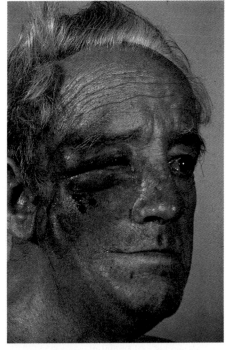

Lymphedema due to recurrent cellulitis

Mastocytosis

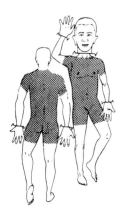

▪ **Morphology**
Papules and plaques are diffuse, doughy, and leatherlike. Vesicles are large and follow trauma.

▪ **Distribution**
Generalized, with accentuation in groin and axillae.

▪ **Patient Profile**
Any age, both sexes. In children, multiple coalescing papules that may evolve into blisters. Lesions usually resolve by early adulthood. Adults have infectious, yellow to tan plaques that may be focal or generalized and do not resolve. Lesions very pruritic. Frequently fatal and associated with systemic mast cell infiltration.

▪ **Diagnosis**
Production of erythema and edema within a few minutes after stroking the plaque is diagnostic. Biopsy with special stains (toluidine blue) demonstrates mast cells.

▪ **Treatment**
Ultra-high-potency topical steroids with occlusion overnight for 6 weeks. PUVA therapy. Systemic antihistamines may be needed.

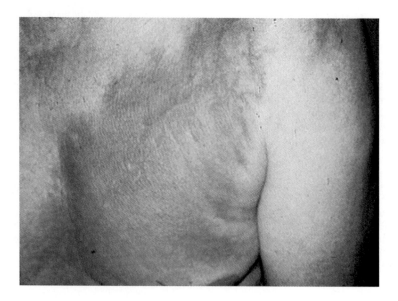

Pachydermoperiostosis

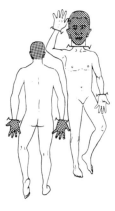

▪ Morphology
Skin is thickened and coarse folds and furrows are present. Seborrhea and hyperhidrosis may occur. Fingers are clubbed; body hair may be sparse.

▪ Distribution
Face, scalp, hands, and feet.

▪ Patient Profile
Both sexes. Familial form begins at puberty and is autosomal dominant. Sporadic form occurs in older age group and is associated with intrathoracic malignancy.

▪ Diagnosis
X-rays reveal periostitis in diaphysis of long bones and metacarpals. In cutis verticis gyrata, the coarse folds are limited to the scalp.

▪ Treatment
Surgical removal of excess tissue.

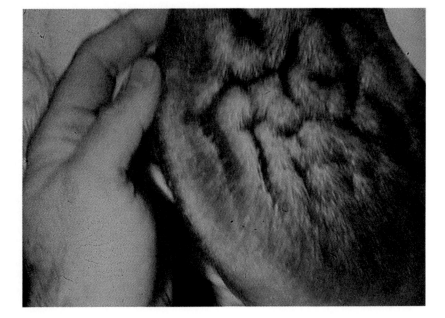

Scleredema

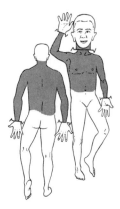

▪ **Morphology**
Diffuse, slightly erythematous induration of skin.

▪ **Distribution**
Chest and back. Occasionally face and extremities but almost always spares hands and feet.

▪ **Patient Profile**
Older children, young adults of both sexes. Lesions appear after severe streptococcal sore throat in about one half of cases.

▪ **Diagnosis**
Biopsy reveals mucopolysaccharide infiltration of the skin without sclerosis or loss of skin appendages. In debilitated, premature newborns, sclerema neonatorum should be considered.

▪ **Treatment**
Treatment of underlying disease. Long-term systemic antistreptococcal therapy often useful.

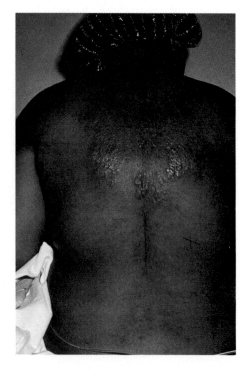

Scleroderma

■ Morphology
Diffuse, poorly defined induration and thickening of skin. Lesions are frequently devoid of hair. Diffuse hyperpigmentation and mottled hyperpigmentation and hypopigmentation are common. Periungual telangiectasia, ulcerations of finger tips, and calcinosis cutis are frequently seen.

■ Distribution
Most prominent acrally; begins as hand and finger swelling. Sclerosis progresses to involve entire skin, especially anterior chest, trunk, and face.

■ Patient Profile
Older children and adults of both sexes. Patients may exhibit Raynaud's phenomenon, dysphagia, arthritis, enteropathy, myopathy, fatigue, and shortness of breath.

■ Diagnosis
Biopsy demonstrates epidermal atrophy, dermal-epidermal junction mononuclear cells, loss of skin appendages, increased collagen, and fibrosis of the subcutaneous fat. Laboratory studies that help to confirm the diagnosis include antinuclear antibody (nucleolar or speckled pattern), abnormal esophageal motility, and decreased carbon monoxide diffusion capacity. Eo-

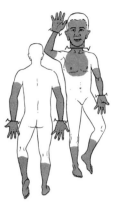

sinophilic fasciitis (Shulman's syndrome) resembles scleroderma, and patients manifest edema and marked induration of the extremities, eosinophilia, and minimal systemic problems. Sclerodermatous changes may also be seen in mixed connective tissue disease.

■ Treatment
Avoidance of low temperatures. Penicillamine, systemic steroids, and extracorporeal chemo-photopheresis have been used with some success. Laser for telangiectases.

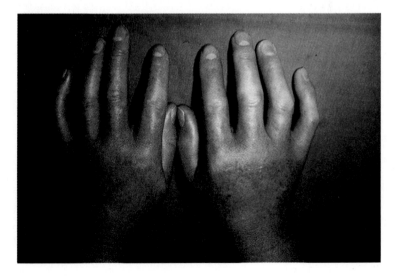

Rare Scleroderma-like Diseases

Diffuse, indurated areas of skin that mimic scleroderma may be seen in a variety of disorders, including:

Acromegaly: Diffuse thickening and coarseness of the skin, large hands and feet, enlargement of the jaw, and gigantism suggest this diagnosis, which is confirmed by finding increased levels of growth hormone.

Amyloidosis: This disease may be associated with induration of the face and papules that become purpuric with minor trauma. Biopsy reveals amyloid.

Ataxia-telangiectasia: Patients may demonstrate sclerodermatous change on the bridge of the nose.

Carcinoid syndrome: This syndrome is characterized by induration of the face associated with flushing, diarrhea, and increased urinary 5-hydroxyindoleacetic acid.

Congenital generalized fibromatosis: This disease is chracterized by poorly circumscribed, fibrous nodules in the subcutaneous tissue and viscera. Infants with this disease fail to thrive and die in early childhood.

Diffuse infiltrating carcinoma *(peau d'orange):* This form of cancer may be associated with localized areas of induration. Breast carcinoma often has a peau d'orange appearance.

Erythropoietic protoporphyria: Children with marked photosensitivity may have sclerodermatous change on the bridge of the nose and dorsum of the hands.

Graft-versus-host reactions: Sclerodermatous change is associated with fever, hepatitis, and diarrhea in a patient with a history of bone marrow or thymus transplant.

Leprosy: This disease is associated with facial infiltration; the biopsy is diagnostic and demonstrates acid-fast organisms.

Lipoid proteinosis: Diffuse thickening of the skin is associated with scarring, hoarseness, oral and periorbital papules, tongue enlargement, and intracranial calcification. Biopsy shows PAS-positive material around capillaries and blood vessels.

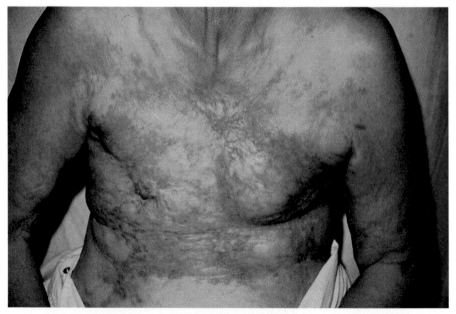

Infiltrating breast carcinoma

Mucopolysaccharide storage disorders (Hurler's syndrome, Hunter's syndrome): Diffuse thickening of the skin, hirsutism, and discrete papules accompany the retardation, hepatomegaly, and corneal changes. Mucopolysaccharides are in the urine.

Myxedema: This condition is associated with generalized thickening of the skin, most commonly on pretibial areas; exophthalmos; acropachy; and abnormal thyroid function tests. Biopsy stained for mucin and blood tests of thyroid function establish the diagnosis.

Phenylketonuria: Sclerodermatous change is associated with mental retardation, light hair and skin color, and eczema.

Porphyria cutanea tarda: Sclerodermatous change in sun-exposed areas is associated with photosensitivity, blistering, scarring, hyperpigmentation, hypertrichosis, and increased excretion of uroporphyrin and coproporphyrin in the urine.

Progeria: Diffuse sclerodermatous change is associated with dwarfism, alopecia, birdlike facial features, and generalized arteriosclerosis. This disease starts in childhood, whereas Werner's syndrome, which has similar features, begins in the second and third decades.

Scleromyxedema: Diffuse, persistent thickening of the skin, especially prominent on the face, in middle-aged adults, suggests this possibility. Biopsy reveals mucin deposition in the upper dermis, and the serum contains an abnormal paraprotein (usually λ light chain).

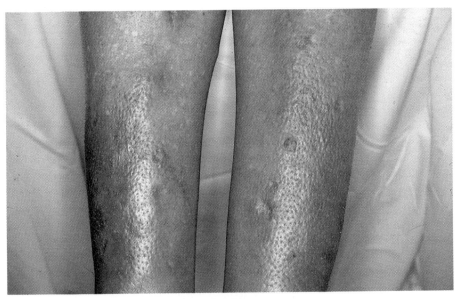

Myxedema

ATROPHY

Lichen sclerosus et atrophicus
Lupus erythematosus
Lupus vulgaris
Morphea
Necrobiosis lipoidica diabeticorum
Poikiloderma
Porphyria cutanea tarda
Striae
Trauma or injection
Varioliform or chickenpox scarring
Rare causes of subcutaneous atrophy

Lichen Sclerosus et Atrophicus
(Balanitis Xerotica Obliterans)

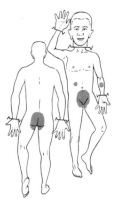

▪ Morphology
Ivory white, flat or depressed, sharply circumscribed lesions that begin as several millimeters in diameter and may coalesce into plaques. The skin is wrinkled, slightly scaly, and hairless. The openings of the sweat glands and sebaceous glands are dilated. Blisters and hemorrhage may occur in lesions.

▪ Distribution
Symmetric. Genitalia, especially vulva (lichen sclerosus) and glans penis in uncircumcised males (balanitis xerotica obliterans). Less commonly, lesions are found on trunk and flexor surfaces of arms.

▪ Patient Profile
Female-male ratio of 10:1. Lesions occur in older age group but can occur before puberty. Lesions may itch and burn and are slowly progressive.

▪ Diagnosis
Slightly scaly, atrophic white lesions on genitalia in the older age group suggest this diagnosis. Biopsy reveals hyperkeratosis, thinning of the epidermis with hydropic degeneration of the basal layer, edema of the papillary dermis, and a bandlike lymphocytic infiltrate. Leukoplakia and squamous cell carcinoma occur with increased frequency in this disease. Sometimes associated with morphea within the lesion.

▪ Treatment
Topical corticosteroids (class III or IV); topical testosterone may be effective (2% to 5% ointment). Aggressive therapy with UVB has also been effective in some cases.

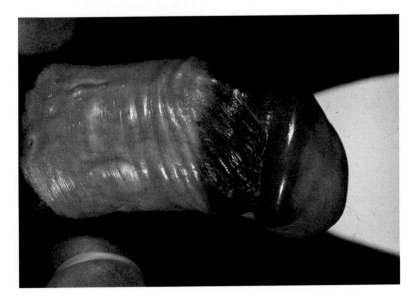

Lupus Erythematosus
(Discoid Lupus Erythematosus)

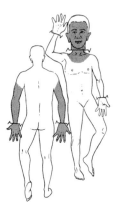

▪ Morphology
Atrophic, sharply circumscribed, hyperpigmented and hypopigmented plaques. Lesions frequently are scaly, red, and have prominent telangiectasia. Scalp lesions have loss of hair with scarring and decrease in hair follicles. Elevated red plaques, especially in sun-exposed areas, diffuse thinning of hair, palmar erythema, periungual telangiectasia, and oral lesions may also be present.

▪ Distribution
Sun-exposed areas: most often scalp, inside external ear, and palms and soles.

▪ Patient Profile
Most common in young women and older men but can occur at any age, including newborns. Lesions are worse with exposure to sunlight. Lesions may be associated with systemic lupus erythematosus.

▪ Diagnosis
Biopsy reveals hyperkeratosis, thinning of the epidermis, liquefaction of the basal cells, and a perivascular and periadnexal round-cell infiltrate. Immunofluorescent examination of biopsies reveals deposition of immunoglobulin and complement at the dermal-epidermal junction. All patients must be evaluated for systemic lupus erythematosus. On occasion, squamous cell carcinoma arises in lesions of lupus. Atrophic forms of lichen planus (see p. 139) may mimic lupus erythematosus; the biopsy usually differentiates these two diseases. Pseudopelade is hypopigmented scarring alopecia of the scalp.

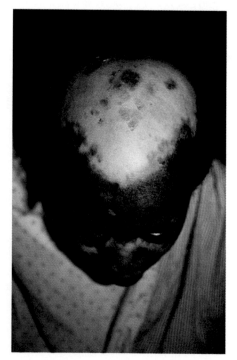

▪ Treatment
Systemic evaluation mandatory. Therapies include antimalarials, UVA and UVB sunscreens; systemic steroids and antimetabolites for patients with more systemic involvement; sun-protective clothing. Isotretinoin and thalidomide have been used for more resistant cutaneous lupus.

Lupus Vulgaris

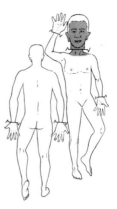

▪ Morphology
Red-brown plaque with central scarring and peripheral yellow papules and nodules. Lesions may scale, ulcerate, destroy cartilage, or develop papillary overgrowth. Lesions are most commonly single and slowly progressive.

▪ Distribution
Head and neck are most common and may involve nasal, ocular, and oral mucosae.

▪ Patient Profile
Three times more common in females than in males. Any age but lesions most often begin in childhood. Patients have tuberculosis.

▪ Diagnosis
Biopsy reveals classic caseation necrosis and very sparse acid-fast bacteria. Culture of lesions may not grow *Mycobacterium tuberculosis*. PCR may be helpful in establishing the diagnosis. The histologic picture and a positive tuberculin skin test differentiates this disease from tertiary syphilis, leishmaniasis, yaws, blastomycosis, sarcoidosis, and vasculitis, which can simulate this appearance. Squamous cell carcinoma may occur in these chronic, scarred lesions.

▪ Treatment
Systemic antituberculous agents.

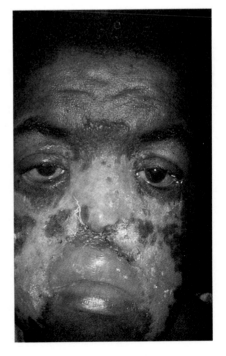

Morphea

▪ **Morphology**
Circumscribed white to yellow atrophic plaque, which may have a purple border. Droplike generalized lesions may occur.

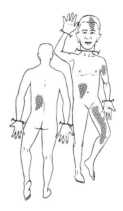

▪ **Distribution**
Trunk, proximal extremities, often linear when it involves the face and scalp.

▪ **Patient Profile**
Female-male ratio of 3:1. More common in whites than in blacks. Ages 20 to 40 years. Linear morphea more common in children. These patients do not have systemic scleroderma and rarely progress to that disease. Sometimes associated with lichen sclerosus et atrophicus.

▪ **Diagnosis**
Biopsy reveals epidermal atrophy, dermal fibrosis, loss of skin appendages, and inflammatory cells.

▪ **Treatment**
Potent topical corticosteroids under occlusion. Systemic corticosteroids, phenytoin (Dilantin), penicillamine have been used with minimal success. POTABA reported to be useful.

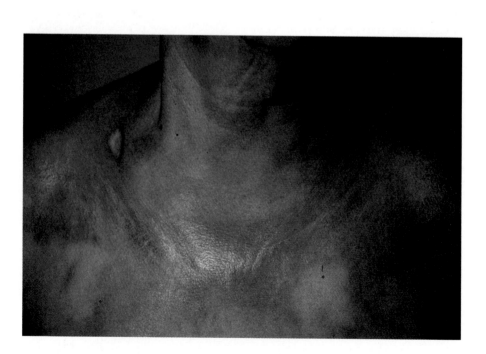

Necrobiosis Lipoidica Diabeticorum

■ **Morphology**
Red-yellow plaques with dilated blood vessels and depressed atrophic areas showing loss of skin markings. Lesions may ulcerate. Borders are often scalloped.

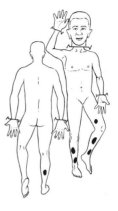

■ **Distribution**
Often symmetric on shins but can occur anywhere.

■ **Patient Profile**
Both sexes; any age, more common in adulthood. Over half of patients have or will have diabetes mellitus. Painful when ulcerated.

■ **Diagnosis**
Yellow color with prominent superficial vessels in an atrophic plaque is diagnostic. Biopsy shows necrobiosis; inflammatory cells, including giant cells; fibrosis; and increased mucin. Studies to exclude diabetes are necessary. Rarely, lupus vulgaris and other granulomatous diseases may appear similar to necrobiosis.

■ **Treatment**
Potent (class I or II) topical corticosteroids and sometimes intralesional corticosteroids.

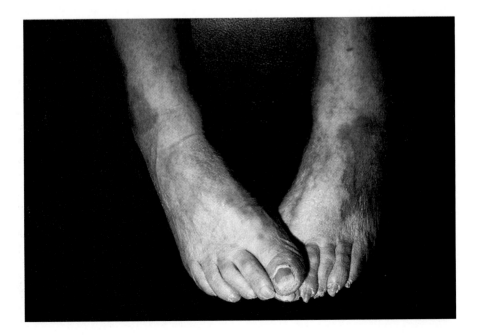

Poikiloderma

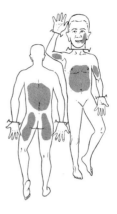

▪ Morphology
Atrophic, slightly scaly, mottled lesions that wrinkle like cigarette paper when pinched and have hyperpigmentation, hypopigmentation, and telangiectasia.

▪ Distribution
Symmetric on face, neck, trunk, and flexors. Lesions rarely involve mucosa.

▪ Patient Profile
Young children and older adults of both sexes. Lesions are asymptomatic and slowly progressive.

▪ Diagnosis
Biopsy reveals hyperkeratosis, thinning of nucleated epidermis, hydropic degeneration of basal cells, and a dense, bandlike infiltrate of mononuclear cells.

Young children: It is often associated with Bloom syndrome, Cockayne's syndrome, dermatomyositis, progressive systemic sclerosis, dyskeratosis congenita, erythropoietic rotoporphyria, hereditary poikiloderma, Rothmund-Thomson syndrome, and Werner's syndrome.

Adults: Poikiloderma may be associated with sun exposure (especially on neck: poikiloderma of Civatte), dermatomyositis, Hodgkin's disease, lupus erythematosus, and mycosis fungoides. Sharply circumscribed, geometric-appearing poikiloderma should suggest thermal burn or x-ray damage. Patients with these latter forms of poikiloderma may develop squamous cell carcinoma. Poikilodermatous changes may be secondary to chronic use of potent topical steroids.

▪ Treatment
Treatment of underlying disease. In most instances, the poikiloderma is irreversible.

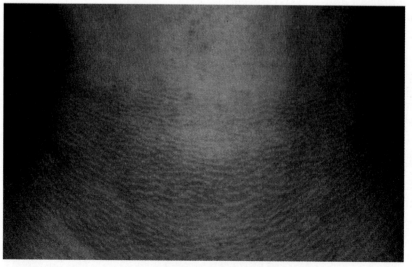

Poikiloderma of Civatte

Porphyria Cutanea Tarda

■ **Morphology**
Atrophic. Scaly plaques with hemorrhage, blisters, crusting. Milia are papules that are white, smooth, 2- to 4-mm epidermal inclusion cysts at the site of old blisters.

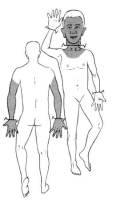

■ **Distribution**
Vesicles and milia are usually on sun-exposed or traumatized areas, especially on the dorsum of the hands. Hyperpigmentation may be generalized but is accentuated in sun-exposed areas. There may be purple discoloration around the eyes and hypertrichosis of the face. Sclerodermatous changes usually occur in sun-exposed areas. No oral lesions, but conjunctival injection may occur.

■ **Patient Profile**
Usually adults (30 to 60 years of age) with a slight male preponderance. Insidious onset with duration of several months to a few years. Burning in affected sites.

■ **Diagnosis**
Excess liver uroporphyrin production, the metabolic basis of this disease, is most commonly precipitated by chronic ethanol use or drugs (estrogen, birth control pills, griseofulvin, iron). Urine fluoresces pink with an ultraviolet light if more than 1 mg/L of uroporphyrin is present. A 24-hour urine collection for uroporphyrin is more sensitive and should be obtained when this diagnosis is suspected. Skin biopsy reveals subepidermal bullae and deposition of PAS-positive amorphous material in the dermis.

■ **Treatment**
Remove inciting agent, if present. Phlebotomy or low-dose antimalarials usually effective. Sunscreens.

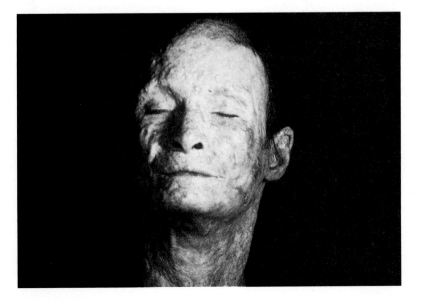

Striae

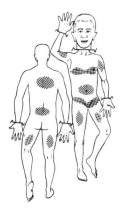

▪ **Morphology**
Linear, slightly depressed areas of thin skin. New lesions are red; older lesions, white. Lesions may vary in length and width.

▪ **Distribution**
Bilateral; thighs, abdomen, breasts, lower back, and intertriginous areas are most common sites.

▪ **Patient Profile**
More frequent in females than in males. May occur in early adolescence, after period of intensive weight lifting, and during pregnancy. Cushing's syndrome, oral corticosteroids, or occlusive topical corticosteroid therapy may cause striae.

▪ **Diagnosis**
Linear pattern of lesions.

▪ **Treatment**
Treatment with 12% lactic acid, topical Retin-A, or laser after parturition.

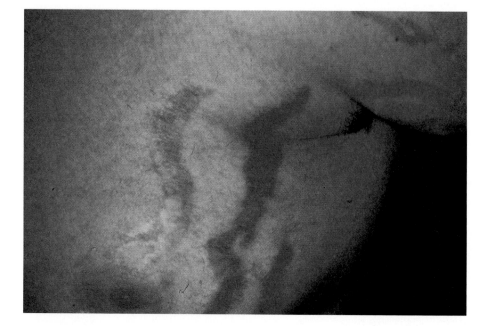

Trauma or Injection

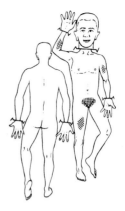

■ **Morphology**
Depressed area of skin with normal epidermis.

■ **Distribution**
Proximal extremities and trunk.

■ **Patient Profile**
Patient has been undergoing injections, most commonly insulin, corticosteroids, or Talwin. Old trauma can result in depressed scars.

■ **Diagnosis**
History of injection or trauma. Biopsy may reveal granulomatous inflammation and evidence of foreign bodies with polarization microscopy and special stains.

■ **Treatment**
Corticosteroid atrophy resolves spontaneously but slowly, except for dilated vessels.

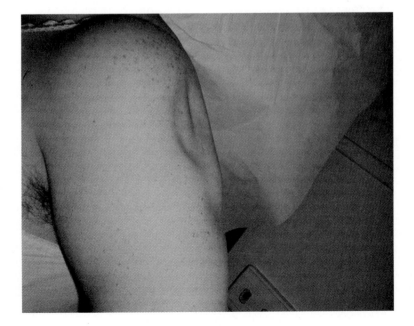

Varioliform or Chickenpox-like Scarring

Sharply marginated, depressed, hypopigmented lesions with loss of normal skin markings may be seen in several diseases.

Postinflammatory causes: These are the most common causes of varioliform scars. Acne, chickenpox, smallpox, herpes zoster, rickettsialpox, and lipid proteinosis produce these lesions, but any excoriated dermatoses may produce varioliform scarring.

Lymphomatoid papulosis: Erythematous papules and nodules suggest this diagnosis. Lesions may ulcerate and heal with atrophic scars. Biopsy shows atypical lymphocytes that are CD30-positive.

Malignant atrophic papulosis (Degos' disease): Porcelain, white, atrophic circular scars, 5 mm to 2 cm, are associated with red papules, vasculitis, and perforation of abdominal viscera.

Pityriasis lichenoides et varioliformis acuta: Varioliform scars are associated with red, sometimes vesicular or hemorrhagic, scaly, symmetric, pruritic papules in young adults. Biopsy reveals a lymphocytic vasculitis.

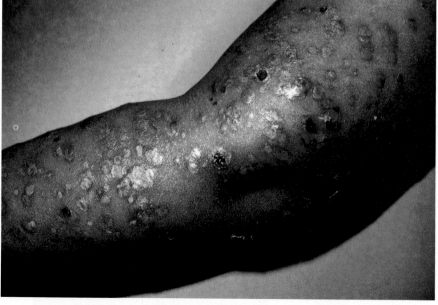

Lymphomatoid papulosis

Rare Causes of Subcutaneous Atrophy

Deeply depressed areas with normal-appearing overlying skin characterize this group of disorders. The skin can be moved easily over the atrophic area. Prominent superficial veins may be present.

Acrodermatitis chronica atrophicans: A patient is bitten by a tick and develops acral plaques that rapidly become atrophic owing to infection with *Borrelia.*

Acrogeria: Young females develop thin, transparent skin on the dorsum of hands and feet.

Anetoderma: Small, sharply circumscribed circular lesions with underlying loss of skin substance. A discrete hole under the epidermis can be felt.

Facial hemiatrophy (Parry-Romberg syndrome): Atrophy of subcutaneous tissue, muscle, and bone on one side of the face characterizes this syndrome. The dermis is soft and nonadherent, which distinguishes this syndrome from linear scleroderma (see p. 379).

Focal dermal hypoplasia (Goltz's syndrome): Small, sharply circumscribed, very soft yellow papules that are herniations of subcutaneous fat into the dermis. There are associated perioral papillomas; eye, dental, and bone defects.

Gower's panatrophy: Subcutaneous and dermal atrophy beginning in adult life in circumscribed areas that seem to be noninflammatory.

Partial lipodystrophy: Lipoatrophy limited to the upper part of the body. Glomerulonephritis and hypocomplementemia are commonly present.

Progeria: Premature aging that begins at age of 6 months, results in alopecia, atrophy of skin, birdlike appearance, cardiovascular disease, and death by age 20 years.

Total lipoatrophy (Lawrence-Seip syndrome): This generalized disease begins at birth or in early childhood and has associated acanthosis nigricans, hirsutism, clitoral or penile enlargement, insulin-resistant diabetes, hepatomegaly, and hypertriglyceridemia. Biopsy shows absence of signet-type fat cells.

Weber-Christian disease (see p. 434): This and other forms of panniculitis may heal with deeply depressed scars.

Werner's syndrome: Adolescents develop aged appearance of face, scleroderma-like plaques, calcinosis, diabetes, hypogonadism, premature atherosclerosis.

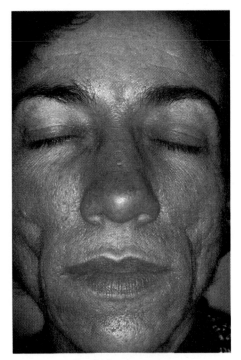

Partial lipodystrophy

Chapter 9

■ ■

Nodules and Cysts

DIAGNOSTIC OBSERVATIONS

These lesions are located in the deep dermis and subcutaneous tissue. The most important clinical characteristic of these nodules is that the epidermis and superficial dermis can be visibly moved over the lesion. These lesions resemble icebergs in that most of their substance is deep in the skin. Infections may begin with single nodules, which are followed by the appearance of new lesions that progress proximally on an extremity. Systemic mycosis and atypical mycobacteria (see pp. 412, 459–460) may cause single painful nodules. Biopsy and culture demonstrate the organism. Suppurative adenitis (see p. 429), in its initial stage, may present with a single lesion or several lesions. Diagnosis often requires biopsy of the lesion; examination of tissue by polarizing microscopy; and culture of the tissue for bacteria, mycobacteria, and fungi. Firm cysts mimic nodules.

MAJOR CATEGORIES

Cysts
Flesh-colored to red nodules
Purple nodules
Tender red nodules

CYSTS

DIAGNOSTIC OBSERVATIONS
Cysts are sharply circumscribed, often movable, compressible lesions (Table 9–1). They may have a central punctum from which foul-smelling material can be expressed.

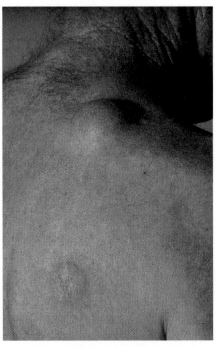

Epidermoid cyst

TABLE 9–1. **Differential Diagnosis of Cysts**

Type	Number of Lesions	Location	Patient Profile	Histology of Cyst
Epidermoid cyst	Single or several, occasionally multiple	Face, trunk, scalp	Older age group.	Normal keratinizing epithelium.
Pilar cyst	Single or several, occasionally multiple	Scalp	Older age group.	No granular layer of epithelium.
Dermoid cyst	Single	Midline, often face	Congenital.	Keratin, bone, tooth, nerve tissue.
Steatocystoma multiplex	Multiple	Sternum, proximal arms, scrotum	Puberty, males more common, autosomal dominant.	Epidermal adnexal structure, especially sebaceous glands.
Parasitic cyst	Multiple	Anywhere	Any age. Patient has appropriate exposure.	Biopsy reveals parasite. Organisms are *Echinococcus* and *Taenia*.

FLESH-COLORED TO RED NODULES

DIAGNOSTIC OBSERVATIONS

The surface skin over these flesh-colored to red nodules is normal unless otherwise noted. These lesions are usually single or few and often are nontender. Any constituent of the deep dermis and subcutaneous tissue can develop neoplasms. There are subtle points in physical diagnosis that favor the possibility of one tumor over another. Diagnosis rests on biopsy of the lesion.

Deep nodules peculiar to newborns
Dermatofibrosarcoma protuberans
Eccrine poroma
Eccrine spiradenoma (see p. 180)
Fibromatosis
Foreign body
Gummatous syphilis
Hemangioma: blanching with pressure
Juxta-articular nodules
Lipoma: common
Lupus profundus
Malignancies and metastatic carcinoma
Phlebolith
Prurigo nodularis
Sarcoidosis
Systemic mycosis or mycobacterial disease
Vasculitis: often tender lesions (see p. 420)

Deep Nodules Peculiar to Newborns

Sclerema neonatorum is characterized by deep, nonpitting induration in premature, debilitated, hypothermic newborns. Sclerema is diffuse, in contrast to subcutaneous fat necrosis of the newborn, which presents with discrete, painless plaques in an otherwise healthy child.

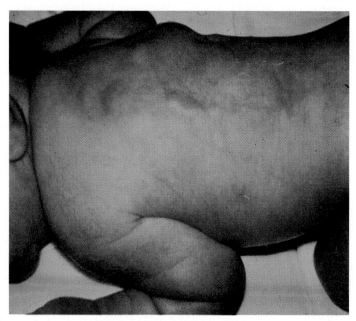

Subcutaneous fat necrosis in a newborn

Dermatofibrosarcoma Protuberans

■ **Morphology**
Erythematous, firm nodule. Some lesions have overlying skin atrophy.

■ **Distribution**
Most common on the trunk.

■ **Patient Profile**
More common in males than in females. Lesions recur if not excised totally, but metastasis is rare.

■ **Diagnosis**
Biopsy shows a cartwheel-like arrangement of spindle-shaped cells with varying amounts of collagen. Must be differentiated from a benign dermatofibroma, which clinically is much smaller than a dermatofibrosarcoma protuberans.

■ **Treatment**
Wide local excision.

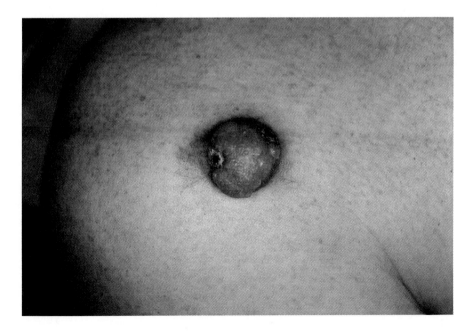

Fibromatosis

▪ **Morphology**
Firm, flesh-colored nodules with normal overlying epidermis.

▪ **Distribution**
Nodules may occur anywhere. Fibrous hamartoma of infancy occurs on the trunk and shoulder, fibromatosis colli develops on the lower third of the sternocleidomastoid muscle, and infantile digital fibromatosis often occurs on the knuckles or distal digits. Infantile myofibromatosis may be solitary or multiple and involve skin, muscle, bone, and underlying organs.

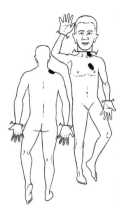

▪ **Patient Profile**
Nodule usually arises spontaneously in infants or children. An aggressive form (multifocal aggressive infantile fibromatosis) may extend into muscle and recur after surgical excision.

▪ **Diagnosis**
Deep dermal and subcutaneous lesions that show a mixture of fibroblasts and collagen.

▪ **Treatment**
Surgical excision, but lesions may recur.

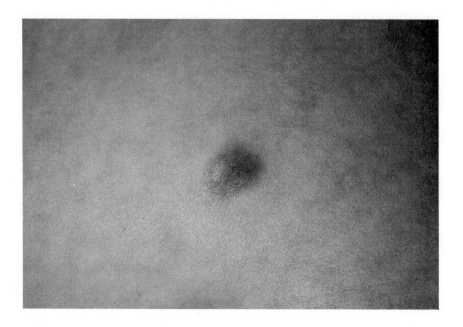

Foreign Body

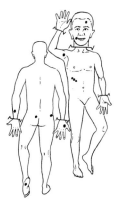

▪ Morphology
Light pink to red nodules that may drain.

▪ Distribution
Anywhere but most common on exposed, traumatized areas. If lesions are multiple, they are often grouped.

▪ Patient Profile
Any age, both sexes. Patient has a history of trauma or had a surgical procedure weeks to months before noticing lesions.

▪ Diagnosis
Deep, indurated lesions appearing in areas of previous trauma should suggest the diagnosis of foreign body. Suture material or oily substances, such as paraffin used for augmentation in plastic surgery, are not uncommon iatrogenic causes. Sea urchin spines and coral spicules may induce foreign-body granulomas in skin divers. Insect stingers may provoke foreign body granulomas. Silica, talc, zirconium, and asbestos may enter the cutis through damaged skin and induce granulomas. Numerous other materials have also been suggested as causative agents for foreign-body reactions. Biopsy reveals granlomatous inflammation. All tissue should be examined by polarization microscopy for foreign material.

▪ Treatment
Surgical removal.

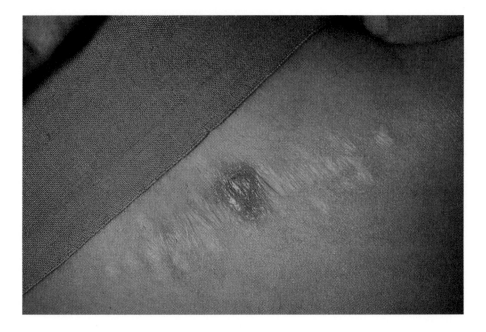

Gummatous Syphilis

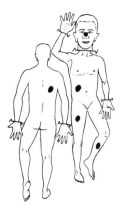

▪ **Morphology**
One or several nontender, rubbery nodules that may ulcerate and heal with non-contractile scarring. Incomplete annular lesions are seen.

▪ **Distribution**
Anywhere, including mucosae. Grouping of lesions is common.

▪ **Patient Profile**
Patient has tertiary syphilis.

▪ **Diagnosis**
Serologic test, especially the fluorescent treponemal antibody-absorption (FTA-ABS) test, is positive. Biopsy reveals granulomatous dermatitis, especially rich in plasma cells.

▪ **Treatment**
For late syphilis, see Table 14–12.

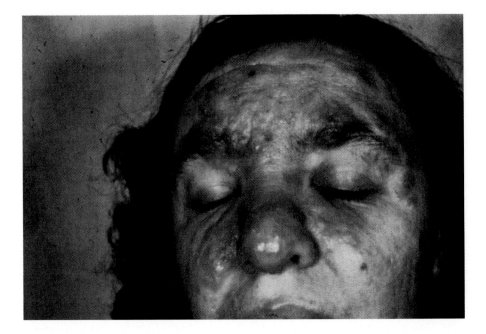

Hemangioma

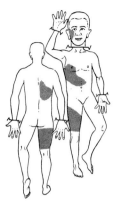

▪ Morphology
Single or multiple red to blue-purple nodules that blanch dramatically with pressure. Diffuse redness, increased hair growth, and scaling may occur in lesions.

▪ Distribution
Anywhere; lesions may appear in a dermatomal distribution.

▪ Patient Profile
Lesions may be present at birth and frequently increase in size during the first few months of life. Lesions may spontaneously regress and may be associated with underlying neurologic or skeletal abnormalities.

▪ Diagnosis
A blue to purple plaque that blanches with pressure suggests the diagnosis of hemangioma. Biopsy reveals vascular proliferation. Lymphangioma may simulate hemangioma.

▪ Treatment
Laser in selected cases.

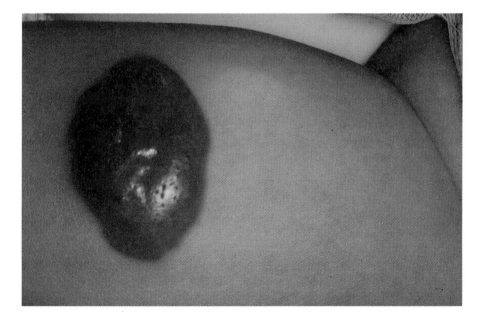

Juxta-Articular Nodules

DIAGNOSTIC OBSERVATIONS
These are deep subcutaneous lesions that appear near joints. They are usually flesh-colored and nontender. Diagnosis is established by clinical presentation, associated diseases, and biopsy (Table 9–2).

TABLE 9–2. **Differential Diagnosis of Juxta-Articular Nodules**

Disease	Number of Lesions	Location	Duration	Associated Diseases
Rheumatoid arthritis	Multiple, symmetric	Elbows, hands, knees, ankles.	Months to years	Severe rheumatoid arthritis with high titer rheumatoid factor
Rheumatic fever	Multiple, symmetric	Elbows over olecranon, hands.	Weeks	Rheumatic fever
Gout	Multiple, symmetric, may drain	Hands, elbows, ears.	Weeks to months	Gout, elevated uric acid
Calcinosis cutis	Multiple, symmetric, may drain	Hands, elbows, ears.	Weeks to months	Tumoral calcinosis, dermatomyositis, scleroderma
Granuloma annulare	Several, asymmetric	Tibia, elbow, scalp.	Weeks to months	Often associated with other lesions of granuloma annulare (see p. 161)
Synovial cysts or ganglion	Single or several, asymmetric	Distal interphalangeal joint or wrist. Attached to tendon sheaths or joint capsule. Associated with joint disease.	Months to years	None
Intrajoint pathology: chondroma, osteoarthritis (Heberden's node). Billo-nodular synovitis	Multiple, asymmetric	Associated with joint disease.	Months to years	Arthritis
Multicentric reticulohistiocytosis	Multiple, symmetric	Distal interphalangeal joints, associated with destructive arthritis.	Months to years	Arthritis
Xanthoma	Multiple, symmetric	Elbows, knees, ankles, hands.	Months to years	Hyperlipidemia

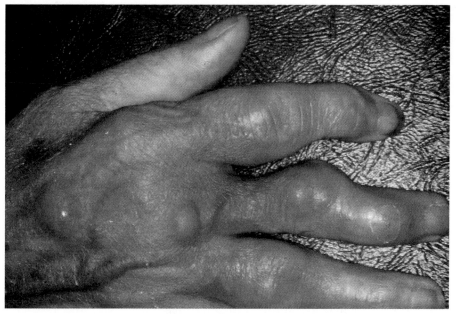

Gout

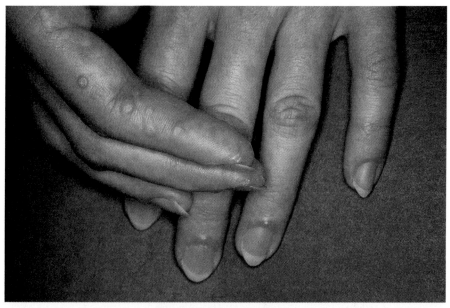

Multicentric reticulohistiocytosis

Lipoma

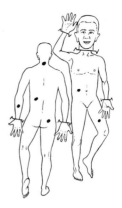

▪ Morphology
Usually single, sharply marginated mass that is soft and movable with palpation. Lesions may vary in size from several millimeters to many centimeters. Overlying skin is completely normal.

▪ Distribution
Posterior neck, trunk, abdomen, forearms, buttocks, and thighs.

▪ Patient Profile
Single lesions usually appear in women between ages of 40 and 60 years. Multiple hereditary (autosomal dominant) lipomas are most common in men. Tender lipomas suggest the possibility of angiolipoma.

▪ Diagnosis
A soft, movable, subcutaneous mass in adults should suggest this diagnosis. Biopsy reveals an encapsulated mass of normal-appearing subcutaneous tissue. Prominent vascular elements histologically suggest angiolipoma.

▪ Treatment
Surgical excision, liposuction. Dercum's disease may respond symptomatically to intermittent intravenous lidocaine therapy.

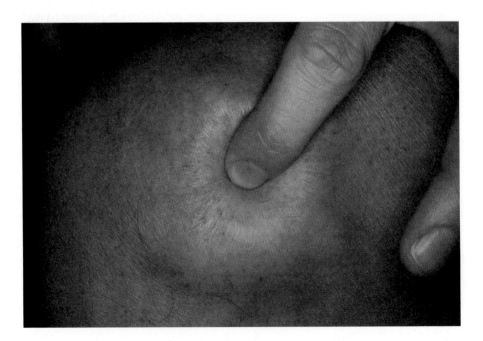

Lupus Profundus

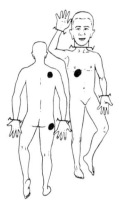

■ Morphology
Deep pink nodules that occasionally ulcerate and heal with depressed scarring. Calcification of lesions may occur.

■ Distribution
Asymmetric; hip and shoulder girdle.

■ Patient Profile
Adults, often women.

■ Diagnosis
Lesions may underlie a plaque of cutaneous lupus or occur by themselves in patients with systemic lupus erythematosus. Biopsy reveals panlobular panniculitis. IgG and complement are usually found at the dermal-epidermal junction in biopsies studied by immunofluorescence.

■ Treatment
Intralesional steroids, antimalarials.

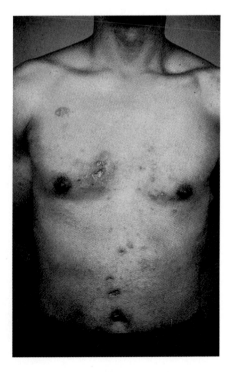

Malignancies and Metastatic Carcinoma

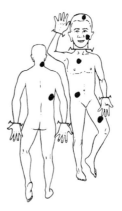

▪ Morphology
Flesh-colored to red, rock-hard nodules.

▪ Distribution
Anywhere, but especially chest, scalp, and abdomen.

▪ Patient Profile
Adults of both sexes.

▪ Diagnosis
Lesions grow quickly. May be fixed to underlying tissues and not movable. In women, the most common primary malignancies are breast, colon, lung, ovary, and melanoma. In men, the most common ones are lung, colon, melanoma, oral cavity, kidney, and stomach. Histologic findings on biopsy depend on the site of the primary. Other tumors to consider:

Adnexal tumors: apocrine hidrocystoma, hidradenoma; sebaceous epithelioma; spiradenoma; and carcinoma of sebaceous glands, eccrine glands, or apocrine glands

Fatty tumors: embryonic lipoma, hibernoma, liposarcoma

Fibrous tumors: desmoid, pseudotumor of Ehlers-Danlos, keloid, atypical fibroxanthoma, nodular pseudosarcomatous fasciitis, dermatofibrosarcoma protuberans, fibrosarcoma; lymphomas: histiocytic lymphoma and lymphocytic lymphoma, myxosarcoma, nodular fasciitis

Lymphoma and leukemia

Merkel cell carcinoma

Metastatic carcinoma (see p. 220)

Metastatic melanoma (see p. 173)

Muscle tumors: leiomyoma, leiomyosarcoma, rhabdomyoma

Neural tumors: neurofibroma, neurilemoma, neuroma, granular cell myoblastoma, glioma

Vascular tumors: lymphangioma, hemangioma

▪ Treatment
Treatment of primary process. Surgery or radiation therapy of metastatic site.

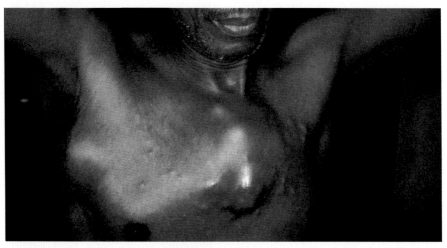

Sarcoma

Phlebolith

■ **Morphology**
Small, shotlike, hard nodules that are freely
movable under the skin. Lesions occasionally have a blue tint.

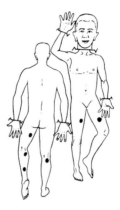

■ **Distribution**
Along course of veins. Lower extremities
most common but can occur anywhere.

■ **Patient Profile**
Both sexes. Most common in older patients with prominent varicose veins but
can occur in anyone.

■ **Diagnosis**
Hard, small nodules along the course of a
vein suggest this diagnosis. Biopsy reveals
calcified scarring in a vein.

■ **Treatment**
Usually unnecessary.

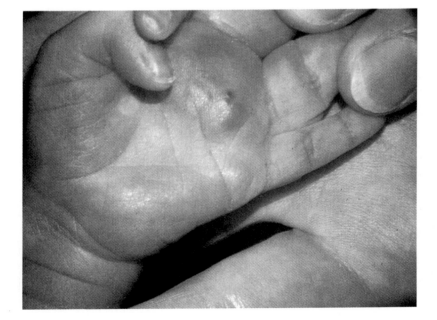

Prurigo Nodularis

▪ **Morphology**
Single or multiple dome-shaped lesions several centimeters in diameter with a central excoriation. Scaling and erythema are frequently present.

▪ **Distribution**
Lower legs, extensor aspect of arms most common sites.

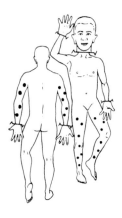

▪ **Patient Profile**
Most frequently middle-aged women. Lesions are very pruritic. They may persist for years.

▪ **Diagnosis**
Biopsy shows irregular epidermal hyperplasia and nerve fiber proliferation.

▪ **Treatment**
Class I or II topical steroids with Cordran tape; for intralesional corticosteroids, one month may be necessary. Cryotherapy. Combined UVA and UVB for generalized disease. More potent antihistamine-like drugs, such as doxepin, are often needed. Thalidomide has been used for its antipruritic effects. If lesions are related to delusions of parasitosis, pimozide often effective.

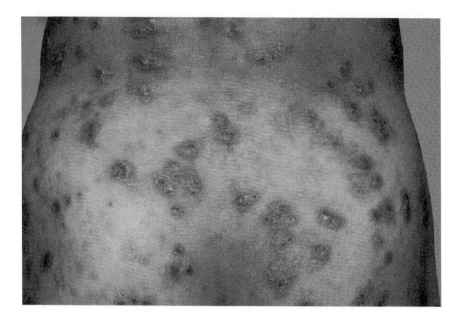

Sarcoidosis

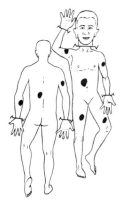

▪ Morphology
Single or multiple flesh-colored, brown, or pink nontender nodules.

▪ Distribution
Trunk, proximal extremities but can occur anywhere. Lesions may arise in scars.

▪ Patient Profile
Young adults, more common in blacks. Patients often have adenopathy, hepatosplenomegaly, and pulmonary disease.

▪ Diagnosis
Biopsy reveals noncaseating granulomas.

▪ Treatment
Small lesions may respond to class I topical steroids or intralesional steroids. Deforming skin lesions may require hydroxychloroquine or, rarely, systemic steroids.

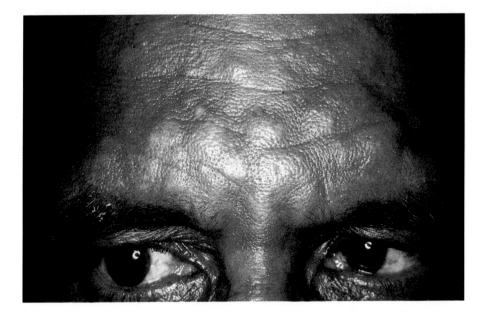

Systemic Mycosis or Mycobacterial Disease

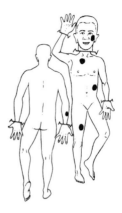

▪ **Morphology**
Pink to red nodules that develop pustules, drain purulent material, and form sinuses.

▪ **Distribution**
Anywhere, usually trunk.

▪ **Patient Profile**
Any age, both sexes. Patient is usually systemically ill with such fungal diseases as coccidioidomycosis, nocardiosis, blastomycosis, or typical or atypical mycobacteria. Patients with AIDS have developed cutaneous atypical and *Mycobacterium hominis* skin lesions.

▪ **Diagnosis**
Biopsy and culture demonstrate organism.

▪ **Treatment**
Systemic antibiotic therapy depending on organism's sensitivity.

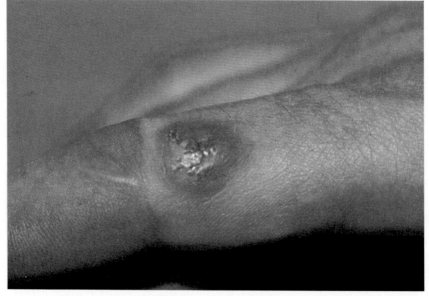

Atypical mycobacterial infection

PURPLE NODULES

DIAGNOSTIC OBSERVATIONS
These lesions are blue to purple, deep, nodular "iceberg" lesions.

Hemangiomas (see p. 403): on unusual occasions, may present as deep blue nodules
Kaposi's sarcoma
Lymphoma, leukemia, mycosis fungoides
Melanoma

Kaposi's Sarcoma

▪ Morphology

Purple-blue nodules that decrease in size with firm pressure and return to original size over a period of 10 to 15 seconds. Lesions may have mild scaling and often progress to ulceration and bleeding. In patients with HIV, lesions often are linear and erupt rapidly.

▪ Distribution

Lower extremity in older patients. Anywhere, including the face and trunk, in HIV-positive patients.

▪ Patient Profile

Most common in older males and HIV-positive patients. Older patients often have bilateral edema of legs, adenopathy, gastrointestinal hemorrhage, and leukemia. In Africa, Kaposi's sarcoma may be seen in a younger population.

▪ Diagnosis

Biopsy reveals proliferation of blood vessels that are lined with neoplastic endothelial cells. Lymphangiosarcoma, bacillary angiomatosis, malignant angioendothe-

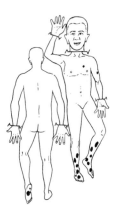

lioma, and hemangiopericytoma may mimic Kaposi's sarcoma.

▪ Treatment

Cryotherapy, bleomycin, or x-ray therapy. For systemic therapies, consult appropriate sources.

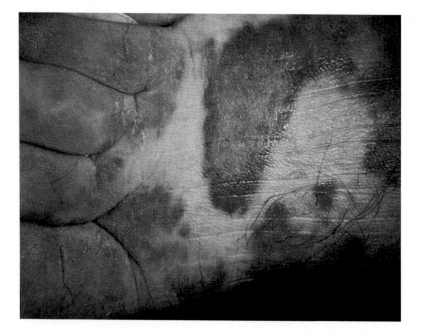

Lymphoma, Leukemia, Mycosis Fungoides

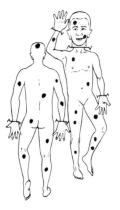

■ **Morphology**
Purple-blue to red brown nodules deep in the skin.

■ **Distribution**
Anywhere.

■ **Patient Profile**
Both sexes, older age group. Lesions often erupt in crops and grow rapidly. Patients usually have stigmata of underlying neoplasm, such as purpura, as well as constitutional symptoms, organomegaly, and adenopathy. Lesions may develop over days.

■ **Diagnosis**
Diagnosis is made by biopsy, and histologic findings depend on the primary tumor.

■ **Treatment**
Systemic chemotherapy for lymphoma and leukemia. Local x-ray for disease limited to the skin. For mycosis fungoides: topical treatments consist of corticosteroids, nitrogen mustard, BCNU, and PUVA; systemic treatments consist of interferon, photopheresis, and methotrexate.

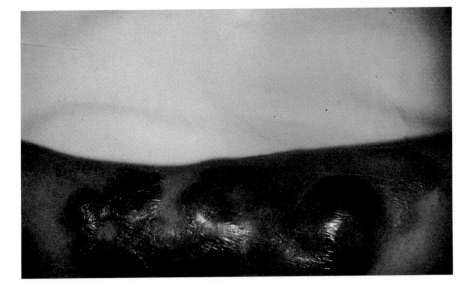

Melanoma

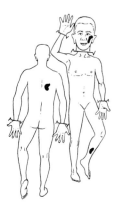

▪ Morphology
Blue, black, or brown nodules that may have areas of white and red pigmentation. Borders of the lesions are irregular and there may be notches. Skin markings are altered.

▪ Distribution
Light-exposed areas, palms, and soles but can occur anywhere.

▪ Patient Profile
Usually older patients of both sexes. Uncommon in blacks but does occur.

▪ Diagnosis
Histologic examination demonstrates melanoma.

▪ Treatment
Systemic chemotherapy and immunotherapy used for advanced disease.

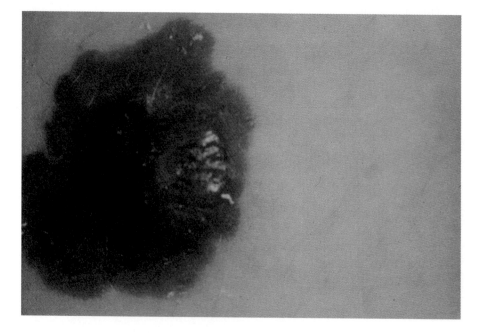

TENDER RED NODULES

DIAGNOSTIC OBSERVATIONS
These are deep nodules that appear in groups over hours to days and are often tender.

- Calcinosis cutis
- Carbuncle (boil)
- Erythema induratum
- Erythema nodosum
- Hidradenitis suppurativa
- Leishmaniasis
- Lymphogranuloma venereum
- Nodules peculiar to tropical or subtropical areas
- Panniculitis with pancreatic disease
- Polyarteritis nodosa
- Subacute migratory panniculitis
- Suppurative adenitis
- Systemic mycosis or mycobacterial disease
- Temporal arteritis
- Thrombophlebitis
- Trauma or cold
- Weber-Christian disease

Calcinosis Cutis

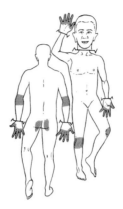

▪ Morphology
Single or multiple erythematous to flesh-colored nodules that may progress to drain chalky material.

▪ Distribution
Symmetric, bilateral, juxta-articular; around shoulder and hip girdle and tips of digits.

▪ Patient Profile
Any age, both sexes. Lesions may be tender.

▪ Diagnosis
Aspiration of chalky material reveals calcium apatite crystals. Biopsy demonstrates deposition of calcium phosphate on bone and chronic inflammatory cells. Uric acid nodules in gout may simulate calcinosis (see p. 405). Causes of calcinosis include abnormalities of parathyroid function, calciphylaxis, chronic Ehlers-Danlos syndrome, hypervitaminosis D, milk alkali syndrome, myositis ossificans, paraplegia, parasitic infection, polymyositis (including dermatomyositis), scleroderma, tumoral calcinosis, and Werner's syndrome.

▪ Treatment
Controlling underlying diseases. Surgical excision.

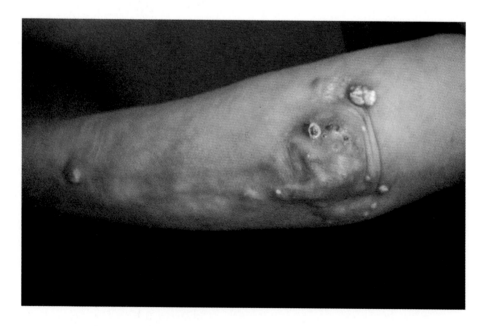

Carbuncle (Boil)

■ **Morphology**
Erythematous, hot nodule that may become fluctuant and spontaneously discharge pus.

■ **Distribution**
Hairy areas exposed to trauma and maceration, especially buttocks, neck, face, and axillae.

■ **Patient Profile**
Any age, both sexes. Lesions are tender, and patient may be febrile. Lesions develop over days.

■ **Diagnosis**
Incision of the fluctuant lesion releases creamy pus. Gram's stain demonstrates numerous organisms, the most common being *Staphylococcus aureus*.

■ **Treatment**
Incision and appropriate systemic antibiotics.

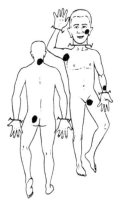

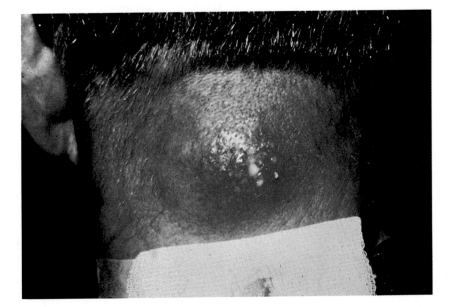

Erythema Induratum
(Nodular Vasculitis)

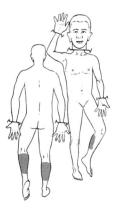

▪ Morphology
Deep nodules and ulcers with infiltration beyond the lesion characterize this disease. The ulcer edge is frequently irregular. A netlike vascular pattern (see livedo reticularis, p. 78) is commonly seen on the legs. Atrophic hyperpigmented scars from healed ulcers may be present. Frequently the legs are diffusely swollen.

▪ Distribution
Most common on posterior calves.

▪ Patient Profile
Middle-aged women. Lesions are precipitated by cold and last months to years.

▪ Diagnosis
Nodules and ulcers on the posterior calves of a middle-aged woman are very suggestive of this diagnosis. This disease can be associated with local or systemic tuberculosis. Biopsy shows vasculitis, fat necrosis, caseation necrosis, inflammatory cells, and granulomas. Tuberculin testing with very dilute reagents initially. PCR can establish diagnosis of tuberculosis.

▪ Treatment
Systemic antituberculosis therapy if sufficient evidence for tuberculosis. Systemic steroids, SSKI in other cases.

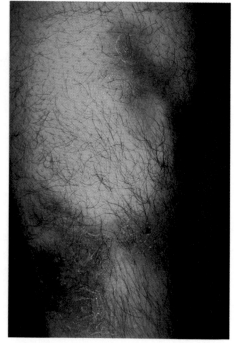

Erythema Nodosum

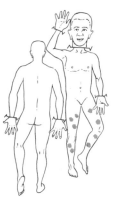

▪ Morphology
Crops of red to blue tender nodules, 1 to 5 cm in diameter, with normal epidermis. Purpura is commonly present. Lesions heal without scarring. Individual lesions may be in different stages of development.

▪ Distribution
Symmetric lesions on pretibial areas. Rarely occurs elsewhere.

▪ Patient Profile
Young adults; most common in women. Individual lesions last from 3 weeks to 2 months. Recurrent crops of lesions may occur. Fever, polyarthralgias, thrombophlebitis, or hilar adenopathy may be present. Sarcoidosis, progesterone in birth control pills, drug allergy, streptococci, coccidioidomycosis, ulcerative colitis, and tuberculosis are common causes of erythema nodosum.

▪ Diagnosis
Crops of tender, slightly purpuric lesions on the anterior lower legs suggest this diagnosis. Biopsy shows septal inflammation and broadened fibrous septae with multinucleated giant cells. More generalized lesions with ecchymoses, pancytopenia, coagulation defects in histiocytic cytophagic panniculitis.

▪ Treatment
While underlying cause is being determined, symptomatic treatment with leg elevation, salicylates, and NSAIDs appropriate.

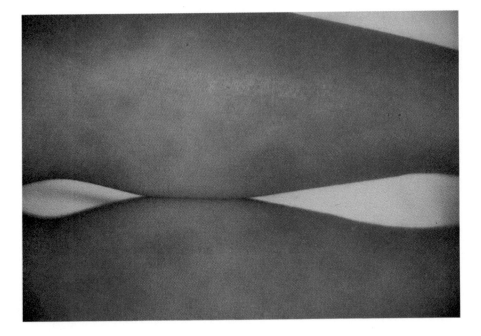

Hidradenitis Suppurativa

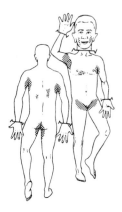

■ Morphology
Erythematous, indurated lesions that often form sinus tracts. Double comedones, pustules, and abscesses are associated with this condition.

■ Distribution
Bilaterally symmetric; axillae, groin, occasionally anterior abdomen.

■ Patient Profile
Postpubertal young adults of both sexes. Lesions are tender. Patients may have severe cystic acne and cellulitis of the scalp.

■ Diagnosis
Biopsy reveals inflammation of the apocrine glands.

■ Treatment
Systemic broad-spectrum antibiotics, especially minocycline, metronidazole. Isotretinoin (Accutane) sometimes helpful. Extensive excisional surgery may be necessary.

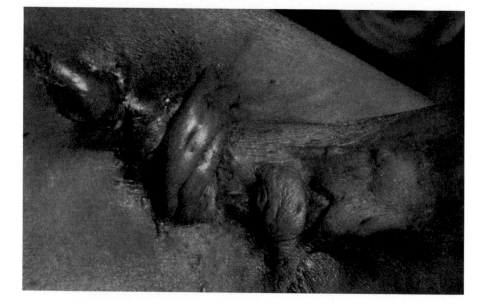

Leishmaniasis

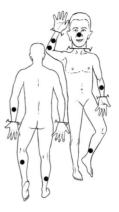

■ Morphology
Erythematous papule that slowly enlarges to become a crusted nodule. Satellite papules may be present. Ulcer formation at the site of the lesion is followed by scar formation.

■ Distribution
Lesion develops at the site of sandfly bite.

■ Patient Profile
History of travel to Asia, Africa, or Middle East. Multiple lesions may occur with *Leishmania major.* Cutaneous leishmaniasis, diffuse cutaneous leishmaniasis (DCL), mucocutaneous leishmaniasis (MCL), and visceral leishmaniasis (VL) are the different forms of the disease.

■ Diagnosis
Diagnosis is established by demonstrating the parasite on direct smear from the lesion. Staining the smear with Giemsa shows pale-blue, oval amastigotes within tissue macrophages.

■ Treatment
Cutaneous leishmaniasis is self-limited; DCL, MCL, and VL may require intralesional sodium stibogluconate or systemic pentamidine.

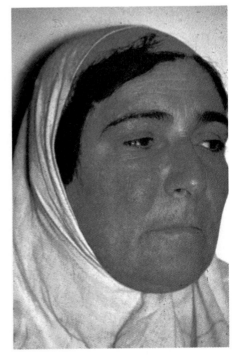

Lymphogranuloma Venereum

■ **Morphology**
Tender, red lymph nodes that may ulcerate and drain. Lesions are often above and below the inguinale ligament, producing a groove sign. Genital elephantiasis may occur.

■ **Distribution**
Groin, unilateral or bilateral.

■ **Patient Profile**
Sexually active adults. More common in blacks. Transmitted by sexual contact. Patient develops an asymptomatic papule on the genitalia that heals. Several weeks later, the characteristic adenopathy occurs. Lesions may persist for years.

■ **Diagnosis**
A positive serologic test for *Chlamydia* organisms confirms the diagnosis of lymphogranuloma venereum.

■ **Treatment**
Sulfisoxazole or tetracycline as in STD protocol (see Table 14–12).

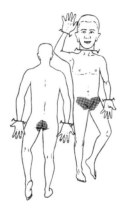

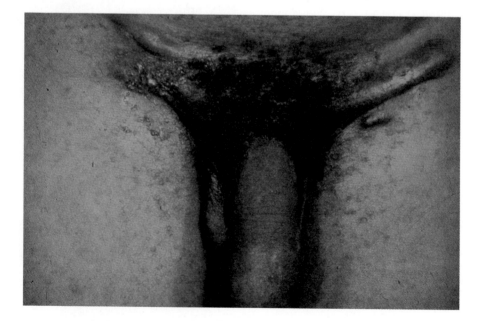

Nodules Peculiar to Tropical or Subtropical Areas
(See Ulcers, p. 461)

■ Morphology
Single but more frequently multiple, deep, indurated nodules that may progress to drain pus and ulcerate.

■ Distribution
Frequently exposed areas.

■ Patient Profile
Any age, both sexes. The skin has frequently been bitten by an insect or traumatized while the patient was in a tropical area.

■ Diagnosis
Biopsy and culture of lesion discloses the diagnosis. A pathologist should use special stains for organism in the biopsy. Diseases include deep fungi and especially South American blastomycosis, Buruli ulcer (atypical mycobacteria), leishmaniasis (protozoa), leprosy, myiasis (insect larvae), nematodes (round worms, flat worms), rhinoscleroma, and yaws.

■ Treatment
After identifying organism, see standard infectious disease texts for specific treatment.

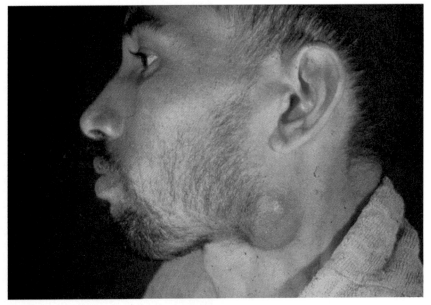

South American blastomycosis

Panniculitis (with Pancreatitis)

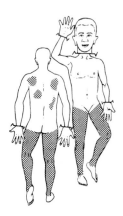

▪ **Morphology**
Tender nodules that may become fluctuant and drain creamy or oily material. Lesions heal with scarring and hyperpigmentation.

▪ **Distribution**
Inside of legs and thighs and on wrists and digits but can occur anywhere.

▪ **Patient Profile**
Most common in middle-aged men. Fever, arthritis, abdominal pain, leukocytosis, increased serum lipase and amylase may be present. Pancreatitis and adenocarcinoma of the pancreas cause this condition. Arthritis and synovitis often present.

▪ **Diagnosis**
Biopsy is diagnostic and demonstrates fat necrosis (ghost cells) and deposition of calcium soaps. Markedly elevated serum lipase and amylase.

▪ **Treatment**
Treatment of underlying disease. Somatostatin effective in some patients.

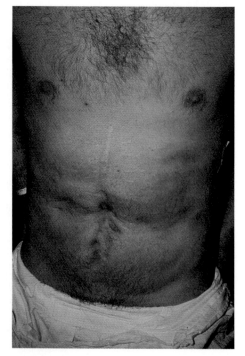

Polyarteritis Nodosa

■ **Morphology**
Nodules are 5 to 10 mm, clustered along arteries, and may ulcerate. May be associated with netlike livedo pattern.

■ **Distribution**
Anywhere, especially on legs and at branching points of arteries.

■ **Patient Profile**
Both sexes, more common in adults. Lesions may be limited to the skin or associated with asthma, arthritis, neuropathy, renal disease, and hypertension.

■ **Diagnosis**
Biopsy reveals necrosis and inflammation in walls of muscular arteries.

■ **Treatment**
Systemic corticosteroids; immunosuppressives are often necessary. Therapy requires a complete medical evaluation. There are cutaneous forms of polyarteritis limited to skin and joints that are treated with NSAIDs.

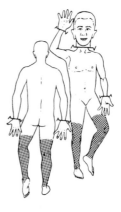

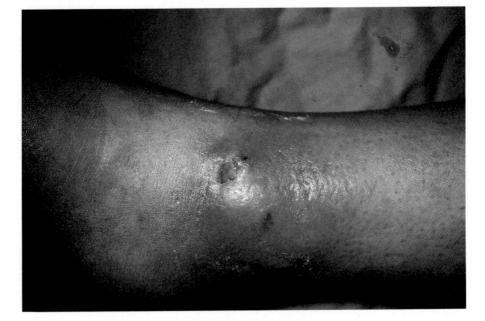

Subacute Migratory Panniculitis

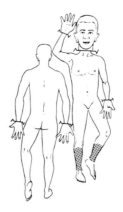

■ **Morphology**
Red to blue tender nodules with scalloped borders that migrate over days to weeks and leave yellowish hyperpigmented areas. Usually not more than three lesions are present.

■ **Distribution**
Anterior legs near ankles or knees.

■ **Patient Profile**
Most common in middle-aged women. Lesions last 2 to 8 months.

■ **Diagnosis**
Biopsy demonstrates vasculitis, vascular proliferation, and granulomatous infiltration of the septae. Lesions often regress with iodide therapy.

■ **Treatment**
Treatment with SSKI until inflammation resolves. Class I or II steroids, sometimes with occlusion. NSAIDs often successful.

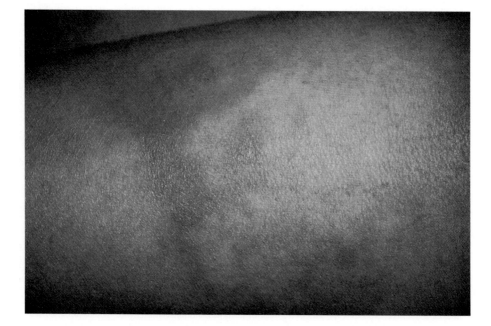

Suppurative Adenitis

▪ Morphology
Linear 1- to 3-cm deep nodules that proceed proximally along a lymphatic vessel and that are pink to red in color. Lesions may ulcerate and drain purulent material. Initial site of inoculation may be present.

▪ Distribution
Upper and lower extremities.

▪ Patient Profile
Adults of both sexes. Patient usually has a history of traumatic lesions followed in weeks to months by development of subcutaneous nodules proceeding proximally up an extremity or on the perineum. May persist for months. Constitutional symptoms may be present.

▪ Diagnosis
Biopsy and culture of lesion establish the etiology. Possible etiologies include sporotrichosis, atypical mycobacteria, cat scratch fever, tularemia, lymphopathia venereum, and deep fungal infection.

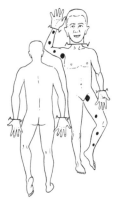

▪ Treatment
Systemic antibiotics for the underlying disease.

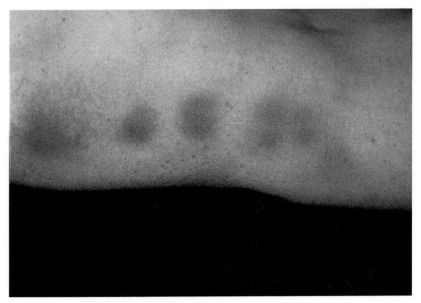

Sporotrichosis

Systemic Mycosis or Mycobacterial Disease

▪ **Morphology**
Deep pink to red nodules that may develop pustules, drain purulent material, and form sinuses.

▪ **Distribution**
Anywhere, usually trunk.

▪ **Patient Profile**
Any age, both sexes. Patient is usually systemically ill with such fungal diseases as coccidioidomycosis, histoplasmosis, nocardiosis, blastomycosis, or typical or atypical mycobacteria. All patients should be tested for HIV.

▪ **Diagnosis**
Biopsy and culture demonstrate organism.

▪ **Treatment**
Depending on organism (see infectious disease texts).

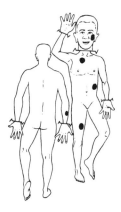

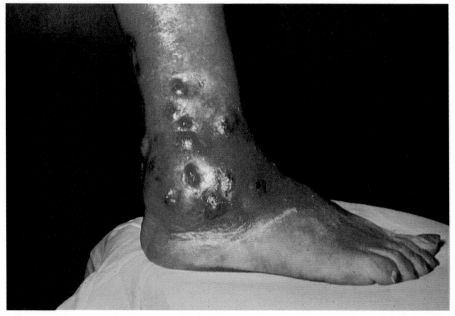

Nocardiosis

Temporal Arteritis
(Cranial Arteritis)

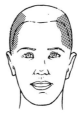

■ **Morphology**
Tender cords along tortuous temporal arteries. Scalp gangrene may be present.

■ **Distribution**
Over temporal and occipital arteries.

■ **Patient Profile**
Both sexes, adults older than 55 years. Fever, weight loss, neuropathy, muscular pain in proximal muscles, unilateral headaches, temporomandibular pain, and decreased vision may be associated.

■ **Diagnosis**
Erythrocyte sedimentation rate is frequently elevated. Biopsy of temporal arteries shows granulomas and giant cells.

■ **Treatment**
Systemic corticosteroids and immunosuppressives.

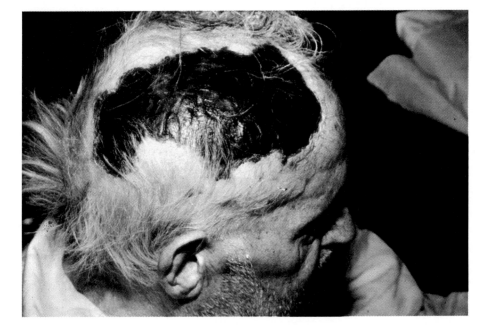

Thrombophlebitis

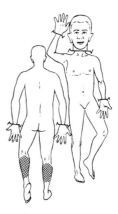

▪ Morphology
Red, painful nodules with tenderness of the overlying skin. Linear, sausagelike areas corresponding to underlying veins may be present. Marked edema may be present. A change in extremity may be present (pale, phlegmasia alba dolens; or cyanotic and cold, phlegmasia cerulea dolens).

▪ Distribution
Legs, especially calves.

▪ Patient Profile
Adults of both sexes. Predisposing causes include blood dyscrasia, thromboangiitis obliterans, malignancy, varicosities, vasculitis, septic infections, and trauma.

▪ Diagnosis
In thrombophlebitis of the calf, dorsiflexion of the foot induces calf pain. Venograms confirm the diagnosis.

▪ Treatment
Hospitalization and anticoagulation as described in medicine texts.

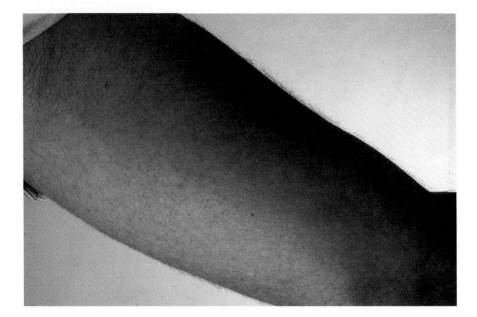

Trauma

■ **Morphology**
One or several deep, indurated, flesh-colored to red or purple nodules.

■ **Distribution**
Asymmetric, grouped; in area of trauma or cold injury.

■ **Patient Profile**
Patient has had trauma or localized cold exposure. May follow sucking on a popsicle.

■ **Diagnosis**
Diagnosis is based on history. Biopsy reveals resolving inflammatory infiltrate.

■ **Treatment**
Spontaneous resolution. Avoidance of precipitating events.

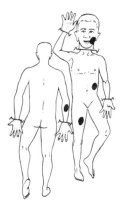

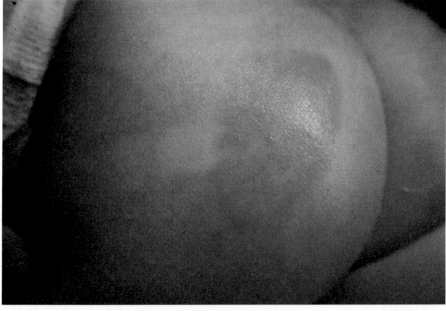

Cold-induced panniculitis in a newborn

Weber-Christian Disease

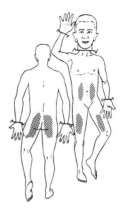

▪ **Morphology**
Crops of red-blue, tender nodules that evolve into depressed and hyperpigmented scars. Nodules rarely ulcerate.

▪ **Distribution**
Symmetric; trunk, thighs, buttocks, and internal fat.

▪ **Patient Profile**
Most common in middle-aged women. Disease lasts months to years. Fatigue, fever, abdominal pain, and leukocytosis accompany the crops of skin lesions.

▪ **Diagnosis**
Biopsy shows panniculitis with lipid-laden macrophages forming granulomas. Patient should be studied for alpha$_1$-antitrypsin deficiency.

▪ **Treatment**
Systemic steroids have been used with some success.

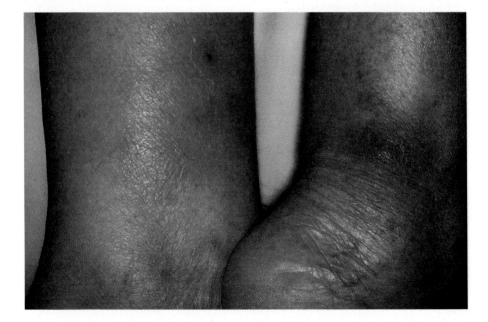

Chapter 10

■ ■

Ulcers

DIAGNOSTIC OBSERVATIONS

An ulcer is a depressed lesion in which both the epidermis and dermis are lost. Ulcers heal with scarring.

The diagnostic approach to ulcer disease is as follows:

1. Remove crust from the ulcer.
   a. Observe whether the base of the ulcer is purulent.
   b. Note whether there is an underlying nodule or tumor.
2. Define the nature of the ulcer border (see drawing at right).
3. Observe surrounding skin for primary dermatologic disease.
4. Palpate margin for subcutaneous induration.
5. Determine whether the area around the ulcer has decreased pain sensation.
6. Note exact location of ulcer: lateral versus medial aspect of leg, genitals, and so forth.
7. Check for associated adenopathy.
8. Determine whether the ulcer is spontaneously painful and tender. Neuropathic ulcers are usually painless.
9. If there is any doubt about the diagnosis of an ulcer or if the base is purulent, biopsy the rim of the ulcer. Divide the biopsy in half, and send one part for histologic examination and the remaining tissue for culture for aerobic and anaerobic bacteria, fungi, and mycobacteria, including mycobacterial culture at 33°C. Culture of the skin biopsy is usually more useful than culture of the exudate. Pyogenic bacteria can infect damaged skin. Abscesses can go on to ulceration and drainage. Staphylococci commonly infect ulcers.

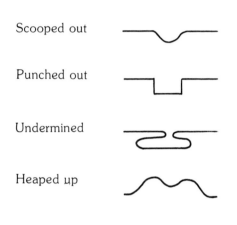

Scooped out

Punched out

Undermined

Heaped up

MAJOR CATEGORIES

Anesthetic ulcers
Painful and ischemic ulcers
Ulcers in areas of primary dermatologic disease
Purulent ulcers
Ulcers in specific locations

ANESTHETIC ULCERS

Neuropathic Ulcers, Mal Perforans

■ **Morphology**
Sharply marginated, painless ulcers. The area around the ulcer is frequently anhidrotic, heaped up, scaly, and hyperpigmented. The base is usually clean. On the face, the ulcer may have an angular outline. The lesion and surrounding skin are anesthetic to pinprick, but deep pain may be present.

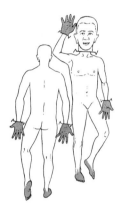

■ **Distribution**
Soles of feet, especially over bony prominences, face, and alae nasae are common sites.

■ **Patient Profile**
Age of patient depends on etiology; both sexes. Lesion is usually completely painless. Sometimes familial.

■ **Diagnosis**
Ulcer is secondary to trauma in a patient with neurologic disease, which may be at any level of the neuraxis. Specific diagnoses to be considered include diabetes

mellitus, tabes dorsalis (syphilis), leprosy, syringomyelia, polyneuropathy (familial and heavy metals). Ulcers in the area of the alae nasae follow alcohol injection of the trigeminal nerve for tic douloureux, brain stem disease, or Parkinson's disease.

■ **Treatment**
Prevention of trauma and pressure on anesthetic sites. Hydrocolloid dressings, soaks, and topical antibiotics.

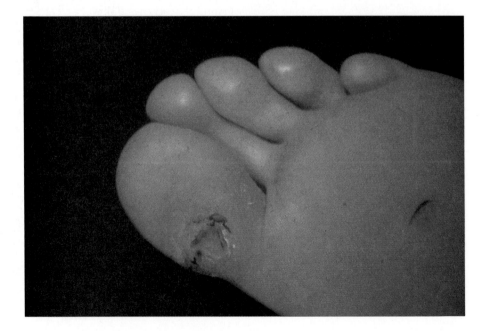

PAINFUL AND ISCHEMIC ULCERS

DIAGNOSTIC OBSERVATION
Ischemic ulcers are punched out, sharply marginated, tender, and often spontaneously painful. They frequently occur on the legs and favor the anterior shin, lateral malleolus, and acral portions of the toes.

Arteriosclerosis
Atrophie blanche
Bacterial emboli
Cholesterol emboli
Consumption coagulopathy
Cryoglobulinemia
Cutaneous polyarteritis nodosa
Diabetes mellitus
Dysproteinemia
Ergotism
Giant cell arteritis
Hemoglobinopathy
Hyperparathyroidism
Hypertensive cardiovascular disease
Insect bites (especially of the brown recluse spider)
Lupus erythematosus
Midline lethal granuloma
Polyarteritis nodosa
Polycythemia rubra vera
Raynaud's disease
Rheumatoid vasculitis
Scleroderma
Thromboangiitis obliterans
Thrombotic thrombocytopenic purpura
Wegener's granulomatosis

Ischemic Ulcers with Chronic Arterial Disease

■ **Morphology**
Painful ulcers have a rapid onset, are sharply marginated, and have little peripheral extension or undermining. Hemorrhagic bullae may precede the infarctive stage. Extremities demonstrate stigmata of chronic arterial disease, such as cold, pallor on exertion or elevation, redness on dependency, decreased pulses, and shiny, hairless, atrophic skin.

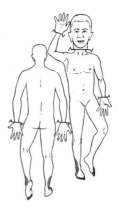

■ **Distribution**
Lower extremities, most commonly above lateral malleolus.

■ **Patient Profile**
Usually middle-aged or elderly patients of both sexes. Lesions are painful, especially at night. There may be a history of intermittent claudication for months to years preceding the ulcer.

■ **Diagnosis**
History of vascular symptoms and signs of chronic vascular disease suggest arterial ulcer. Among the causes of ischemic ulcers with chronic arterial disease are:

Arteriosclerosis and atherosclerosis: Bruits can be heard; arteriograms should be obtained.

Atrophie blanche: Lesions on lower legs are extremely painful. Healed lesions appear as white atrophic macules with telangiectases. Patients often have venous incompetence.

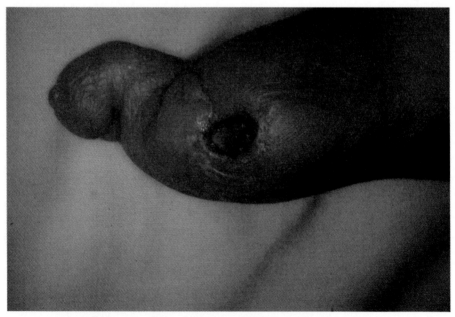

Diabetic ulcer

Diabetes mellitus: There may be evidence of older scarred lesions and hyperpigmented macules (diabetic dermopathy).

Livedo reticularis with ulceration (cutaneous polyarteritis): Lower legs have a prominent netlike purple pattern.

Thromboangiitis obliterans (Buerger's disease): Small-vessel disease in middle-aged men who are heavy smokers.

▪ Treatment

Unna boots to decrease edema, hydrocolloid dressings such as Vigilon and Ace bandages, daily soaks to keep clean, topical antibiotics. Surgical intervention when appropriate. Calcium channel blockers, pentoxifylline, ASA. Avoidance of smoking.

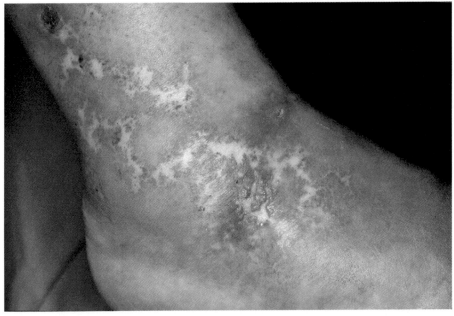

Atrophie blanche

Ischemic Ulcers without Preceding Vascular Disease
(Vasculitic Ulcer)

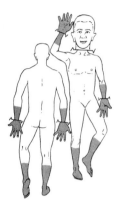

▪ Morphology
Painful, sharply marginated ulcers that have little peripheral extension or undermining. Hemorrhagic bullae frequently precede the ulcer. Ulcers are often covered with black, adherent crust. Gangrene may be present. Scattered areas, palpable purpura, or petechiae may be present.

▪ Distribution
Extremities, especially distally. Ears, nose, mucous membranes may be involved. Purpuric lesions are often symmetric, but the ulcers are not. Livedo reticularis may be present.

▪ Patient Profile
Any age, both sexes. Systemic complaints such as arthralgia and fever are common.

▪ Diagnosis
Sudden onset of palpable purpuric lesions that may ulcerate are diagnostic of vasculitis. Etiologies of clinical vasculitis include:

Bacterial emboli: Septic emboli may be present as pustules that become superficial ulcerations.

Cholesterol emboli from atherosclerosis: Usually there is evidence of chronic arterial disease and recent anticoagulation. Most common on legs. Cholesterol clefts are seen in alcohol-fixed biopsy tissue. Thromboembolism, tumor emboli, or oxalosis may rarely cause similar lesions.

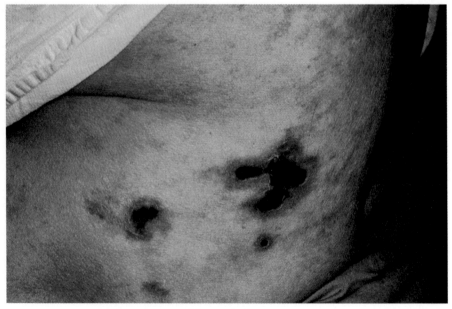

Atheroembolism

Consumption coagulopathy (purpura fulminans): Large purpuric areas with blistering, gangrene, and superficial hemorrhage. Low platelet count and the presence of fibrin split products confirm this diagnosis. Warfarin (Coumadin) may produce similar lesions in the first 2 to 10 days of administration, frequently involving the breast, buttocks, and thighs.

Cryoglobulinemia, dysproteinemia, macroglobulinemia, and cryofibrinogenemia: Hemorrhagic ulcers (up to 6 to 10 cm in length) on ankles, hands, and ears after exposure to cold. Distal areas of purpura are frequent. Extensive hemosiderin in the skin of the lower extremities is common. Cryoglobulins, macroglobulins, and cryofibrinogens can be measured in plasma. Biopsy of ulcer edge reveals vessels plugged with eosinophilic material; leukocytoclastic angiitis may be seen along with vascular thrombi.

Ergotism: Raynaud's phenomenon, ulceration, and gangrene may be produced by administration of ergots for migraine headaches or in accidental mushroom poisoning.

Hereditary anemia (sickle cell disease, thalassemia, hereditary spherocytosis): This form of anemia should be considered in younger patients with leg ulcers. Study of the blood smear, red cell indices, and hemoglobin electrophoresis should be done to make this diagnosis.

Giant cell arteritis (temporal): Hemorrhagic ulcers especially on the scalp, tongue, and legs. This disease is associated with headache, arthritis, visual changes, difficulty opening mouth, pain on chewing, weakness. Temporal artery biopsy shows fibrosis and giant cells.

Hyperparathyroidism: Livedo and purpura are common. Occurs in patients with chronic renal failure. Ulcers may be either proximal or distal. High serum calcium, low serum phosphorus, and calcified small vessels on biopsy or x-ray suggest this diagnosis.

Lupus erythematosus (see p. 252): Skin, oral, and nasopharyngeal ulcerations may occur.

Midline lethal granuloma: Adults with edema, hemorrhage, and extensive destruction of nose and sinuses. Endothelial swelling and the absence of frank vasculitis and granulomas permit this histologic diagnosis.

Polyarteritis (see p. 427): Lesions begin as erythematous nodules, which become hemorrhagic and ulcerate. Livedo reticularis is common in this disease.

Polycythemia rubra vera: Increased hemoglobin levels and increased white blood cell and platelet counts confirm this diagnosis in an adult with erythromelalgia, leg ulcers, and pruritus induced by warm showers.

Raynaud's phenomenon or scleroderma (see pp. 106, 379): Ulcers are usually acral and arise in sclerotic skin; calcinosis cutis may be present. Werner's syndrome should be considered when sclerodermatous ulcers arise in a young male patient with cataracts.

Rheumatoid vasculitis: This disease is characterized by high titer rheumatoid factor, rheumatoid nodules, and mononeuritis multiplex. Felty's syndrome may be associated with this disease; splenomegaly and leukopenia, in addition to high titer rheumatoid factor, are features of this syndrome.

Thrombotic thrombocytopenic purpura: Low platelet count, hemolytic anemia, and systemic vasculitis distinguish this from other causes of vasculitis.

Wegener's granulomatosis: Adults with hemorrhagic perinasal, perioral, laryngeal, and nasopharyngeal ulceration. Lung and kidney are frequently involved. Granulomatous reaction with necrosis of superficial vessels is seen on biopsy.

■ Treatment

Treatment of underlying disorder.

ULCERS IN AREAS OF PRIMARY DERMATOLOGIC DISEASE

DIAGNOSTIC OBSERVATIONS

This group of ulcerating diseases is characterized by the preexistence of a chronic dermatologic disease. Papules and nodules that may ulcerate are discussed in the next section. The crust should always be removed from an ulcer and the presence of an underlying papule or nodule should be determined. Whether the nodule goes deeply into the subcutaneous tissue should be determined by palpation. Purulent ulcers may have induration at the base and are discussed later in this section. On occasion, the panniculitis of lupus erythematosus and Weber-Christian disease ulcerates. Undermined ulcers extend beyond the ulcer rim under the skin. A probe can be passed several centimeters beyond the ulcer rim. These lesions often progress rapidly.

Bites
Calcinosis cutis
Decubitus ulcer
Erythema induratum
Factitial ulceration
Gout
Leishmaniasis
Milker's nodule (see p. 309)
Necrobiosis lipoidica diabeticorum
Nodular liquefying panniculitis
Orf (see p. 309)
Pyoderma gangrenosum
Radiodermatitis
Stasis dermatitis
Trauma
Tumor nodules

Bites

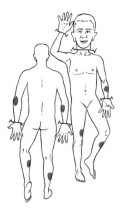

■ **Morphology**
Small puncture ulcerations conforming to teeth arrangement. Crusting may be present.

■ **Distribution**
Anywhere; hands and face common.

■ **Patient Profile**
Children and adults. Children often bitten by dogs.

■ **Diagnosis**
Presence of puncture wounds establishes the diagnosis.

■ **Treatment**
Irrigate and wash area thoroughly. Antibiotics.

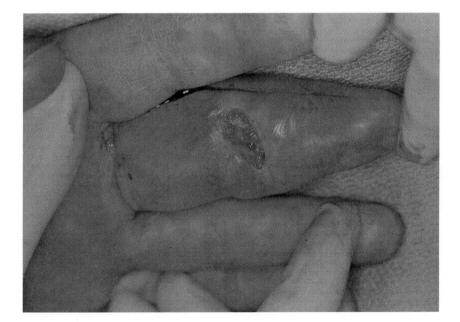

Calcinosis Cutis

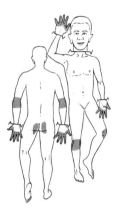

▪ Morphology
Ulcers occur in papules and nodules, which drain white to yellow chalky material. Lesions often become infected.

▪ Distribution
Around joints, buttocks, trunk, and tips of fingers.

▪ Patient Profile
Any age, both sexes.

▪ Diagnosis
Biopsy reveals deposition of calcium and chronic inflammatory cells. The calcium phosphate deposits are radiopaque on x-ray. Calcinosis cutis is associated with increased calcium and phosphate levels, dermatomyositis, scleroderma, tumoral calcinosis, and myositis ossificans.

▪ Treatment
Excision of lesion.

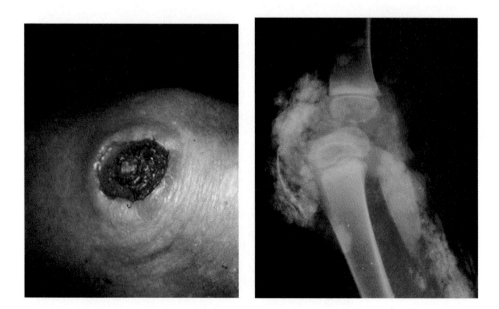

Decubitus Ulcer

■ **Morphology**
Ulceration with marked peripheral under-mining that can spread in diameter and depth very quickly. Ulcers can extend down to bone.

■ **Distribution**
Areas of pressure and trauma, usually over bony prominences in bedridden patients. Characteristic regions are presacral, scapular, and over the ischial tuberosities and heels.

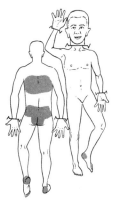

■ **Patient Profile**
Patients are confined to bed and do not move about. Ulcers occur most commonly in older patients, but young patients with neurologic disease can be affected.

■ **Diagnosis**
Deep ulcers over bony prominences in bedridden patients suggest this diagnosis. Although the lesion is undermined, the edges are not ragged and red-purple, as in pyoderma gangrenosum. X-rays are necessary to rule out osteomyelitis. Biopsy is not diagnostic.

■ **Treatment**
Removal of pressure; treatment of infection with systemic antibiotics; surgical treatment with muscle flaps.

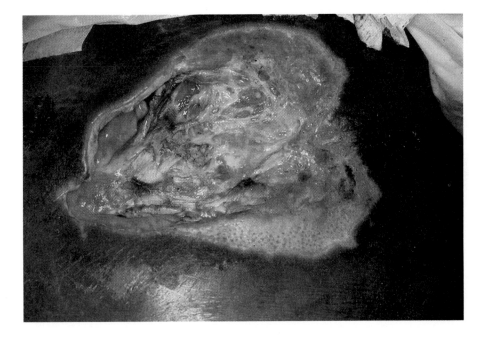

Erythema Induratum

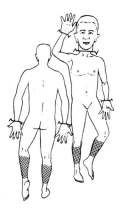

▪ Morphology
Nodules are blue to reddish brown, deep in subcutaneous fat, and firmly attached to overlying skin. Nodules frequently ulcerate. The ulcer margin may be jagged and blue. The leg may be cyanotic with a netlike fine vascular pattern. Ulcers heal with depressed atrophic scars.

▪ Distribution
Posterior calves and thighs.

▪ Patient Profile
Commonly a disease of middle-aged women (female-male ratio of 10:1), but it can occur at any age. The course is prolonged (years), with remissions and exacerbations.

▪ Diagnosis
Lesions often start in winter, possibly precipitated by cold. Rare cases are associated with active tuberculosis. Nodules on the back of the leg, which ulcerate in middle-aged women, are suggestive of this diagnosis. Biopsy shows vasculitis, granulomatous inflammation, and caseation necrosis of fat. Acid-fast stains and cultures for mycobacteria are usually negative. PCR of some patients has shown human mycobacterial DNA.

▪ Treatment
Antimycobacterial systemic therapy. SSKI useful in some patients.

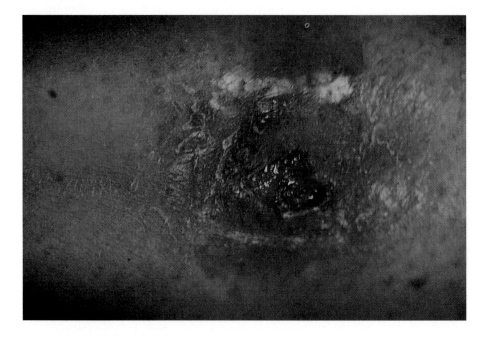

Factitial Ulceration

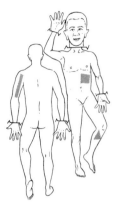

▪ Morphology
Ulcerations have unusual geometric, linear, or rectangular conformations. Lesions may have black adherent crusts, and they frequently heal with scarring.

▪ Distribution
Lesions are located at sites accessible to self-induced trauma. For example, lesions on right-handed patients are easily accessible to the right hand. Lesions are most frequent on arms and face.

▪ Patient Profile
Usually adolescents or adult women. Patients usually deny inducing lesions, and they are relatively indifferent to the lesion. Injection of drugs, especially pentazocine, may produce factitial ulceration and fibrosis. Insect bites may simulate factitial ulceration.

▪ Diagnosis
Unusual ulcerations without obvious cause should suggest this diagnosis. Therapy left to the patient does not result in improvement. Applications of occlusive dressings or casts frequently lead to healing. Biopsy is not specific. This diagnosis is one of exclusion and often difficult to prove.

▪ Treatment
Psychiatric consultation is warranted, and if self-induced disease is established, the psychiatrist should play a major role in patient management.

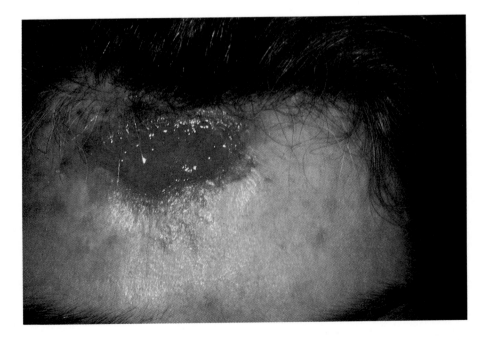

Gout

■ Morphology
Ulcerated papules and nodules are flecked with yellow and have a firm, chalky, noninflammatory base.

■ Distribution
Helix of ears; over elbows, hands, and feet.

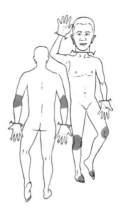

■ Patient Profile
More common in middle-aged men. A childhood form with self-mutilation and retardation occurs in boys (Lesch-Nyhan syndrome).

■ Diagnosis
Chalky material at base of ulcer has characteristic pattern of sodium urate crystals on polarizing microscopy. Deposits are not radiopaque, differentiating urates from calcium deposits.

■ Treatment
Disease resolves slowly with long-term allopurinol therapy. Very large lesions may require excision.

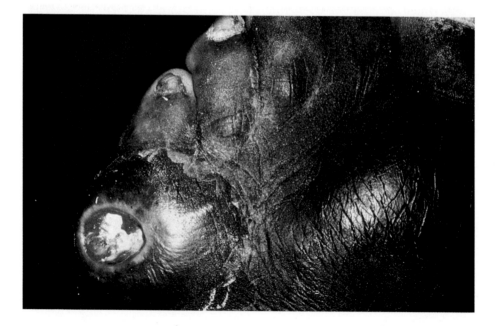

Leishmaniasis

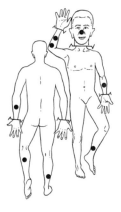

■ Morphology
Erythematous papule that slowly enlarges to become a crusted nodule. Satellite papules may be present. Ulcer formation at the site of the lesion is followed by scar formation.

■ Distribution
Lesion develops at the site of sandfly bite.

■ Patient Profile
History of travel to Asia, Africa, or Middle East. Multiple lesions may occur with *Leishmania major*. Cutaneous leishmaniasis, diffuse cutaneous leishmaniasis (DCL), mucocutaneous leishmaniasis (MCL), and visceral leishmaniasis (VL) are the different forms of the disease.

■ Diagnosis
Diagnosis is established by demonstrating the parasite on direct smear from the lesion. Staining the smear with Giemsa shows pale-blue, oval amastigotes within tissue macrophages.

■ Treatment
Cutaneous leishmaniasis is self-limited; DCL, MCL, and VL may require intralesional sodium stibogluconate or systemic pentamidine.

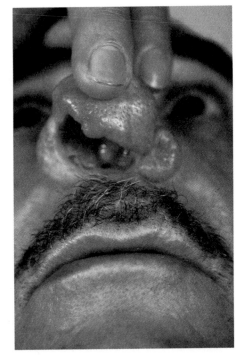

Necrobiosis Lipoidica Diabeticorum

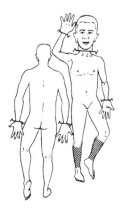

▪ Morphology
Ulcer arises in sharply circumscribed plaque. The plaque is shiny, atrophic, yellow-tan in color, and has prominent telangiectasia.

▪ Distribution
Lesions are most common pretibially and are often multiple and bilateral; they may occur anywhere.

▪ Patient Profile
More common in females than in males. In diabetics, lesions occur in childhood and in adults older than 40 years. In nondiabetics, lesions occur between 20 and 40 years of age. Chronic use of potent topical corticosteroids, especially in intertriginous areas, may result in a condition mimicking ulcerating necrobiosis.

▪ Diagnosis
Most patients have diabetes mellitus. Biopsy reveals necrobiosis, granulomatous inflammation, and thickening of vessel walls.

▪ Treatment
Occlusive dressings; potent steroids sometimes effective.

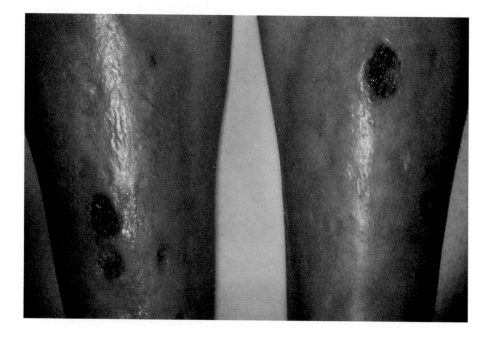

Nodular Liquefying Panniculitis
(Panniculitis with Pancreatitis)

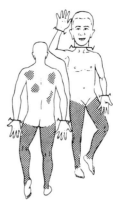

▪ Morphology
Nodules are red to violaceous and a few millimeters to many centimeters in diameter. They become fluctuant, ulcerate, exude creamy white or oily material, and heal with depressed, hyperpigmented scars. Vasculitic-like lesions may be present.

▪ Distribution
Legs, wrists, and fingers.

▪ Patient Profile
Most frequent in middle-aged men. Lesions are very tender, may occur in crops, and can be associated with fever, abdominal pain, synovitis arthritis, and polyserositis. Noncutaneous fat may be involved.

▪ Diagnosis
Pancreatitis and pancreatic adenocarcinoma cause this condition. Leukocytosis, increased serum amylase, and increased serum lipase are frequently found. Biopsy is diagnostic and shows fat necrosis (ghost cells) and deposition of calcium soaps.

Oil injections: Injections of oil into the penis and breasts may cause nodules, plaques, and ulcerations. Biopsy reveals many cavities resembling Swiss cheese and foreign-body giant cells containing refractile material.

Silicon injections can ulcerate.

Pentazocine injections: Pentazocine injections cause panniculitis with extensive fibrosis and ulceration. Fibrosis frequently extends beyond the margin of the ulceration.

▪ Treatment
Treat underlying pancreatic disease.

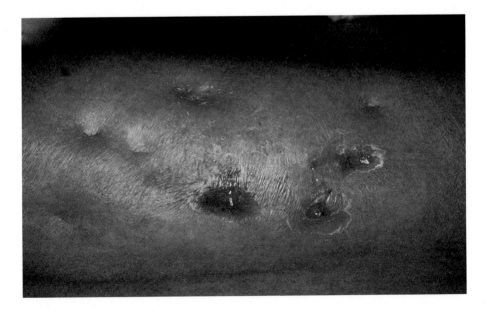

Pyoderma Gangrenosum

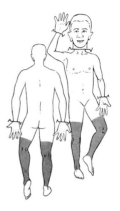

■ Morphology
Ulcers have a raised, tender, red-purple border that is undermined. The base of the ulcer is ragged, irregular, and purulent. Lesions begin as tender, red papules that progress to ulceration. Ulcers heal with atrophic, cribriform scarring. There may be an associated diffuse, pustular eruption.

■ Distribution
Most common on the lower legs but may occur anywhere. Lesions are usually single but may be multiple.

■ Patient Profile
Usually adults of both sexes. Ulcers are usually spontaneously painful and very tender. Ulcers may be induced by minimal trauma (pathergy). Pyoderma gangrenosum is associated with ulcerative colitis, granulomatous colitis, leukemia, dysglobulinemia, delayed hypersensitivity defects, rheumatoid arthritis, systemic lupus erythematosus, and chronic active cirrhosis.

■ Diagnosis
The rim of the ulcer should be biopsied for histologic examination and culture to rule out the possibility of atypical mycobacterial infection, amebiasis, deep fungal infection, blastomycosis, and cryptococcosis. Studies to rule out chronic bromide ingestion, syphilis, collagen vascular disease, and Wegener's granulomatosis should be obtained. Biopsy reveals acute and chronic inflammation and occasionally vasculitis.

■ Treatment
Treatment of underlying disease, if identified. If not (as in half of cases) or if patient is not responding to that therapy, treatments include systemic corticosteroids, using pulsed steroids intravenously; dapsone; clofazimine; or cyclosporine.

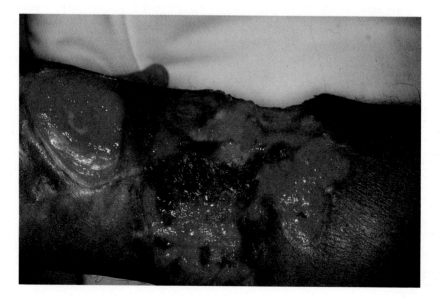

Radiodermatitis

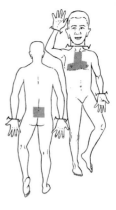

▪ Morphology
Ulceration occurs in an area of exposure to x-ray. Acute ulcerations are seen 6 to 8 weeks after radiation therapy. Lesions begin with bullae, which develop shaggy, dirty-appearing, painful ulcerations. Chronic ulcerations are sharply circumscribed and occur years after radiation in areas of radiodermatitis, which is characterized by atrophy, loss of hair, thinning, mottled hyperpigmentation and hypopigmentation, and telangiectasia.

▪ Distribution
Any area that has been irradiated.

▪ Patient Profile
Any age, both sexes. Patient gives a history of irradiation with x-rays.

▪ Diagnosis
Painful ulceration in a sharply circumscribed geometric area of radiodermatitis suggests this diagnosis. The ulcer must be biopsied to rule out the possibility of cutaneous carcinoma. Biopsy in radiodermatitis reveals epidermal atrophy, loss of appendages, fat fibroblasts, increased collagen, and thromboses of blood vessels.

▪ Treatment
Initially, occlusive dressings. If not effective, skin grafting.

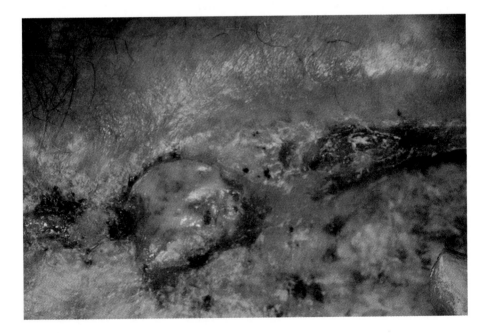

Stasis Ulcers

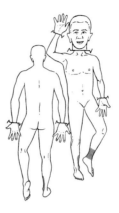

▪ Morphology
Ulcers are superficial, scooped out, 1 to 4 cm in diameter, and are found in areas of obvious venous insufficiency and stasis dermatitis. Stasis dermatitis is characterized by mottled, red-purple to brown hyperpigmentation, scaling, thinning of the epidermis, and presence of dilated superficial veins. There is often pitting edema, varicosities, and evidence of venous insufficiency.

▪ Distribution
Lesions most common over the medial malleoli. Pure venous ulcers are less frequent on the shin or over the lateral malleoli.

▪ Patient Profile
Usually adult women. This syndrome is most frequently associated with a history of deep leg vein thrombosis. Lesions commonly itch. They are not usually painful but can become tender when they are infected.

▪ Diagnosis
Ulceration over the medial malleolus in an area of hyperpigmentation and dermatitis with a history of deep vein thrombosis is diagnostic. Similar lesions may be seen in patients with lymphedema. On rare occasions, arteriovenous fistula may mimic stasis ulcers. Stasis ulcers in children and young adults should suggest the possibility of hemoglobinopathy or hereditary anemia.

▪ Treatment
Elevation of extremity to decrease edema. Systemic antibiotics for infected lesions, occlusive dressings, and pressure wraps, including Unna boots to prevent edema. Skin grafting in selected instances. Preventive therapy with supportive stockings.

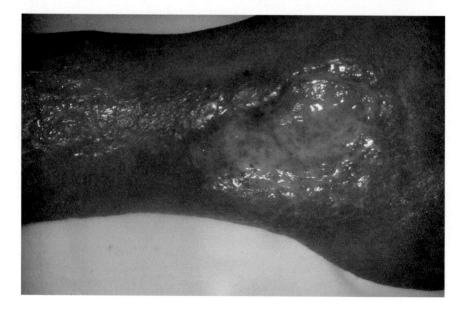

Trauma
(Mechanical Trauma, Thermal Burn,
Electrical Burn, Frostbite)

Mechanical trauma, thermal burns, electrical burns, microwave burns, exposure to chrome, and cold injuries may produce gangrene and ulceration. Geometric configuration and history of trauma suggest this diagnosis.

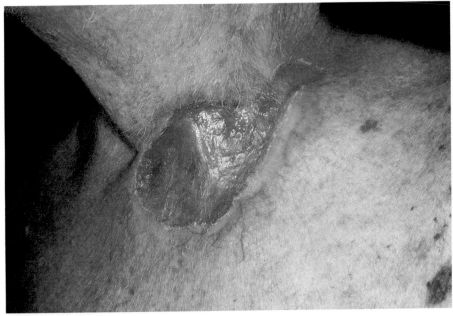

Traumatic ulcer

Tumor Nodules

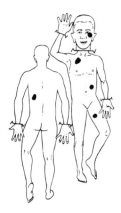

▪ Morphology
Deep. Single or multiple hard nodules that break down and ulcerate. Lesions are flesh-colored, red, brown, or blue.

▪ Distribution
Anywhere.

▪ Patient Profile
Patient has tumor. Most common tumors are basal cell carcinomas, squamous cell carcinoma, keratoacanthoma, melanoma, metastatic breast and gastrointestinal carcinoma, and Kaposi's sarcoma.

▪ Diagnosis
Biopsy demonstrates tumor.

▪ Treatment
Excision of lesion.

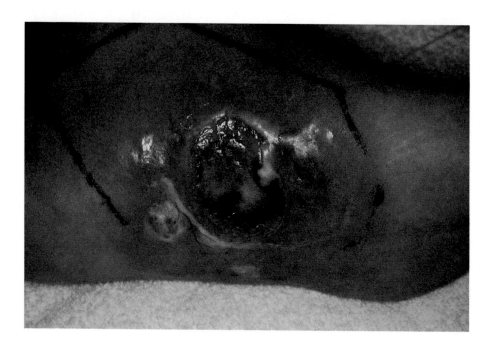

PURULENT ULCERS

DIAGNOSTIC OBSERVATIONS

Purulent ulcers have indurated bases that may be yellow, brown, white, or gray. Satellite pustules, sinuses, and papules may be seen. Evaluation of these ulcers requires:

1. Gram's stain
2. Fungal stain
3. Culture for aerobic and anaerobic bacteria
4. Culture for acid-fast organisms, including mycobacterial culture at 33°C
5. Fungal cultures

These lesions must be biopsied and the biopsy material ground for complete and adequate cultures. Patients require thorough examination for systemic disease.

MAJOR CATEGORIES

Purulent ulcers without marked adenopathy (nongenital)

Purulent ulcers with marked, often painful adenopathy

Purulent ulcers peculiar to tropical and subtropical areas

Purulent Ulcers without Marked Adenopathy (Nongenital)

Pyogenic bacteria can infect damaged skin. Abscesses can go on to ulceration and drainage. All ulcers should be carefully cultured (Table 10–1). Staphylococci commonly infect ulcers and may not be the primary pathogens.

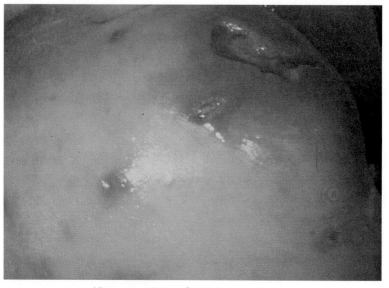

Ulcer secondary to *Staphylococcus aureus*

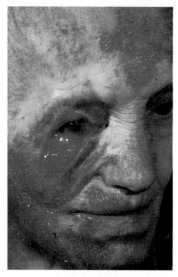

Lupus vulgaris

TABLE 10–1. **Purulent Ulcers without Marked Adenopathy in Nongenital Locations**

Disease	Systemic Symptoms	Morphology	Location	Organism
Anthrax (see p. 363)	Fever and chills	Large pustule that ulcerates and is covered with black eschar.	Anywhere; usually face and extremities.	*Bacillus anthracis.*
Atypical mycobacteria	Usually none	Warty nodule that may ulcerate.	Extensor extremities.	Atypical acid-fast bacteria. Special attention should be paid to culturing at various temperatures.
Blastomycosis	Pulmonary and urogenital disease	Indurated plaques with pustules and ulceration.	Face.	*Blastomyces dermatitidis*, bromoderma, and iododerma simulate this disease.
Botryomycosis	Fever, host usually compromised	Multiple purulent ulcers with sinus tracts containing colonies of *Staphylococcus aureus.*	Anywhere.	Exuberant growth of *S. aureus.*
Coccidioidomycosis	Meningeal, bone, and pulmonary disease	Papule or nodule that ulcerates (especially in blacks and Filipinos).	Anywhere.	*Coccidioides immitis.*
Cryptococcosis	Meningitis and pulmonary disease in immunosuppressed host	Ulcerated cellulitis plaque with bullae and hemorrhage.	Anywhere.	*Cryptococcus neoformans.*
Diphtheria	Occasional neuropathy and carditis	Ulcer with very adherent crust and decreased sensation around lesion.	Legs and flexors.	*Corynebacterium diphtheriae.*
Herpes simplex	Usually none	Shallow, clean ulcer; hemorrhagic, heaped up. May go on to chronic ulceration with heaped-up borders.	Anywhere, but often on buttocks.	*Herpesvirus hominis.*
Lupus vulgaris	Occasional weight loss and fever	Yellow-brown, atrophic scaly plaque that ulcerates.	Head and neck most common. May have painless adenopathy.	*Mycobacterium tuberculosis.*
Pasteurella multocida infection	Usually none	Inflammatory ulcer with discharge at the site of a dog or cat bite.	Extremities.	*Pasteurella multocida.*
Progressive bacterial synergistic gangrene	Fever and septicemia	Tender gangrene with zone of erythema around wound.	Perineum, abdomen.	*Streptococcus* and *Staphylococcus.*
Pseudomonas infection	Fever and septicemia in a compromised host	Sharply marginated ulcer covered by sweet-smelling, adherent eschar.	Axillary and anogenital areas.	*Pseudomonas aeruginosa.*
Tuberculosis orificialis	Moribund patient with fever	Rapidly spreading, painful, nonhealing ulcers.	Mouth, nose, and rectum.	*Mycobacterium tuberculosis.*

Purulent Ulcers with Marked, Often Painful Adenopathy

TABLE 10–2. **Purulent Ulcers with Prominent and Painful Adenopathy***

Disease	Constitutional Symptoms	History	Location	Organism
Atypical mycobacteria	None	Trauma in fresh water, especially involving fish tanks	Extremities with nodules along lymphatics	Atypical mycobacterium on biopsy and in culture (best grown at 33°C)
Cat scratch fever	+/−	Trauma from cat	Arms, hands, head, and neck	*Chlamydia* (*Bedsonia*)
Glanders	+	Exposure to horse or donkey	Mucous membranes	*Pseudomonas mallei*
Plague	++	Exposure to rat fleas	Trunk	*Pasteurella pestis* in lymph nodes
Sporotrichosis	+/−	Trauma from plants (rose bush) or timber	Nodules along lymphatics on extremities	*Sporothrix schenckii*
Tularemia	++	Exposure to rodents or ticks from rodents	Face, eyes, and extremities	*Francisella tularensis* on biopsy and culture

+/− = Inconstant; + = often present; ++ = prominent.
*These ulcers are often painful.

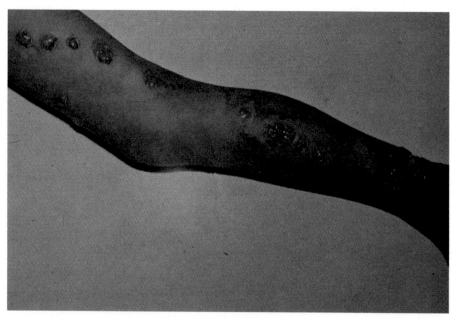

Sporotrichosis

Purulent Ulcers Peculiar to Tropical and Subtropical Areas

TABLE 10–3. **Ulcers Peculiar to Tropical and Subtropical Areas**

Disease	Constitutional Symptoms	Morphology	Location	Organism
Amebiasis	Mild	Painful ulcers with heaped-up borders, may be multiple.	Penile, perineal, or around hepatic or colonic fistulae	*Entamoeba histolytica*
Blastomycosis (South American)	Mild with adenopathy	Ulcerating warty nodule.	Around nose and mouth	*Paracoccidioides brasiliensis* (yeast with multiple buds)
Buruli ulcer	None	Undermined, immense, deep ulcers. Frequently found in children.	Legs and arms	*Mycobacterium ulcerans* (atypical mycobacterium best grown at 33°C)
Chromomycosis	None	Purulent ulcer associated with warty plaques.	Usually on shins	Fungus, *Phialophora*, or *Cladosporium* genus
Leishmaniasis	Mild symptoms with fever and weight loss	Ulcerating warty nodule that oftens heals spontaneously with scarring.	Primarily face and mucocutaneous junctions	*Leishmania tropica* or *Leishmania brasiliensis* intracellularly in macrophages
Leprosy	Mild	Neurotrophic ulcer.	Neuropathic areas, nose, and mouth	*Mycobacterium leprae* on smear or biopsy
Yaws	Occasional fever, bone lesions, and arthritis	Heaped-up, exuberant ulcer with drainage. Lesions may be single or multiple.	Anywhere	*Treponema pertenue*

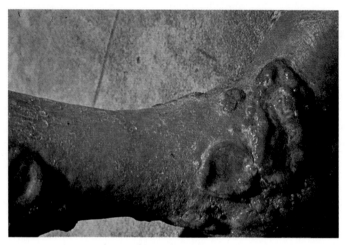

Chromomycosis

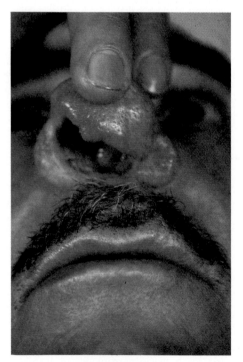

Leishmaniasis

ULCERS IN SPECIFIC LOCATIONS

Ulceration of Nasal Septum

Ulceration of the nasal septum is an uncommon but unique physical finding. Diagnosis almost always requires a thorough history, physical examination, and biopsy. Causes include:

Collagen Vascular Disease
Granulomatosis, lupus erythematosus, midline lethal granuloma, mixed connective tissue disease, relapsing polychondritis

Infection
Bacterial: noma, mycobacterial infection, tuberculosis, leprosy
Treponemal disease: syphilis, yaws
Deep fungal: blastomycosis, histoplasmosis, mucormycosis, rhinosporidiosis, sporotrichosis
Parasitic: leishmaniasis

Trauma
Inhalation of chrome or cocaine, arsenic ingestion, self-induced.

Tumor
Squamous cell carcinoma, lymphoma, chondrosarcoma, vascular neoplasm

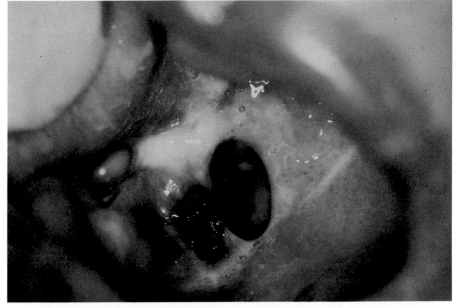

Mucormycosis

Genital Ulcers

Syphilis
(Chancre)

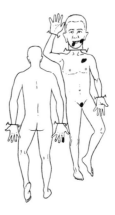

▪ Morphology
Ulcerated, pink papule or nodule with a clean, firm base and regional, nontender lymphadenopathy. Lesions usually single and relatively nontender, but on occasion may be multiple, tender, or purulent. (See Table 10–4 for more information about genital ulcers.)

▪ Distribution
Genital lesions are most common, but lesions can occur anywhere. Cervical lesions in females and perirectal lesions in males are easily overlooked. Oral lesions appear as erosions.

▪ Patient Profile
Any age, both sexes. Patient is usually exposed approximately 4 weeks before onset, but incubation period can vary from 2 weeks to 3 months. Lesion begins as a firm, nontender papule that ulcerates; spontaneously clears over days to weeks.

▪ Diagnosis
Firm, ulcerated, nontender ulcer on genitalia with regional adenopathy is diagnosed as syphilis until proven otherwise. Diagnosis can be confirmed by dark-field examination. Dark-field examination of oral lesions is not recommended, because oral spirochetes in normal flora may be difficult to differentiate from the syphilis spirochete. A positive serologic test supports the diagnosis. Serology may be negative in early lesions; in suspected cases, blood studies should be repeated weekly for 1 month, then monthly for 2 months. The fluorescent treponemal antibody-absorption serology (FTA-ABS) becomes positive earlier and is more specific than other serologic studies.

▪ Treatment
Systemic antibiotics using Centers for Disease Control and Prevention protocol.

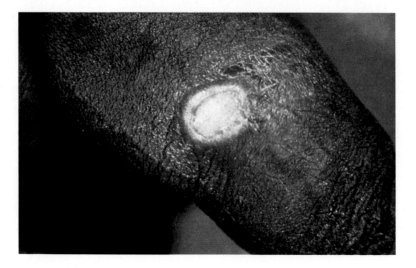

Chancroid

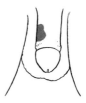

■ **Morphology**
Single or multiple ragged ulcers with yellow-gray exudate. Begin as pustules.

■ **Distribution**
Genitalia, perirectal area.

■ **Patient Profile**
Ulcers very painful. Painful unilateral inguinal adenitis (bubo) in 50% of patients.

■ **Diagnosis**
Gram-negative bacilli can be seen on Gram's stain of purulent ulcer material. Organisms can be cultured, but specimens must be plated early for best results.

■ **Treatment**
Ceftriaxone sodium 250 mg IM or erythromycin 500 mg PO qid for 7 days.

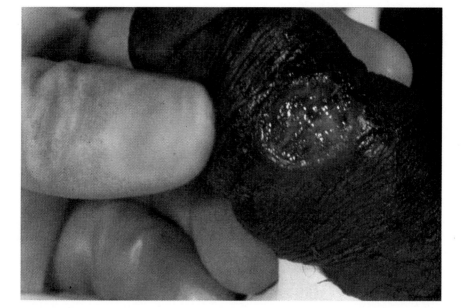

TABLE 10–4. **Genital Ulcers**

Disease	Adenopathy	Constitutional Symptoms	Morphology	Diagnosis
Aphthae	+/−	+/−	Sharply marginated, tender ulcers with a ragged base. Frequently recurrent and two to four in number. May be associated with Behçet's syndrome.	No distinctive bacteriology or biopsy.
Balanoposthitis	None	None	Inflammation and ulceration of mucosa between glans and prepuce.	Bacteria, *Candida*.
Chancroid	+, painful	+/−	Painful, multiple, nonindurated, undermined ulcers.	Extracellular, gram-negative rods in groups (*Haemophilus ducreyi*).
Chemical (quaternary amine, dequalinium)	+	None	Tender with multiple erosions and abundant white exudate.	History of topical quaternary amine.
Gonorrhea	None	+/−	Multiple, small erosions and abundant white exudate.	Gram-negative intracellular diplococci (*Neisseria gonorrhoeae*).
Granuloma inguinale	None	+/−	Nontender ulcer with a raised border. Lesion is not undermined.	Twenty times more common in males. Gram-negative rod within macrophages (*Donovania granulomatis*).

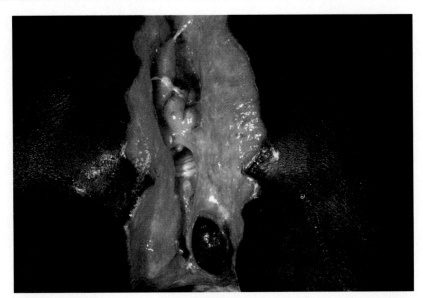

Granuloma inguinale

TABLE 10–4. **Genital Ulcers** (Continued)

Disease	Adenopathy	Constitu-tional Symptoms	Morphology	Diagnosis
Primary herpes simplex	+, may be tender	+	Multiple umbilicated vesicles with erosions going on to ulceration.	Positive Tzanck smear and culture for herpes simplex virus.
Primary syphilis (chancre)	+, painless	None	Usually single, clean, sharp punched-out ulcer with indurated base.	Positive dark-field examination, positive serology for syphilis (*Treponema pallidum*).
Recurrent herpes simplex	None	None	Groups of umbilicated vesicles with erosions going on to ulceration.	Positive Tzanck smear and culture for herpes simplex virus.
Trauma	+	+	Superficial or deep erosions.	History.
Tuberculosis	+	+	Tender, indurated papules with ulceration.	Acid-fast bacillus on smear and in culture (*Mycobacterium tuberculosis*).
Tumor	+/−	+/−	Tumor nodule with induration and ulceration.	Biopsy reveals underlying tumor. Squamous cell carcinoma most frequent.
Wart	None	None	Heaped-up cauliflower-appearing growth with ulceration.	Biopsy demonstrates papillomatosis and vacuolated cells.

+ = Common finding; +/− = inconstant finding.

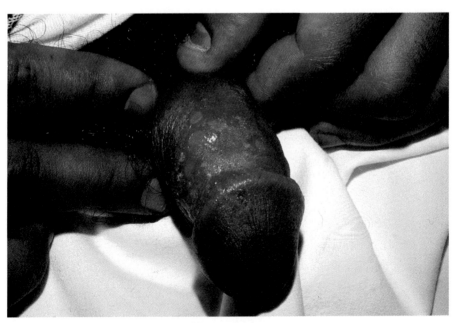

Herpes simplex

Chapter 11

■ ■

Hair and Scalp Diseases

MAJOR CATEGORIES

Acquired hair loss: normal scalp, scarred scalp
Congenital and genetic disorders: alopecia, abnormal hair
Abnormal color of hair
Increased hair growth
Scalp and hair scaling

EXAMINATION OF THE SCALP AND HAIR

General Examination

The skin of the scalp should be carefully examined. The physician observes for any abnormality, especially for signs of atrophy. These include loss of hair follicles (enhanced by side lighting, see p. 11), follicular plugging, loss of skin markings, wrinkling of the epidermis, increase or loss of pigment, telangiectasia, and sclerosis.

Potassium Hydroxide Preparation and Gram's Stain

Many infectious diseases (pyogenic bacteria and fungi) cause scalp disease and hair loss. Gram's stain and potassium hydroxide preparation and culture of the scales and extracted hairs are necessary to diagnose these causes of alopecia.

Wood's Lamp Examination

Wood's lamp examination (see p. 11) may reveal green fluorescence in alopecia caused by *Microsporum canis.*

Hair Pluck Test

The hair pluck test is essential for evaluation of any patient with diffuse alopecia. The 100 to 200 hairs that a normal individual loses every day are resting (telogen) hairs and have a small white sac at their base. With a sturdy hemostat or with a hemostat on which rubber or plastic tubing has been placed on the jaws of the clamp, the physician firmly plucks about 20 hairs from the scalp. Hairs can be examined using good light and a hand lens or the lower power of a microscope. The physician can distinguish growing (anagen) hairs, which have long, translucent root sheaths and a pigmented base, from resting hairs, which lack sheaths and have a small white sac at the base. Usually there are 85% to 90% growing hairs and 10% to 15% resting hairs. The percentage of resting hairs is markedly increased in telogen effluvium (see p. 479).

Looking at fewer than 20 hairs decreases the statistical reliability of the test; looking at more than 20 increases reliability. If hairs are not forcibly plucked or if the hemostat slides along the hairs, there will be an increased number of resting hairs in the sample, because telogen hairs are most easily removed from the scalp. Very twisted or curly hairs may break during plucking.

Morphologic Examination of Hair

Hair varies in size and color among individuals and increases in diameter during childhood. Under the 10× and 40× objective of the microscope, the physician may see abnormal morphologic findings:

Monilethrix: Hair with multiple beadlike variations in diameter. This should be verified with a binocular microscope.

Pili torti: Twisted hairs resembling ribbons. This should be verified under a binocular microscope, because the two-dimensional view of twisted hair resembles hair with varying diameters. Pili torti may be difficult to diagnose in a patient with naturally curly hair.

Trichorrhexis nodosa: Frayed hairs with ends resembling a broomstick. This is often mechanically induced by rubbing or other trauma. Rarely, this is associated with argininosuccinicaciduria, an inborn error of metabolism.

Polarizing Microscopy

Abnormalities of hair are accentuated when hairs are examined with a polarizer on a normal light microscope. Transverse alternating bands of birefringence allow a morphologic diagnosis of the trichothiodystrophy (see p. 498).

Special Chemical Studies of Hair

Hair amino acid analysis: This analysis is essential to diagnose trichothiodystrophy.

Urinary amino acids: This study is necessary only if there is a very high clinical suspicion of argininosuccinicaciduria.

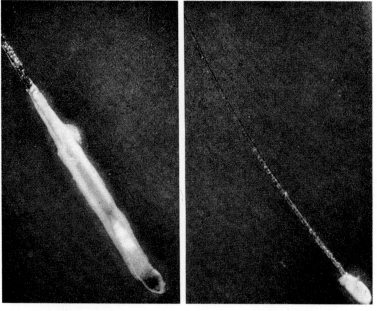

Anagen hair   Telogen hair

ACQUIRED HAIR LOSS

NORMAL SCALP
Alopecia areata
Androgenetic alopecia
Dermatophyte infection (tinea capitis)
Follicular mucinosis
Traumatic alopecia
Trichotillomania

**Hair Loss with Systemic
Diseases/Medications**
Telogen effluvium

SCARRED SCALP
Congenital scalp defect
Discoid lupus erythematosus
Folliculitis decalvans
Hot comb alopecia
Infections: bacterial, fungal, and viral
Kerion (dermatophyte infection)
Lichen planopilaris
Linear morphea
Necrobiosis lipoidica diabeticorum
Neoplasia
Nevus sebaceous
Radiodermatitis
Trauma and rarer causes

Acquired Hair Loss with Normal Scalp

Alopecia Areata

▪ Morphology
Hair loss is sharply marginated and discrete but may become confluent. The scalp is normal. Thin, often hypopigmented hairs, discrete follicles with a black stub of hair, and sparse hairs of normal length may be seen. At the edge of lesions, hairs with irregular diameters (*exclamation point hairs*) may be appreciated. This disease may involve total scalp (*alopecia totalis*) or entire body (*alopecia universalis*).

▪ Distribution
Multiple sites are common; all parts of body, especially scalp, eyebrows, eyelids, beard, trunk, and extremities may be involved. Nails may show a fine stippling of the nail plate. Vitiligo may be present.

▪ Patient Profile
Any age, both sexes. Sometimes familial. Emotional trauma may precipitate this illness.

▪ Diagnosis
The exclamation point hairs at the periphery of a lesion, which have a shaggy, broken-free tip and a tapering end in an atrophic bulb, are highly suggestive of this disease. The generally uniform pattern of hair loss excludes trichotillomania and inflammatory diseases such as syphilis. The lack of scarring excludes lupus erythematosus, scleroderma, and so forth. Hairs plucked away from involved areas show normal telogen-anagen ratios. Biopsy shows a heavy lymphocytic infiltrate in the dermis.

▪ Treatment
Topical (class I or II) or injectable corticosteroids, topical anthralin, PUVA therapy, and topical minoxidil in some cases may be helpful. Frequent spontaneous remissions complicate evaluation of therapies. Topical sensitizers under investigation.

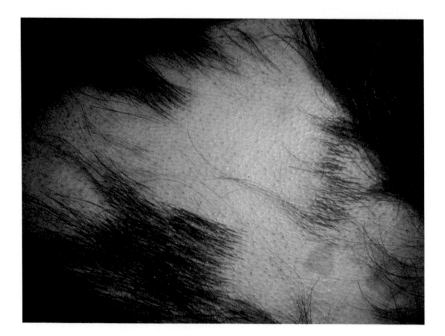

Androgenetic Alopecia

▪ Morphology
There is a gradual decrease in the number of coarse terminal hairs and in the diameter of hairs going from normal scalp to the area of alopecia. Tiny lanugo hairs can be seen in the bald areas. The lanugo hairs are thinner and lighter in color than the terminal hairs.

▪ Distribution
Scalp.

▪ Patient Profile
Adult men: Condition begins at any time after puberty. May have bilateral-frontal-temporal-central or vertex (crown) involvement progressing to balding, leaving a peripheral fringe of terminal hairs.

Adult females: Condition begins at any age after puberty and may have a diffuse form of alopecia; frequently both forms of alopecia are common within the same family.

▪ Diagnosis
Women with advanced forms of alopecia should be studied for masculinizing syndromes. Diagnosis is usually by history; biopsy is not required.

▪ Treatment
Topical minoxidil is useful, especially early in the course of the disease. Finasteride, 1 mg qd.

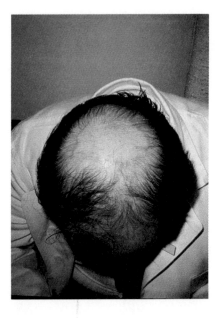

Dermatophyte Infection
(Tinea Capitis)

▪ Morphology
Single or multiple areas of short or absent hair with scaling and prominent follicles on the scalp. Nails and general body skin may be involved.

▪ Distribution
Scalp; beard, eyebrows, or eyelashes may be involved.

▪ Patient Profile
More common in children than in adults. Both sexes.

▪ Diagnosis
Infection with *Microsporum* species and some *Trichophyton* species causes hair to have a bright green fluorescence with a Wood's lamp. *Trichophyton tonsurans* causes a characteristic follicular black-dot pattern and occurs commonly in adults and children. Fungal scrapings and cultures are necessary to establish this diagnosis.

▪ Treatment
Oral griseofulvin or ketoconazole often supplemented with topical selenium sulfide. Infection should be treated until mycologically cured. Examination of other family members for mild forms of disease and treatment, if necessary, are required to eliminate reinfection.

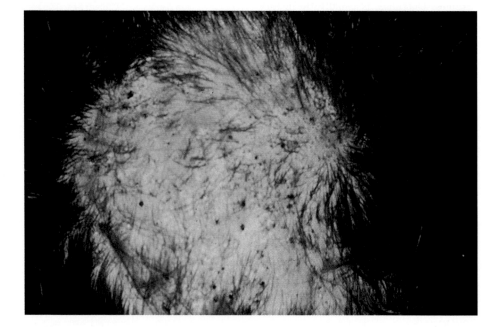

Follicular Mucinosis

■ **Morphology**
Red to blue plaques with prominent follicular openings associated with alopecia.

■ **Distribution**
Most common on scalp and face but can be anywhere.

■ **Patient Profile**
Children and adults of both sexes.

■ **Diagnosis**
In adults, this disease may be associated with lymphoma or mycosis fungoides. Biopsy is diagnostic and shows mucopolysaccharide in the outer root sheath and sebaceous glands. Systemic malignancy should be evaluated clinically.

■ **Treatment**
High-potency (class I) topical steroids or intralesional steroids. Treatment of underlying disease.

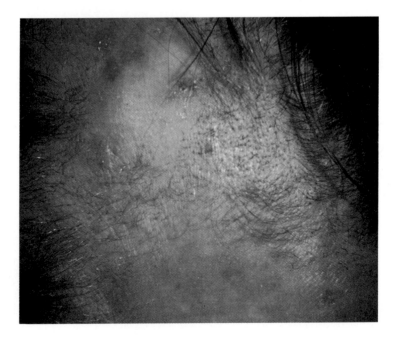

Traumatic Alopecia

▪ **Morphology**
Hairs will be broken off at various levels; scalp is usually perfectly normal.

▪ **Distribution**
Limited to scalp, often bitemporal.

▪ **Patient Profile**
Adults and children of both sexes. Reasonably common, especially in African-Americans. History of using combs, pics, tight hair rollers, braiding, excessive bleaching agents, hair straighteners, hair waving solutions, excessive exposure to ultraviolet light, or vigorous rubbing of hair when wet can lead to scarring alopecia.

▪ **Diagnosis**
Microscopic examination shows irregularly fractured hair with ends that may resemble a straw broom (trichorrhexis nodosa).

▪ **Treatment**
Avoidance of trauma to hair.

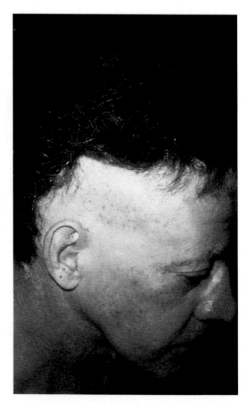

Trichotillomania

■ **Morphology**
Focal areas of thinning with hairs of very irregular lengths. The scalp is perfectly normal. Artificial or linear borders may be present.

■ **Distribution**
Scalp, eyelashes, eyebrows commonly involved.

■ **Patient Profile**
Usually children and adolescents. More frequent in females. There is a history of hair manipulation.

■ **Diagnosis**
Microscopic examination shows broken hairs; there is often a history of rubbing or pulling of the hair. Frequently there are emotional disturbances within the family.

■ **Treatment**
Professional psychiatric consultation should be recommended in severe cases. Pimozide may be useful.

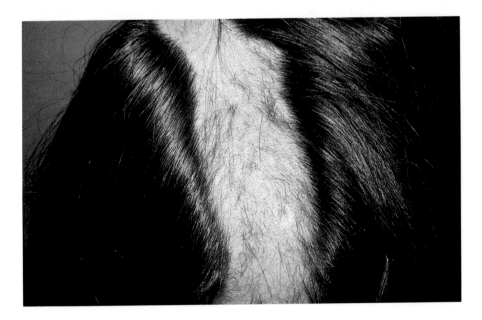

Acquired Hair Loss with Systemic Diseases

DIAGNOSTIC OBSERVATIONS
Drugs, alterations in endocrine metabolism, and generalized diseases can cause diffuse alopecia to occur over days to weeks. In some instances, this is due to telogen effluvium (see p. 479). In other instances (e.g., cytotoxic drugs), it is due to a loss of anagen hairs. Complete evaluation for the various causes listed is required to determine the exact etiology. Telogen effluvium should be considered and a hair pluck test done.

Acquired immunodeficiency syndrome.

Drugs, including methotrexate, cytoxan, and colchicine, thallium, Triparanol, isotretinoin (Accutane), etretinate, and vitamin A.

Endocrine causes: Hypopituitarism, hypothyroidism, and hypoparathyroidism.

Protein malnutrition and severe chronic disease including neoplasia.

Secondary syphilis: Commonly causes multiple areas of mild alopecia (motheaten appearance) affecting the scalp and outer eyebrows.

Systemic lupus erythematosus: Generalized alopecia, especially frontal alopecia, may be present.

Radiation therapy or electron beam therapy: Therapy to localized areas for treatment of malignancies.

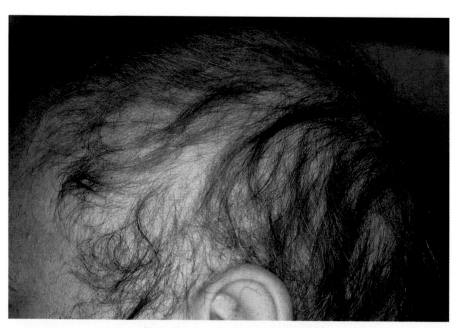

Alopecia secondary to chemotherapy

Telogen Effluvium

▪ Morphology
Hair loss with no scarring, atrophy, or erythema of the scalp. Uniform decrease in hair density. Several hundreds to thousands of hairs may be lost in a day. In areas of hair loss, growing hairs may be seen.

▪ Distribution
Scalp usually only site affected.

▪ Patient Profile
Usually adults of both sexes but does occur in childhood.

▪ Diagnosis
Parturition, stress, surgery, protein or caloric malnutrition, hypothyroidism, iron deficiency, high fever, myocardial infarction, warfarin (Coumadin) or heparin, and β-blockers may trigger this syndrome. Plucking of hair roots reveals 50% to 90% telogen hairs instead of the normal amount (<20%). Biopsy often is not necessary but shows increased numbers of telogen hairs.

▪ Treatment
Treatment of underlying disease or removal of offending drugs.

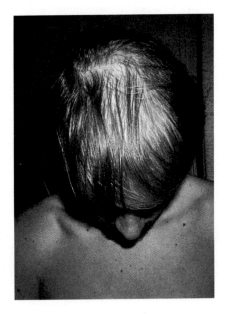

Acquired Hair Loss with Scarred Scalp

Congenital Scalp Defect
(Cutis Aplasia)

▪ Morphology
Usually single hairless area at the vertex.

▪ Distribution
Scalp. Rarely, there are associated defects on the legs.

▪ Patient Profile
Infants of both sexes are born with ulcerating lesions. Sometimes familial. Rarely associated with epidermal dysplasia or underlying cranial abnormalities.

▪ Diagnosis
Characteristic location, sparsity of lesions, and onset at birth suggest this diagnosis. Birth trauma is almost never the cause of this disorder. In extensive disease, forms of epidermolysis bullosa should be considered.

▪ Treatment
Scalp reduction or excision when patient is older.

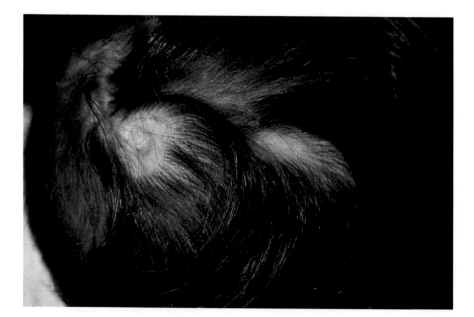

Discoid Lupus Erythematosus

▪ Morphology
Multiple areas of hair loss with thin skin, scaling, hyperpigmentation and hypopigmentation, and dilated blood vessels. Hair follicles may be completely lost. Diffuse or patchy alopecia may be present.

▪ Distribution
Scalp, face, external ear, and sun-exposed areas of body.

▪ Patient Profile
Adults of both sexes.

▪ Diagnosis
Biopsy is diagnostic and shows epidermal atrophy, vacuolar degeneration of the basal cells, and a thickened basement membrane. Immunofluorescent examination shows deposition of immunoglobulin in the basement membrane region in a large number of cases.

▪ Treatment
High-potency (class I) topical or intralesional steroids. Systemic antimalarials. Sunscreens and sun-protective clothing (hats).

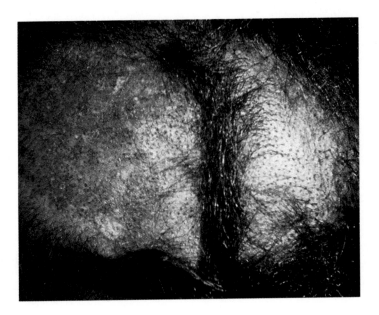

Folliculitis Decalvans

■ **Morphology**
Multiple, scattered areas of scarring (up to 5 cm) with associated perifollicular pustules.

■ **Distribution**
Scalp; rarely eyebrows.

■ **Patient Profile**
Adults of both sexes.

■ **Diagnosis**
Biopsy is nondiagnostic, showing scarring, abscesses, and pustules with polymorphonuclear leukocytes. Bacteriologic cultures should be obtained.

■ **Treatment**
Intralesional or topical corticosteroids (class I or II) may be effective early in the course. When infected, systemic antibiotics should be used; rifampicin often helpful.

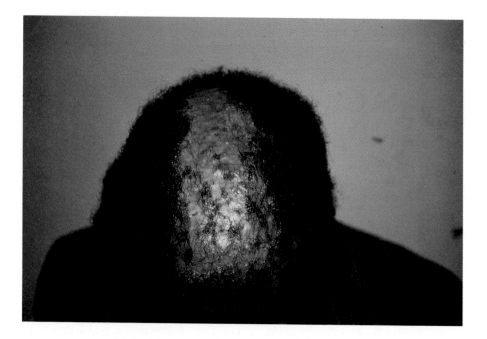

Hot Comb Alopecia
(Follicular Degeneration Syndrome)

■ **Morphology**
Irregularly defined areas with markedly decreased numbers of hairs. Scalp shows thinning of epidermis, loss of pigment, and decreased numbers of hair follicles.

■ **Distribution**
Limited to scalp.

■ **Patient Profile**
Women, blacks with tightly coiled hair. This results from use of a hot comb and petrolatum during hair-straightening process, although this is not established unequivocally.

■ **Diagnosis**
A carefully elicited history is essential for this diagnosis. Biopsy is not diagnostic but will exclude discoid lupus erythematosus and lichen planus.

■ **Treatment**
Avoidance of hot comb; surgical grafting or scalp reduction.

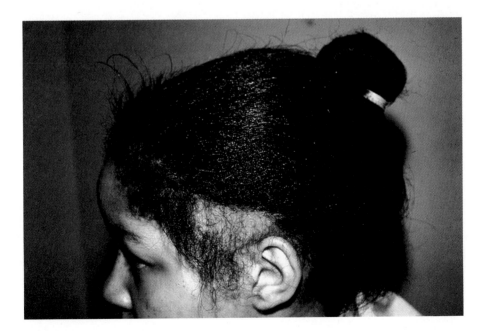

Infections

The morphology, distribution, and patient profile of the scarring alopecias secondary to infectious causes resemble that of the original infection.

Bacterial
Dissecting cellulitis of the scalp (see p. 356)
Leprosy (see p. 380)
Lupus vulgaris (see p. 385)
Pyogenic infections with streptococci and
    staphylococci

Fungal
Deep fungi (see pp. 341, 459)
Dermatophyte infection with inflamma-
    tory kerions

Viral
Varicella zoster (see p. 312)
Variola (see p. 394)

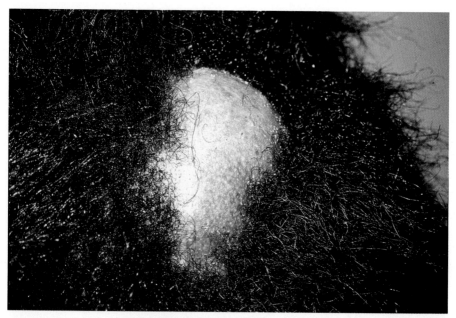

Dissecting cellulitis

Kerion
(Dermatophyte Infection)

■ **Morphology**
Usually single or multiple elevated, red, painful nodules with scarring and sometimes ulceration.

■ **Distribution**
Scalp only.

■ **Patient Profile**
Children of both sexes. Rare in adults.

■ **Diagnosis**
Single areas are called kerions and are a hypersensitivity reaction to *Microsporum* or *Trichophyton* species. Diffuse scarring is caused by *Trichophyton schoenleinii*. Potassium hydroxide preparations and fungal cultures are necessary to establish this diagnosis.

■ **Treatment**
Systemic antifungals and systemic corticosteroids for 4 to 6 weeks to decrease inflammation.

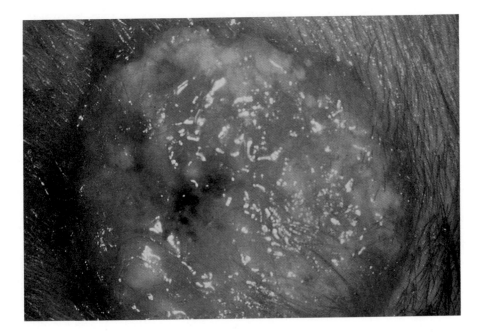

Lichen Planopilaris

▪ **Morphology**
Multiple scarred areas with associated prominent, plugged, raised follicles. Lichen planus lesions (see p. 251) may be present elsewhere.

▪ **Distribution**
Scalp; axillae, pubic area, trunk. Mucosal lesions of mouth and genitalia.

▪ **Patient Profile**
More common in adult women. Pseudopelade may be the terminal scarred stage of this disease.

▪ **Diagnosis**
Biopsy of lichen planopilaris is diagnostic, with a lymphocytic infiltrate around follicles.

▪ **Treatment**
Topical (class I or II) corticosteroids; intralesional corticosteroids, systemic antimalarials, PUVA therapy.

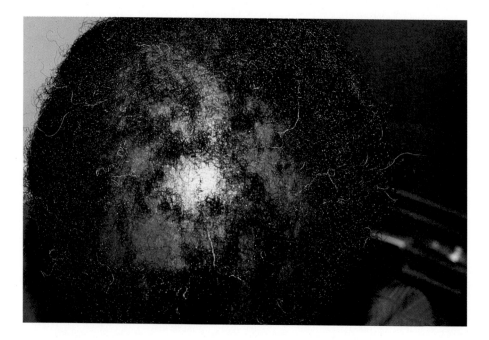

Linear Morphea
(Coup de Sabre)

■ **Morphology**
One or several areas (1 to 10 cm) with no
hair follicles and thickening and sclerosis
of the skin.

■ **Distribution**
Scalp, may extend to face.

■ **Patient Profile**
Children or young adults of both sexes.

■ **Diagnosis**
The linear lesion resembles a saber cut.
Systemic sclerosis is usually not present;
underlying bony defects may be present.
Biopsy reveals thickening of the collagen,
but this is not diagnostic.

■ **Treatment**
High-potency (class I) topical or intralesional steroids may arrest the process.

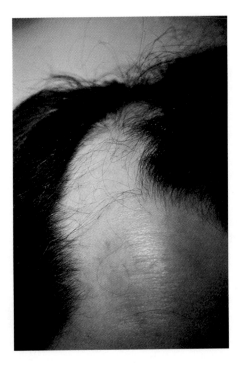

Necrobiosis Lipoidica Diabeticorum

▪ **Morphology**
Sharply circumscribed areas of hair loss confined to atrophic, yellow, telangiectatic plaques.

▪ **Distribution**
Scalp.

▪ **Patient Profile**
Adults of both sexes. Half the patients have diabetes.

▪ **Diagnosis**
Biopsy is diagnostic and shows necrosis, fibrosis, inflammation with giant cells, and increased mucin.

▪ **Treatment**
Potent (class I or II) topical corticosteroids and sometimes intralesional corticosteroids.

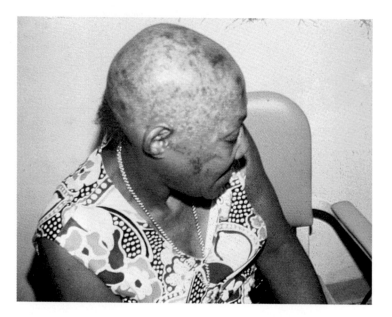

Neoplasia

■ **Morphology**
Usually single discrete area of hair loss on a firm, indurated plaque.

■ **Distribution**
Scalp.

■ **Patient Profile**
Adults of both sexes.

■ **Diagnosis**
Biopsy is essential for diagnosis. Morphea-like basal cell carcinomas; sclerosing carcinomas of the breast; metastatic ovary, stomach, prostate, and renal tumors. Systemic malignancy should be evaluated clinically.

■ **Treatment**
Surgical excision for diagnosis and treatment.

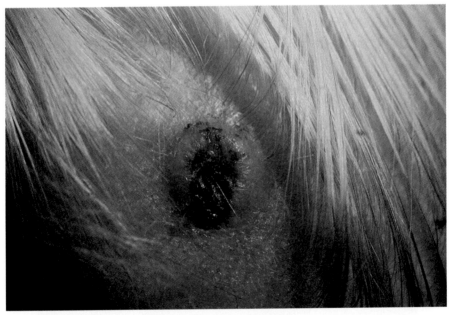

Metastatic squamous cell carcinoma

Nevus Sebaceous

▪ **Morphology**
One or several hairless, raised, yellow velvety lesions that may enlarge with age.

▪ **Distribution**
Scalp and sometimes face.

▪ **Patient Profile**
Disease is present at birth or in early childhood. Extensive lesions may be associated with convulsions and mental retardation. Lesions may develop basal cell–like carcinomas.

▪ **Diagnosis**
Biopsy is diagnostic and shows prominent sebaceous glands and decreased hair follicles at the time of puberty.

▪ **Treatment**
Surgical excision before puberty.

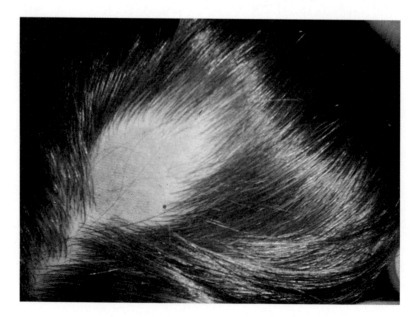

Radiodermatitis

■ **Morphology**
Localized or generalized areas of decreased hair associated with thin epidermis, hyperpigmentation and hypopigmentation, and dilated blood vessels.

■ **Distribution**
Scalp usually.

■ **Patient Profile**
Adults who have been treated with x-ray for fungal infection of the scalp (prior to 1950) or malignancy of the scalp.

■ **Diagnosis**
History of previous radiation confirms this diagnosis. Biopsy reveals radiodermatitis (see p. 453).

■ **Treatment**
Hair transplantation or scalp reduction for cosmetic results.

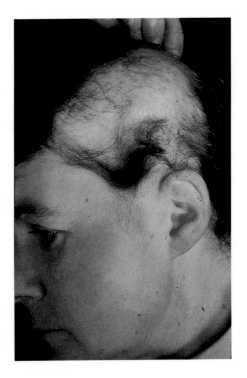

Trauma and Rarer Causes

Trauma and burns are causes of scarring alopecia, and they are evident from history. Several blistering diseases that involve the scalp can scar. These are discussed elsewhere and include dermatitis herpetiformis (see p. 287), bullous pemphigoid (see p. 291), porphyria cutanea tarda (see p. 303), epidermolysis bullosa (see pp. 299, 320–321), and cicatricial pemphigoid (see p. 492).

Inherited dermatologic diseases involving the scalp, especially Darier's disease, lamellar ichthyosis, and X-linked ichthyosis, may be associated with alopecia. *Ulerythema ophryogenes* has associated eyebrow thinning and follicular keratoses. *Keratosis follicularis spinulosa decalvans* has scalp and brow alopecia with extensive follicular keratoses. *Incontinentia pigmenti* (see p. 300) is a blistering disease, occurring predominantly in females, in which scalp scarring may occur. *Conradi's disease* is associated with ichthyosis-like changes with whorl-like markings, bone changes, and, rarely, scarring alopecia.

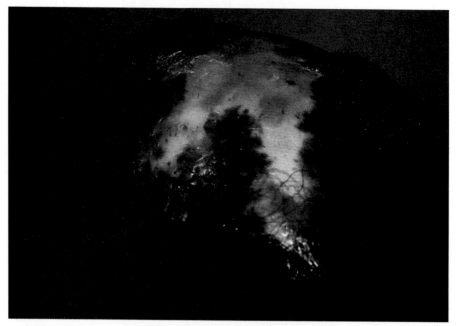

Cicatricial pemphigoid

CONGENITAL OR GENETIC DISORDERS OF HAIR

DIAGNOSTIC OBSERVATIONS
A large number of hereditary disorders have generalized hypotrichosis. Hair with abnormal shape or consistency may fracture easily and the patient may present with a complaint of thinning of the hair or alopecia.

MAJOR CATEGORIES

Alopecia with Normal Hair Shaft
Anhidrotic ectodermal dysplasia
Hidrotic ectodermal dysplasia

Alopecia with Abnormal Hair Shaft
Monilethrix
Pili torti: Menkes' syndrome and uncombable hair syndrome
Trichothiodystrophy
Trichorrhexis nodosa

Other Alopecias

Generalized
Cartilage-hair hypoplasia: dwarfism
Dyskeratosis congenita (see p. 46)
Hallermann-Streiff syndrome: dwarfism, aplastic mandible
Myotonic dystrophy: myotonia, testicular atrophy
Netherton's syndrome: ichthyosis, atopic diathesis
Pachyonychia congenita: palmar and plantar keratoses, nail defects
Rothmund-Thomson syndrome (see p. 100)
Trichorhinophalangeal syndrome: large philtrum, cone-shaped epiphyses
Turner's syndrome: dwarfism, webbed neck, 45,XO karyotype
Unna's hair dystrophy
Werner's syndrome: progeria (see p. 393)

Localized
Congenital skin defects
Poland's syndrome: unilaterally absent axillary hairs, breast, greater pectoral muscle, and brachysyndactyly
Testicular feminization syndrome

Abnormal Hair without Alopecia
Pseudofolliculitis barbae
Ringed hair
Wooly hair nevus

Alopecia with Normal Hair Shaft

Anhidrotic Ectodermal Dysplasia

▪ Morphology
Decreased numbers of hairs are present. Some of the hairs are thinner and some are coarser than normal.

▪ Distribution
Scalp, eyebrows, eyelashes, and other areas of body hair.

▪ Patient Profile
Disease begins in childhood, males more commonly affected than females. Decreased sweating, absent or abnormally shaped teeth (pegged), depressed nasal bridge, hypoplastic maxillae, and atopic dermatitis are often present. Nails are normal.

▪ Diagnosis
Decreased sweating may be elicited by history. Examination of the palms and soles with a binocular microscope or Nin-hydrin sweat test reveals decreased sweat glands. Dental x-rays can be useful for detecting caries. The disease is X-linked and carrier females may be affected significantly. DNA markers on the X chromosome can be used for prenatal or postnatal diagnosis in most familial cases.

▪ Treatment
Avoidance of high temperatures. Wigs for cosmetic improvement. Dental consultation.

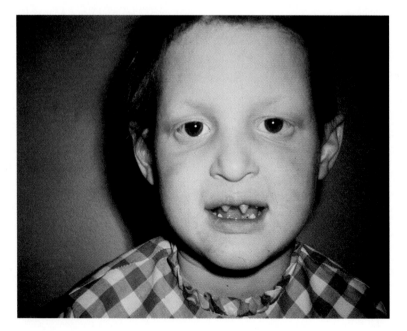

Hidrotic Ectodermal Dysplasia

▪ **Morphology**
Complete or partial absence of hair.

▪ **Distribution**
Scalp; other areas of body frequently affected.

▪ **Patient Profile**
Disease starts in infancy or childhood; both sexes affected equally. Autosomal dominant inheritance. Palmar and plantar hyperkeratosis frequently present. Short nails and marked separation of the nail plate from the nail bed (onycholysis) frequent; normal sweating.

▪ **Diagnosis**
Association of decreased hair with abnormality of nails and palms and soles is diagnostic. Biopsy is not diagnostic. Acrosyringeal hypertrophy on biopsy of nail folds.

▪ **Treatment**
Cosmetic, with wigs.

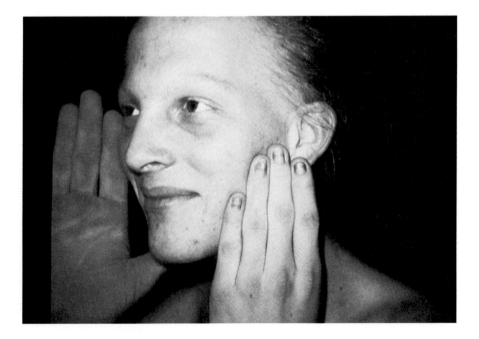

Alopecia with Abnormal Hair Shaft

Monilethrix

▪ **Morphology**
Hair is very short and may have a beaded quality; scaly papules are seen around hair follicles and on the neck.

▪ **Distribution**
Scalp and other portions of the body.

▪ **Patient Profile**
Disease begins in childhood; autosomal dominant trait.

▪ **Diagnosis**
A positive family history coupled with the microscopic examination of the hair, which shows a beaded appearance, confirms this diagnosis.

▪ **Treatment**
None available.

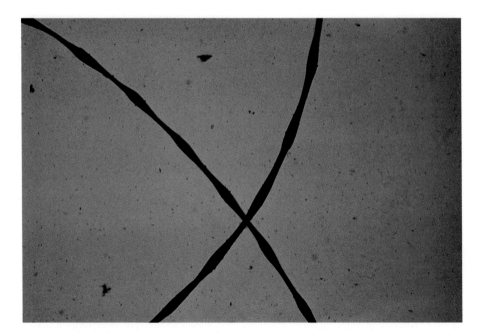

Pili Torti

▪ **Morphology**
The hair is grossly twisted, will not lie flat, and has an irregular, disorderly appearance. Only portions of the scalp may be involved, especially in the acquired forms.

▪ **Distribution**
Scalp and other areas of body hair.

▪ **Patient Profile**
Childhood; young adults in acquired forms.

▪ **Diagnosis**
Microscopic examination, especially with a dissecting microscope, demonstrates twisting of the hair. In the acquired forms of this disease, the individual has progressively larger areas of the scalp involved with coarsely twisted, kinky hairs. The tightly twisted, ribbonlike hair is seen as an isolated, congenital defect, or sometimes associated with deafness or with Menkes' syndrome.

Menkes' syndrome: This syndrome is a disorder of copper metabolism present only in males (X-linked inheritance) and associated with hypothermia, mental and growth retardation, enlargement of bony epiphyses, and low levels of blood copper and ceruloplasmin. The hair in Menkes' syndrome may also be thin. The gene for this syndrome codes for a copper-binding protein present in many tissues. Prenatal diagnosis possible in some cases.

Uncombable hair syndrome: Both sexes involved during childhood with dull, lusterless hair that does not lie flat and has irregular, twisted hair shafts.

▪ **Treatment**
None available.

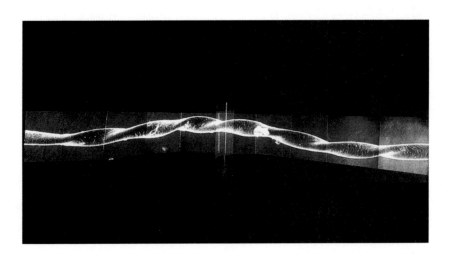

Trichothiodystrophy

▪ **Morphology**
Lusterless, short hair that breaks easily.
The scalp is otherwise normal.

▪ **Distribution**
Scalp.

▪ **Patient Profile**
Disease begins in childhood of both sexes.
Autosomal recessive inheritance, may be
associated with mental retardation, thin
nails, ichthyosis, and decreased fertility.

▪ **Diagnosis**
Examination of hair with a polarizing
microscope shows alternating bands of
birefringence. Chemical examination of
hair shows a low sulfur content and a low
content of the amino acid cysteine.

▪ **Treatment**
No specific treatment available.

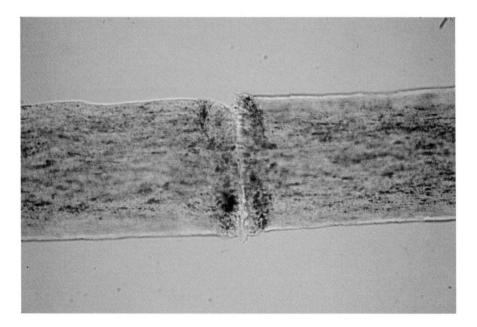

Trichorrhexis Nodosa

■ **Morphology**
Hairs are of irregular length and may have shiny highlights; many hairs may be broken.

■ **Distribution**
Scalp predominantly.

■ **Patient Profile**
Children and adults of both sexes. Usually history of trauma to hair.

■ **Diagnosis**
Microscopic examination shows broomstick fractures of the hair. Children with evidence of mental retardation, seizures, episodic lethargy and ataxia, hepatomegaly, and trichorrhexis nodosa should have their urine analyzed for increased levels of argininosuccinic acid.

■ **Treatment**
Treatment for underlying biochemical defect with arginine supplementation has helped the hair in patients with the liver defect in argininosuccinase. Most patients have no underlying metabolic defect and should be told to avoid excessive rubbing or brushing of the hair when it is wet.

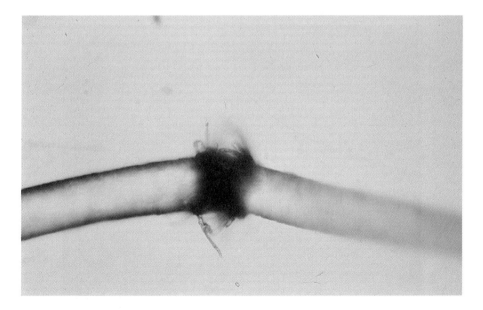

Abnormal Hair without Alopecia

Pseudofolliculitis Barbae

▪ **Morphology**
Multiple, tightly curled hairs that grow into the facial and neck skin, producing red papules and pustules.

▪ **Distribution**
Neck, face, and scalp.

▪ **Patient Profile**
Black-skinned adult men who shave.

▪ **Diagnosis**
Coarse hairs curving back into the skin produce this characteristic disease. Biopsy is nondiagnostic.

▪ **Treatment**
Topical Retin-A, topical antibiotics, medium-potency topical steroids (class III or IV). Growing a beard is therapeutic. If the patient must shave, depilatories, special razors, and not shaving close to avoid re-entry of hair into follicle.

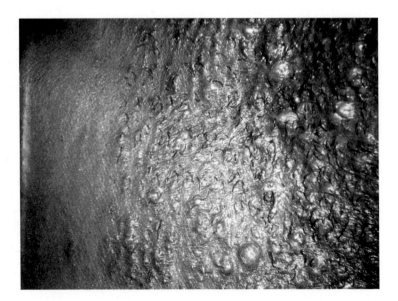

Ringed Hair

■ **Morphology**
Alternating light and dark bands are seen on the hair.

■ **Distribution**
Scalp.

■ **Patient Profile**
Onset during childhood. Both sexes affected. Familial.

■ **Diagnosis**
Microscopy confirms gross banding pattern. This is a normal variant without significant fragility of the hair.

■ **Treatment**
None necessary.

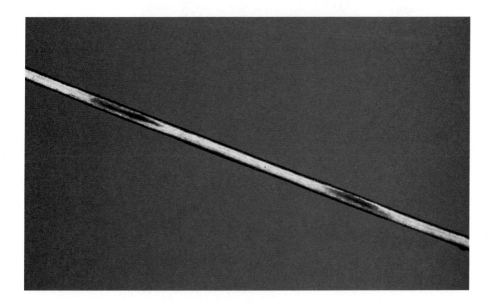

Wooly Hair Nevus

▪ **Morphology**
Discrete areas (1 to 10 cm in diameter) of
abnormally tight, curled hair differing in
consistency and color from surrounding
hair.

▪ **Distribution**
Scalp.

▪ **Patient Profile**
Onset at birth or during childhood. Both
sexes. Acquired pili torti begins focally in
late adolescence.

▪ **Diagnosis**
Discrete patch of abnormal hair is distinctive. Rarely, there are associated defects of
the teeth.

▪ **Treatment**
None available.

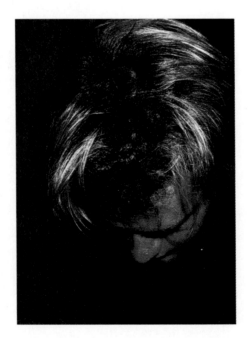

ABNORMAL COLOR OF HAIR

Any patient with a dramatic color change of the hair should be questioned about the use of hair preparations.

Focal areas of white or gray hair may be associated with several disease states, including:

Alopecia areata (see p. 472).

Piebaldism (see p. 114).

Tuberous sclerosis (see p. 115).

Vitiligo (see p. 112).

Vogt-Koyanagi syndrome.

White forelock.

Diffuse diminution in pigment occurs in:

Albinism (see pp. 111–112).

Chédiak-Higashi syndrome (see pp. 111–112).

Gray hair (poliosis), appearing gradually, is most often a function of aging.

Green hair may be associated with copper exposure, especially through water.

Pernicious anemia.

Phenylketonuria (see p. 381).

White hair may appear in blond patients taking chloroquine.

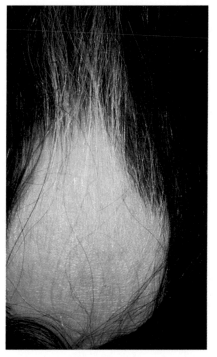

Alopecia areata

INCREASED HAIR GROWTH (HIRSUTISM AND HYPERTRICHOSIS)

DIAGNOSTIC OBSERVATIONS

Hirsutism refers to male hair patterning in women and is androgen induced. Coarse terminal hairs appear on the upper lips, chin, cheeks, trunk, limbs, and male escutcheon. Virilization may or may not be present. Women of different racial groups have different amounts of hair in these body areas, and this must be considered in making the diagnosis of hirsutism. Patients with hirsutism require complete medical evaluations including laboratory tests of pituitary, adrenal, and ovarian function. A description of the complete workup and differential diagnosis in these cases is beyond the scope of this text.

Hypertrichosis is excessive hair growth. It can be generalized or localized, congenital or acquired.

MAJOR CATEGORIES

Acquired

Anorexia nervosa and malnutrition

Dermatomyositis

Drug-related hypertrichosis: diphenylhydantoin, streptomycin, diazoxide, and corticosteroids (systemic or topical), cyclosporine, minoxidil

Epidermolysis bullosa dystrophica (see p. 299)

Hypothyroidism: increased hair, especially in children

Porphyrias: hexachlorobenzene intoxication, erythropoietic porphyria, and porphyria cutanea tarda (hypertrichosis most prominent on face)

Pretibial myxedema: coarse, terminal hairs found within plaque

Sequela of central nervous system disease or injury

Surrounding wounds

Congenital or Genetic

Generalized

Congenital macrogingivae syndrome

Cornelia de Lange's syndrome: cutis marmorata, dwarfism

Hurler's syndrome: coarse facial features, mental and physical retardation

Hypertrichosis lanuginosa: congenital and acquired

Increased mucopolysaccharide in skin and urine

Leprechaunism: redundant skin and abnormal face

Lipodystrophic diabetes: loss of subcutaneous fat, acanthosis nigricans, hypertriglyceridemia, insulin-resistant diabetes

Localized

Becker's nevus (see p. 37)

Faun-tail nevus: over lower spine, associated with spina bifida occulta

Fetal alcohol syndrome: hypertrichosis of eyebrows and across glabella

Giant hairy nevus

Waardenburg's syndrome: increased hair over glabella (see p. 114)

Congenital or Genetic Increased Hair Growth

Hypertrichosis Lanuginosa

▪ **Morphology**
Very long (10 cm), fine, silky hairs are present.

▪ **Distribution**
Generalized: entire body except palms and soles.

▪ **Patient Profile**
Children usually can be diagnosed in infancy. Both sexes. Familial forms exist. Acquired forms starting in adult life associated with internal malignancy.

▪ **Diagnosis**
The clinical appearance is diagnostic. Adults with the acquired form must be studied for internal malignancies.

▪ **Treatment**
Identification of underlying malignancies in adult patients.

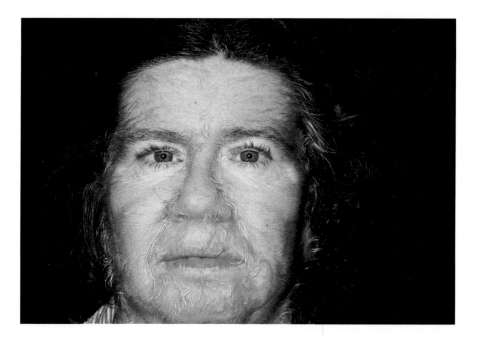

Giant Hairy Nevus

▪ Morphology
One or more lesions up to 30 cm in size with black, brown, and blue hyperpigmented macules, papules, and nodules, often with coarse and prominent terminal hairs.

▪ Distribution
Localized: trunk commonly, but can be anywhere. Leptomeningeal melanosis common, with lesions over spine, and magnetic resonance imaging indicated.

▪ Patient Profile
At birth or in early infancy.

▪ Diagnosis
Lesions, usually large, present at birth, with a characteristic biopsy showing nevus cells infiltrating between collagen bundles, confirm this diagnosis. High incidence of malignant melanoma, especially in large lesions, requires prompt diagnosis and treatment.

▪ Treatment
Lesions should be observed regularly for changes and removal with staged surgical excision.

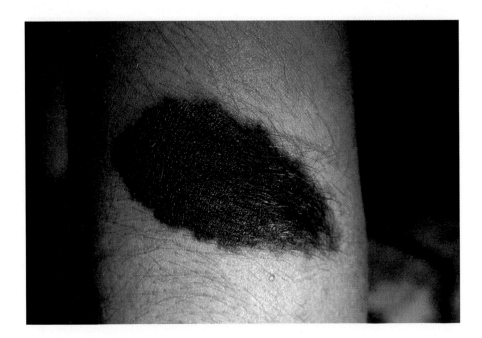

SCALP AND HAIR SCALING

Scaling of the Scalp

Scales on the hair can be easily removed. Scaling of the scalp can be caused by a variety of diseases, discussed elsewhere:

Atopic dermatitis (see p. 243): diffuse scaling

Dandruff (see p. 260): mild form of seborrheic dermatitis

Dermatophyte infection (see p. 246): single or multiple circumscribed plaques

Cutaneous lupus erythematosus (see p. 384): scaling associated with atrophy

Neurodermatitis (see p. 239): scaling of scalp with thickening of skin

Psoriasis (see p. 258): sharply circumscribed plaques anywhere on body

Seborrheic dermatitis (see p. 260): diffuse scaling most prominent around ears

Tinea amiantacea: very thick, asbestos-like scales of the scalp occurring as a result of any of the diseases listed above

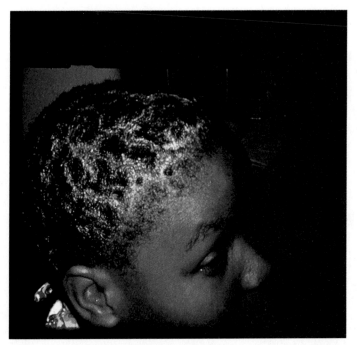

Tinea amiantacea

Firmly Adherent Material on the Hair

Firmly adherent material on the hair suggests several diagnoses:
Pediculosis capitis
Piedra
Trichomycosis axillaris

Pediculosis Capitis

▪ **Morphology**
One or more 1- to 2-mm shiny white egg cases from several millimeters to several centimeters above the scalp. Nits on adjacent hairs are often at the same level above the scalp. Erosions of the scalp and lymphadenopathy occur.

▪ **Distribution**
Scalp, beard, pubic and axillary hairs.

▪ **Patient Profile**
Children and adults of both sexes.

▪ **Diagnosis**
Microscopic examination reveals translucent, double-walled egg cases and *Pedicu-*

lus humanus. Careful examination of playmates and family members.

▪ **Treatment**
Pyrethrin to scalp twice weekly for 2 weeks.

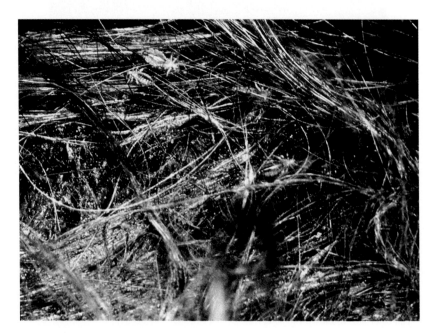

Piedra
(Black and White)

■ Morphology
One or more black or white nodules firmly
adjacent to the hair.

■ Distribution
Scalp or beard.

■ Patient Profile
Adult or children of both sexes. More
common in tropical climates.

■ Diagnosis
Microscopic examination of nodules reveals hyphae with prominent mycelia. Culture of black nodules reveals *Piedraia hor-
tae* (black piedra). Culture of the white
nodules reveals *Trichosporon cutaneum*
(white piedra).

■ Treatment
Topical imidazoles to affected sites.

Trichomycosis Axillaris

▪ **Morphology**
Multiple yellow, red, or black nodules are firmly attached to the brittle hair.

▪ **Distribution**
Axillae, pubic area.

▪ **Patient Profile**
Adults of both sexes.

▪ **Diagnosis**
Potassium hydroxide preparation shows multibranching hyphal elements.

▪ **Treatment**
Topical imidazoles.

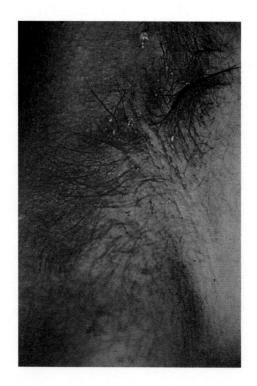

Chapter 12

■ ■

Nail Diseases

DIAGNOSTIC OBSERVATIONS

To properly diagnose disorders of the nails, the physician must decide if the primary disease involves the nail plate, nail bed, or nail folds.

The *nail plate* is the portion commonly called the "nail," which must be trimmed or cut regularly. It is formed predominantly by the *nail matrix*, which is seen as the lunula (half moon) visible at the base of some nails.

The *nail bed* is under the nail plate and makes a small but important contribution to the normal nail plate. The *posterior nail fold* is proximal, at the base of the nail plate; it is contiguous with the epidermis of the dorsum of the distal phalanx. Two *lateral nail folds* are present on the lateral borders of the nail plate and are contiguous with normal epidermis. Diseases of the nail folds and nail bed can interfere with nail plate growth. Compression of the nail plate against the nail bed can determine whether color changes in the nail are in the bed or in the plate. Colors in the plate are unchanged by compression, whereas those in the bed are often altered by compression. To properly diagnose nail disorders, complete examination of the skin and mucous membranes is essential, because many generalized diseases affect the nails. Potassium hydroxide (KOH) scraping and culture should be done in the diagnosis of nail disorders, because dermatophyte and candidal infections of the nails are common. Biopsy of the nail requires good anesthesia, and the technique for this procedure is described in standard texts.

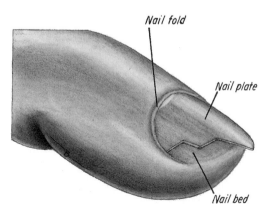

Nail fold

Nail plate

Nail bed

MAJOR CATEGORIES

Nail Plate
Acquired loss
Color changes
Congenital absence
Increase in size
Pits and grooves
Thickening
Thinning

Nail Fold
Acute paronychia
Chronic paronychia
Ingrown nails
Mucous cysts
Papules and cysts of the nail folds
Telangiectasia

Nail Bed
Color changes
Subungual hyperkeratosis
Tumors

DISORDERS INVOLVING THE NAIL PLATE

Loss of the Nail Plate (Acquired)

Major Categories

Permanent Nail Plate Loss (Complete or Partial)

Inflammatory, infiltrative blistering, or vascular diseases of the nail matrix, nail folds, or nail beds may cause permanent loss of portions of the nail plate. These diseases include:

Amyloidosis (see p. 265)

Arterial occlusion, especially scleroderma (see p. 379), Raynaud's phenomenon (see p. 106), and diabetes mellitus

Darier's disease (associated with thin and brittle nail plates)

Dyskeratosis congenita: childhood and adolescence (see p. 46)

Epidermolysis bullosa and other blistering diseases (especially junctional and dystrophic forms) (see pp. 299, 320–321)

Lichen planus

Lupus erythematosus (see p. 252)

Radiodermatitis (see p. 453)

Severe trauma

Temporary Nail Plate Loss

Destruction of the nail plate by dermatologic or infectious disease is usually not permanent.

Candida infections including mucocutaneous candidiasis

Dermatophyte infection

Exfoliative erythroderma of any cause

Psoriasis, pityriasis rubra pilaris, and acropustulosis

Radiation therapy

Reiter's disease

Scabies

Nail Plate Loss Due to Separation of the Nail Plate from the Nail Bed (Onycholysis)

Dermatophyte infection

Dermatitis

Drug-related separation

Hidrotic ectodermal dysplasia

Hyperthyroidism and hypothyroidism

Nail cosmetic treatments

Paronychia

Porphyria cutanea tarda

Psoriasis

Reiter's disease

Trauma: physical or chemical

Weed killers: paraquat and diquat

Permanent Nail Plate Loss

Lichen Planus

▪ Morphology
Thin to absent nail plates with prominent linear markings; posterior nail fold may scar and fuse with nail bed, forming a winglike structure (pterygium). Separation from the nail bed and subungual hyperkeratosis may be present.

▪ Distribution
Toe nails and finger nails.

▪ Patient Profile
Adults of both sexes. Usually evidence of lichen planus (see p. 251) elsewhere.

▪ Diagnosis
Presence of lichen planus elsewhere and biopsy of nail matrix that shows a band-like lymphocytic infiltrate with vacuolization of the basal cells are diagnostic.

▪ Treatment
Topical corticosteroids (class I or II) under occlusion; intralesional corticosteroids.

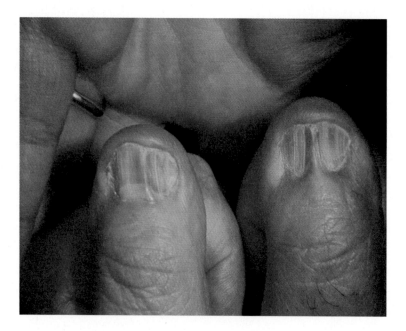

Temporary Nail Plate Loss

Dermatophyte Infection
(Onychomycosis)

▪ Morphology
The plate becomes opaque (white or yellow), frays, cracks, thickens, and develops debris beneath it. The entire plate may be destroyed and replaced by irregular, disorganized debris. The nail folds are normal.

▪ Distribution
More common on feet than on hands. May have all or only one or two nails involved.

▪ Patient Profile
Adults of both sexes. Often evidence of fungal infection on the skin and especially in the finger and toe webs. HIV-infected patients may have unusual patterns of disease.

▪ Diagnosis
Dermatophytes seen on KOH preparation of scrapings taken from beneath the nail plate at the most proximal point in relation to the nail fold. *Trichophyton rubrum* is usual cause.

▪ Treatment
Oral antifungal agents (imidazoles or terbinafine). Intermittent oral agents often effective.

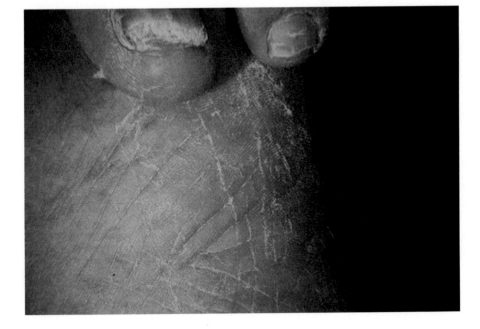

Psoriasis and Pityriasis Rubra Pilaris

▪ **Morphology**

Pitting, separation of the nail plate from the nail bed, subungual splinter hemorrhages, thickening of the plate, brown discoloration of the plate, and partial or complete loss of the plate may occur.

▪ **Distribution**

One to all nails.

▪ **Patient Profile**

All ages (most common in adults), both sexes. Distal phalangeal joint arthritis may be present.

▪ **Diagnosis**

Often psoriasis (see p. 258) or pityriasis rubra pilaris (see p. 256) can be detected elsewhere. Nail changes are not permanent. *Candida* may superinfect psoriatic nails. Biopsy shows epidermal hyperplasia with parakeratosis.

▪ **Treatment**

Topical corticosteroids (class I or II) under occlusion; intralesional corticosteroids. Topical PUVA therapy.

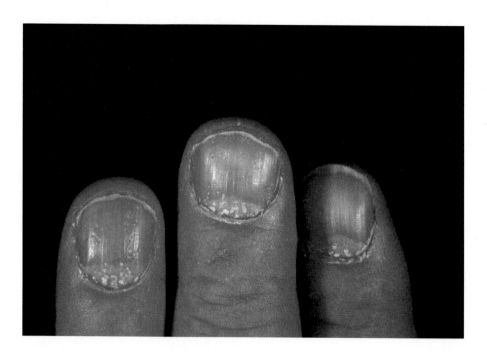

Reiter's Disease

■ **Morphology**
Destruction of the nail plate and pustular lesions of the nail bed and folds occur. Marked erythema of the digits and palmar and plantar pustules may be present in psoriasis and Reiter's disease.

■ **Distribution**
Finger and toe nails.

■ **Patient Profile**
Adults. Reiter's disease is more common in males. Fever, arthritis including sacroiliitis, urethritis, conjunctivitis, and oral lesions common in Reiter's disease. Variants of psoriasis (pustular psoriasis and acrodermatitis continua of Hallopeau) have similar nail changes.

■ **Diagnosis**
Sterile pustules with associated systemic complaints suggest Reiter's disease; patients with this disease are frequently HLA-B27 positive. Psoriasis-like skin lesions are often found on the body. Biopsy shows psoriasiform dermatitis with intraepidermal spongiform pustules.

■ **Treatment**
Topical corticosteroids (class I or II) under occlusion; intralesional corticosteroids. Topical PUVA therapy. Systemic retinoids or methotrexate for severe disabling disease.

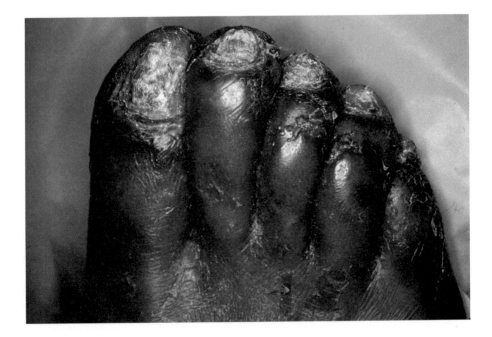

Scabies
(Norwegian Scabies)

▪ **Morphology**
Destruction of the nail plate associated with subungual debris. Scaling, crusts, and redness of the entire skin may be present.

▪ **Distribution**
All finger and toe nails.

▪ **Patient Profile**
Any age, both sexes. Patient is often institutionalized. Lesions are nonpruritic.

▪ **Diagnosis**
Mites (*Sarcoptes scabiei* var. *hominis*) are abundant in scrapings from skin lesions and debris under nails.

▪ **Treatment**
Meticulous application of permethrin (Elimite) over entire body, including under nails, weekly until clear. Nails must be cut short. Ivermectin for difficult-to-treat cases.

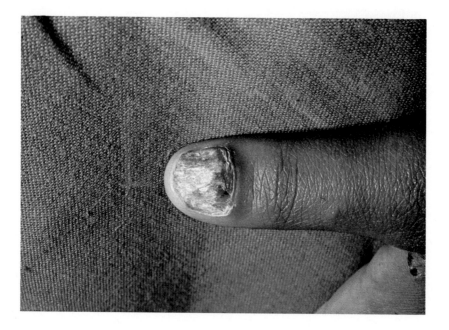

Loss of the Nail Plate due to Separation from the Nail Bed (Onycholysis)

The separated portion of the nail plate is opaque and often has an irregular, attached proximal margin. The separation is usually distal. Proximal separation is a sequela of trauma or an acute paronychial infection (see p. 528). The causes of onycholysis are listed in Table 12–1.

TABLE 12–1. **Causes of Onycholysis**

Disease	Associated Features and Clues to Diagnosis
Dermatitis	Reddish scaling of finger tips or nail folds.
Dermatophyte infection	Rarely is onycholysis the sole sign. Positive scrapings and culture.
Drug-related separation	Tetracyclines and intense sunlight. Psoralens and ultraviolet light A (PUVA). Sudden, painful.
Hidrotic ectodermal dysplasia	Palmar-plantar hyperkeratosis and nonscarring alopecia.
Nail treatments	Nail hardeners with formaldehyde or occlusive artificial nails.
Paronychia	Usually after acute paronychia. Minor degrees of separation with chronic paronychia.
Psoriasis, Reiter's disease	Psoriasis usually elsewhere. May be only nail sign of disease.
Trauma, physical or chemical	Nails may shed after traumatic hematomas. Excessive use of water and detergent may cause separation and splitting of nail plate distally.
Other	Hyperthyroidism and hypothyroidism, hyperhidrosis, yellow nail and shell nail syndromes, paraquat and diquat weed killers, porphyria cutanea tarda.

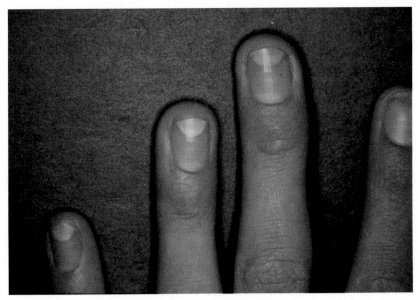

Tetracycline-induced onycholysis

Color Change in the Nail Unit

TABLE 12–2. **Causes of Color Change in Nails**

Color	Morphology	Causes
Black-brown	All nail beds initially	Addison's disease, melanoma with diffuse melanosis, antineoplastic drugs, zidovudine (AZT).
	One or more nails—plate	Nevus, melanoma (common in blacks). Hair dyes, metallic dyes (Grecian Formula).
	One or more nails	Film-developing chemicals, arsenic or gold exposures; psoriasis, chronic malaria.
Green	A few nails	Infection with *Pseudomonas* or *Candida*.
White	All nails—plate	Hereditary (leukonychia totalis).
	Transverse stripes—bed	Trauma, arsenic (Mees' lines); thallium poisoning, associated with systemic illness.
	Stipples—plate	Fungi (*Trichophyton mentagrophytes.*)
	Great toe nails—plate	Fungi (*Scopulariopsis brevicaulis*).
Yellow	All nails—plate	Yellow nail syndrome.
	One or more—plate	*Candida albicans,* nicotine, hair dyes, psoriasis.

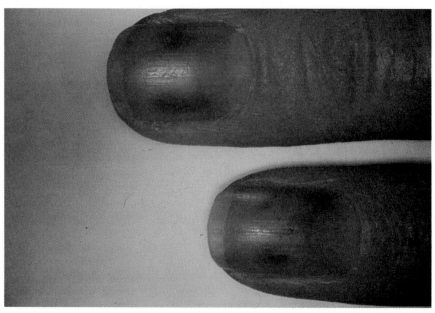

Chloroquine-induced nail color

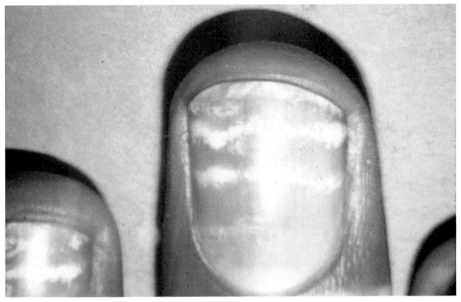

Acquired leukonychial bands after erythema multiforme

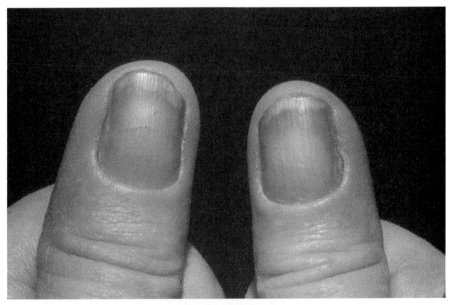

Yellow nail syndrome

Absence of Nail Plate

Congenital Absence

▪ **Morphology**
A portion of the nail plate or the entire nail plate may be absent from birth.

▪ **Distribution**
Finger and/or toe nails; often symmetric.

▪ **Patient Profile**
Congenital; both sexes; familial.

▪ **Diagnosis**
The congenital form has bony abnormalities of the hands and feet. The nail patella syndrome has small or absent nails (invariably involving the ulnar portion of the thumb), absent patella, and posterior bony iliac spines and renal abnormalities. Nail plate may be absent at birth in Hay-Wells syndrome. Epidermal nevus can be associated with decreased and irregular nail plates.

▪ **Treatment**
None.

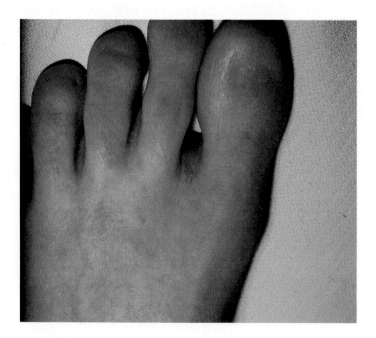

Increase in Size of Nail Plate

An increase in the size of the nail plate accompanies clubbing. The angle between the nail and the posterior nail fold increases, approaching a straight line. Clubbing may be idiopathic, but among its many causes the physician must consider:
Intestinal diseases
Pulmonary and cardiac diseases (including lung carcinoma)
Thyroid acropachy with pretibial myxedema (see p. 381)

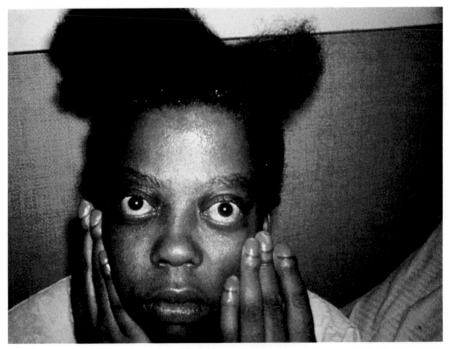

Thyroid acropachy

Pits and Grooves in the Nail Plate

Pits and grooves are caused by alterations in nail growth, which can be due to systemic factors or associated with dermatologic diseases. The dermatologic disease may be generalized or limited to the nails. Many normal people have pits with no apparent cause.

SYSTEMIC CAUSES
Systemic causes include bacterial and viral infections, coronary occlusions, and hypocalcemia. When grooves (Beau's lines) occur, they may not be seen until weeks after the insult.

DERMATOLOGIC CAUSES

Generalized Diseases
Psoriasis (see p. 258): coarse or fine pits, a few to several hundred
Alopecia areata (p. 472): usually multiple fine pits
Dermatitis of posterior nail fold

Localized Diseases
Median nail dystrophy: vertical grooves in most nails with the shape of a fir tree; apex closest to posterior nail fold
Paronychia: especially chronic
Trauma: biting, hitting, occupational trauma, or posthematoma

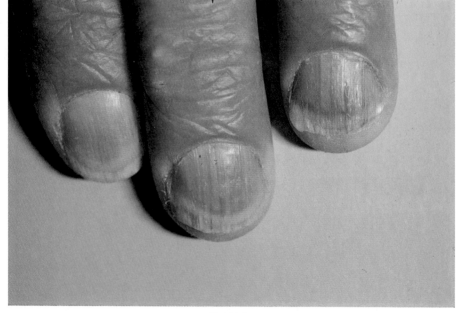

Psoriasis

Increased Thickness of the Nail Plate

Patients with this common complaint need a complete history and physical examination, and careful fungal scrapings and culture. See Table 12–3.

TABLE 12–3. **Causes of Increased Thickness of the Nail Plate**

Disease	Associated Features and Clues to Diagnosis
Dermatophyte infection	Irregular thickening. Toe nails involved more commonly than finger nails. Usually evidence of skin involvement. Positive scrapings and culture. *Trichophyton rubrum* most common cause.
Impaired circulation	Uniform thickening. Secondary bacterial or candidal infection may occur.
Pachyonychia congenita	Subungual debris, sebaceous cysts, palmar and plantar hyperkeratosis, and teeth present at birth.
Psoriasis and pityriasis rubra pilaris	Other signs of these cutaneous diseases.
Yellow nail syndrome	Lymphedema; shell nail may be variant.

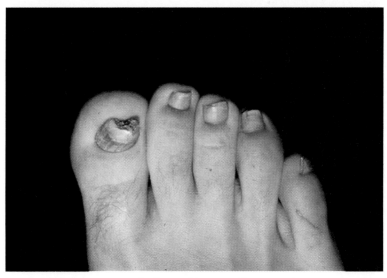

Pachyonychia congenita

Thinning of the Nail Plate

Both systemic and dermatologic diseases must be considered in determining the etiology of thinner-than-normal nail plates. See Table 12–4.

TABLE 12–4. **Causes of Thin Nail Plates**

Diseases	Associated Features and Clues to Diagnosis
Blistering diseases with scarring	Lichen planus and epidermolysis bullosa.
Darier's disease	White and red longitudinal stripes and chipping of nail plate. Associated papular skin lesions.
Dyskeratosis congenita	Reticular hyperpigmentation, telangiectasia, hyperkeratosis of palms and soles, leukoplakia, anemia; usually males.
Familial tendency	No associated disease. Nails also may be spoon-shaped (concave, koilonychia).
Iron deficiency	Often with spooning; family spooning occurs.
Raynaud's disease	History of vasospastic episodes.

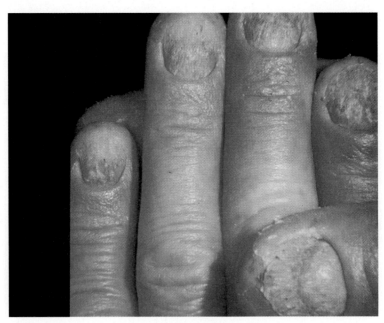

Lichen planus

DISORDERS INVOLVING THE NAIL FOLDS

The main disorders involving the nail folds include:
Acute paronychia
Chronic paronychia
Ingrown nails
Mucous cyst
Papular diseases
Telangiectasia

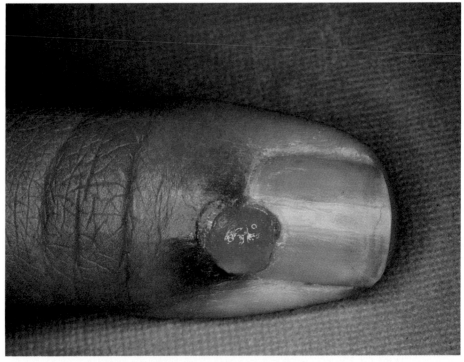

Pyogenic granuloma (see p. 222)

Acute Paronychia

▪ **Morphology**
Red, hot, swollen posterior or lateral nail folds, sometimes with draining pus.

▪ **Distribution**
Nail folds, usually hands.

▪ **Patient Profile**
Any age, both sexes. Painful. Acute onset (1 to 5 days).

▪ **Diagnosis**
Gram's stain and culture are usually positive for staphylococci, *Pseudomonas,* or streptococci. Herpes simplex may involve the nail fold when inoculated by biting; in that case, the giant cell preparation is positive.

▪ **Treatment**
Systemic antibiotics and frequent warm saline or 0.25% acetic acid soaks.

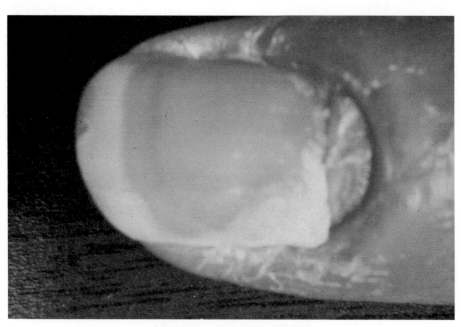

Streptococcus-induced paronychia

Chronic Paronychia

▪ Morphology
Redness and swelling of posterior and lateral nail folds with coarse, irregular ridging and brownish discoloration of the nail plate.

▪ Distribution
Hands, often middle and index finger. Rarely are all nails involved.

▪ Patient Profile
Most common in adult women and in those whose hands are in water a great deal. Lasts weeks to months to years. Often coexists with vaginal candidiasis.

▪ Diagnosis
The nail plate changes are secondary to chronic inflammation. *Candida* is most frequent cause and can be demonstrated by KOH preparation and culture. *Pseudomonas* may also be a cause. Tumors of the nail bed (see p. 537) may present as paronychia and should be considered when the paronychia on a single finger does not respond to therapy.

▪ Treatment
Topical or systemic imidazoles, keeping hands dry.

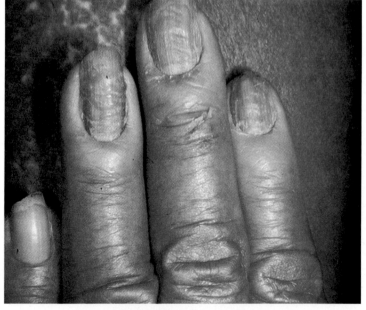

Candida-induced paronychia

Ingrown Nail

▪ **Morphology**
Swelling, redness, and tenderness of the lateral nail fold.

▪ **Distribution**
Big toe nail most commonly involved.

▪ **Patient Profile**
Adults of both sexes. Tight shoes and cutting the nail plate back too far are the contributing causes.

▪ **Diagnosis**
Portions of nail plate can be seen penetrating into the lateral nail fold.

▪ **Treatment**
Surgical removal of ingrowing nail border and possible partial surgical obliteration of lateral portion of nail matrix.

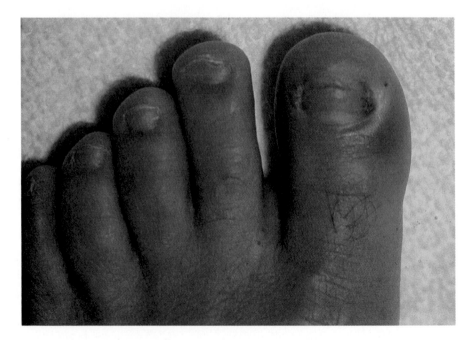

Mucous Cyst

■ **Morphology**
Translucent, cystic swelling just behind the posterior nail fold, often distorting the nail and producing ridges or deep grooves. Usually single lesion.

■ **Distribution**
Usually hands.

■ **Patient Profile**
Adults of both sexes.

■ **Diagnosis**
Viscous fluid can be removed from the lesion, thereby establishing the diagnosis.

■ **Treatment**
Intralesional corticosteroids, cryotherapy, surgical removal of cyst.

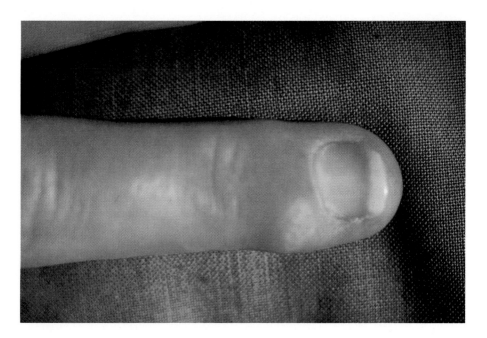

Papular Diseases Involving Nail Folds

Discrete papules may be in the nail folds or under the nails, distorting their growth. These usually represent:

Fibroma of tuberous sclerosis (see p. 000)

Glomus tumor: subungual, painful

Melanoma: blue-black macule, or papule (see p. 000)

Multicentric reticulohistiocytosis (see pp. 000, 000)

Nevi (see p. 000)

Pyogenic granuloma: beefy-red papule, bleeds easily (see illustration, p. 000)

Subungual exostoses: benign tumor, sometimes painful, great toe most commonly involved

Warts (see p. 000)

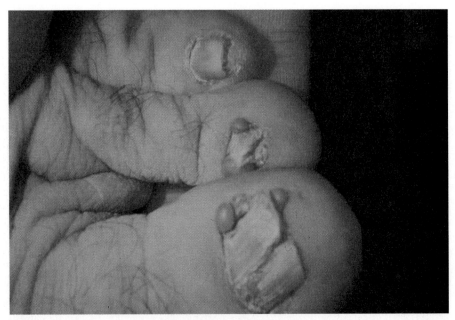

Fibromas of tuberous sclerosis

Telangiectasia

Prominent dilated vessels with their long axes parallel to the axes of the digits are seen on the posterior nail folds of patients with progressive systemic sclerosis, systemic lupus erythematosus, dermatomyositis, rheumatoid arthritis, and Raynaud's disease. The presence of these vessels requires the physician to study the patient for these diseases. Some dilated vessels in this location are a normal finding in older patients.

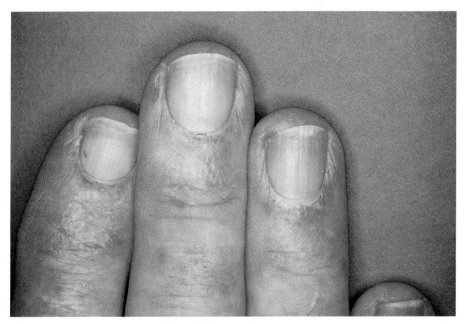

Systemic lupus erythematosus

DISORDERS INVOLVING THE NAIL BED

Disorders of the nail bed include:
Color changes: primarily in the nail bed (Table 12–5)
Subungual hyperkeratosis: often associated with onycholysis

Tumors of the nail bed: displacing the nail plate (Table 12–6)

Nail Bed Color Changes

TABLE 12–5. **Causes of Nail-Bed Color Changes**

Color	Morphology	Causes
Blue	Lunula	Cyanosis, argyria, Wilson's disease, fixed drug reaction, ochronosis, reaction to phenothiazines
Brown	Distal (with proximal white)	Chronic renal disease (half-and-half nails)
	Linear	Nevus and melanoma (common normal variant in African-Americans)
	Diffuse	Addison's disease, melanoma, antineoplastic drugs
Red to brown	Localized	Trauma, glomus tumor (painful)
	Linear	Splinter hemorrhages: trauma, vasculitis, trichinosis, psoriasis, subacute bacterial endocarditis
White	Complete or partial	Chronic renal disease, low plasma albumin, anemia (increased sympathetic activity with vasoconstriction)
	Two transverse lines	Hypoalbuminemia (Muehrcke's lines)

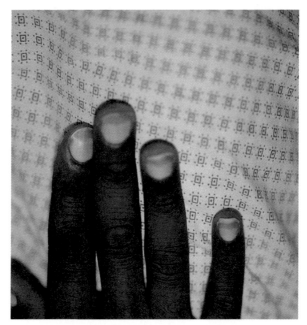

Half-and-half nails of chronic renal disease

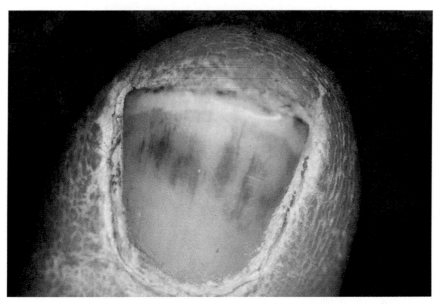

Splinter hemorrhages due to bacterial endocarditis

Subungual Hyperkeratosis

The causes of subungual hyperkeratosis
include:
Bowen's disease of nail bed
Dermatitis of the distal phalanges
Dermatophyte infection (see p. 246)
Epidermal nevi (see p. 265)
Exfoliative erythroderma (see p. 248)
Incontinentia pigmenti (see p. 300)
Lichen planus (see p. 251)
Mycosis fungoides (see p. 253)
Pachyonychia congenita (see p. 525): pas-
    sive leading to a tall, concave nail plate
Parakeratosis pustulosa: first and second
    phalanges in children
Psoriasis and pityriasis rubra pilaris
Squamous cell carcinoma of the nail bed
Tyrosinemia II: palmar and plantar hyper-
    keratosis and keratitis (see p. 280)

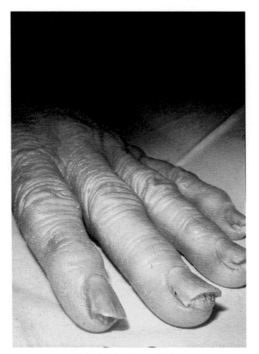

Pityriasis rubra pilaris

Tumors Involving the Nail Bed

These tumors may displace the nail plate.

TABLE 12–6. **Diagnosis of Nail Bed Tumors**

Disease	Clinical Features	Diagnosis
Enchondroma	Paronychia	Radiolucent bone defect on x-ray
Glomus tumor	Bluish, painful	Bone defect on x-ray
Keratoacanthoma	Painful, irregular surface, often ulcerated, paronychia	Bony destruction on x-ray
Melanoma	Linear or diffuse brown color, chronic paronychia	Malignant melanocytes on biopsy
Pigmented nevus	Dense, pigmentation	Nests of nevi cells on biopsy
Squamous cell carcinoma (and Bowen's disease)	Painful, paronychia with irregular surface	Invasive atypical epidermal cells on biopsy
Tuberous sclerosis	Smooth, flesh-colored papule	Fibroma associated with signs of tuberous sclerosis
Warts	Verrucous, heaped-up surface	Paring reveals multiple bleeding points

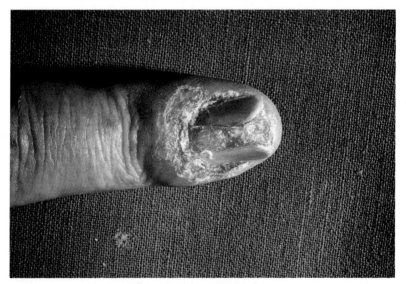

Bowen's disease

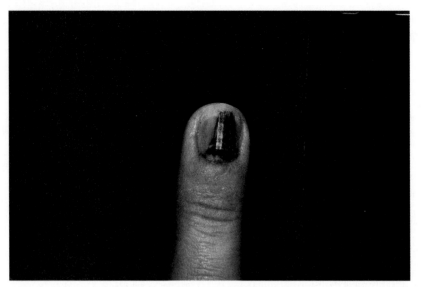

Malignant melanoma

Chapter 13

■ ■

Mouth Lesions

DIAGNOSTIC OBSERVATIONS

To diagnose oral lesions, the physician must use good lighting, a tongue blade, and a gloved hand to judge infiltration and the extent of a lesion. Lesions can be:
Flat or raised
White or pigmented
Compressible, blistered, or ulcerated

MAJOR CATEGORIES

Blistered or Ulcerated
Hypersensitivity-related diseases
Infectious diseases
Neoplastic diseases
Other etiology

Flat or White

Acute
Blistering diseases
Burn
Chemical
Infectious diseases
Mechanical trauma

Chronic

Pigmented

Raised
Cysts
Diffuse thickening of gingivae
Papules and plaques
Vascular lesions

Tongue Lesions
Atrophy
Enlargement

Tooth Defects
Abnormal color
Peg-shaped teeth

BLISTERED OR ULCERATED MOUTH LESIONS

DIAGNOSTIC OBSERVATIONS
Oral blisters will easily erode and ulcerate. Because these two groups of disorders overlap, they are considered together.

Oral ulcers require a complete history, physical examination, and biopsy. The biopsy should be studied histologically for deep fungi, acid-fast organisms, and immunofluorescence. A portion of the biopsy should be cultured. White blood cell counts and serologic tests for syphilis are also mandatory.

MAJOR CATEGORIES

Hypersensitivity-Related Diseases
Benign mucous membrane pemphigoid and other immune blisters
Contact dermatitis
Dermatitis herpetiformis (see p. 287)
Erythema multiforme and toxic epidermal necrolysis
Lupus erythematosus (see p. 252)
Midline lethal granuloma (see p. 441)
Pemphigoid (see p. 291)
Pemphigus (see p. 324)
Wegener's granulomatosis

Infectious Diseases
Aphthous stomatitis
Fungal etiology
   Aspergillosis
   Cryptococcal candidiasis
   Histoplasmosis
   Mucormycosis (in diabetics) (see p. 187)
Mycobacterial infection
   Tuberculosis
   Leprosy
Spirochetal etiology
   Chancre
   Tertiary syphilis (gumma) (see p. 402)

Yaws (see p. 461)
Vincent's stomatitis
Viral etiology
   Herpes simplex
   Herpes zoster
   Other: chickenpox, hand-foot-and-mouth disease, herpangina, smallpox, vaccinia

Neoplastic Diseases
Eosinophilic granuloma
Lymphoma, leukemia (see p. 220)
Squamous cell carcinoma (see p. 472)
Metastatic carcinoma (see p. 220)

Other Etiologies
Agranulocytosis
Antimetabolite therapy (see p. 591)
Epidermolysis bullosa (see p. 330)
Lichen planus (see p. 251)
Parulis (ruptured periodontal abscess)
Reiter's disease
Trauma

Blistered or Ulcerated Mouth Lesions: Hypersensitivity-Related

Benign Mucous Membrane Pemphigoid and Other Immune Blisters

▪ Morphology
Erosions and rarely blisters are found that heal very slowly and sometimes not at all.

▪ Distribution
Anywhere.

▪ Patient Profile
Adults of both sexes.

▪ Diagnosis
Pemphigus (see p. 324) frequently begins as persistent oral erosions and ulcers. In pemphigoid (see p. 291) and dermatitis herpetiformis (p. 287), erosions are usually a minor part of the clinical spectrum. In mucous membrane pemphigoid, oral, eye, and other mucosal involvement is usually more prominent than the skin lesions; lesions go on to scar. Histologic and immunofluorescent studies (see p. 21) of the blisters can be used to confirm these diagnoses.

Blistering and desquamation may be limited to the gingivae; this is called *desquamative gingivitis*. The many causes of this syndrome include lichen planus, bullous pemphigoid, mucous membrane pemphigoid, pemphigus, lichen planus, and sometimes natural or surgically created menopause.

▪ Treatment
Mild or limited cases of the immune-related blistering disease respond to topical (class I or II) corticosteroids or intralesional steroids. More severe cases often have severe skin involvement and require systemic corticosteroids and possibly antimetabolites.

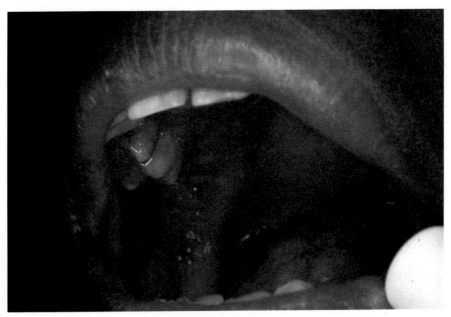

Pemphigus vulgaris

Contact Dermatitis

▪ **Morphology**
Blisters with erythema and crusting.

▪ **Distribution**
Anywhere; often includes lips.

▪ **Patient Profile**
Any age; both sexes. May be recurrent, although each episode self-limited.

▪ **Diagnosis**
Rapid onset related to intake of an offending antigen intraorally. Antigen may be drug, toothpaste, mouthwash, lipstick, lozenges, denture material, or poison ivy leaves.

▪ **Treatment**
Topical (class I or II) corticosteroid ointments or systemic corticosteroids.

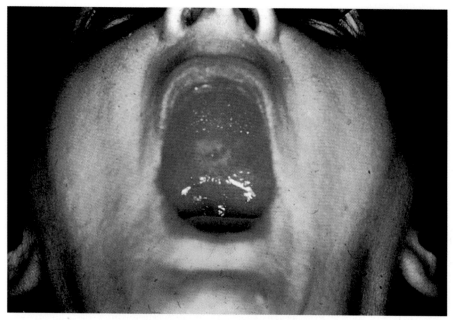

Contact dermatitis related to dentures

Erythema Multiforme and Toxic Epidermal Necrolysis

▪ Morphology
Extensive erosions, which may be hemorrhagic and crusted. Lesions may be discrete or confluent.

▪ Distribution
Anywhere.

▪ Patient Profile
Adults of both sexes. Acute. Skin lesions of erythema multiforme (see p. 288) or toxic epidermal necrolysis (see p. 326) may be present. Fever and malaise may be present. Erythema multiforme is often recurrent and may coexist with and be precipitated by herpes simplex or drug use.

▪ Diagnosis
The systemic toxicity in the disease distinguishes it from aphthous stomatitis. Biopsy shows a destruction of the basal layer in erythema multiforme and extensive mucosal necrosis in toxic epidermal necrolysis.

▪ Treatment
Frequent rinses with hydrogen peroxide mouthwashes. Systemic antibiotics for secondary infection. Use of oral corticosteroids controversial but contraindicated in herpes simplex–induced disease.

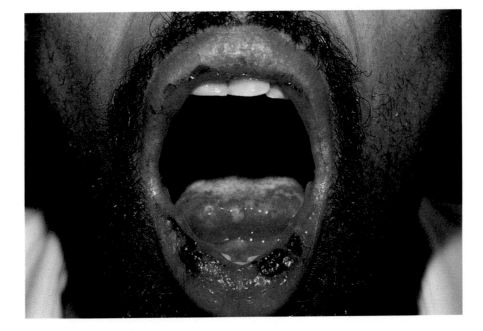

Blistered or Ulcerated Mouth Lesions: Infectious

Aphthous Stomatitis

▪ **Morphology**
One or more vesicles with a gray base and red rim.

▪ **Distribution**
The movable oral mucosa, sparing the hard palate and attached gingivae.

▪ **Patient Profile**
All ages, both sexes. Acute course. Painful lesions that last 7 to 10 days. Frequently recurrent. May recur with measles or trauma.

▪ **Diagnosis**
The small number of lesions and short clinical course suggest this diagnosis. Increased frequency with ileitis; ulcerative colitis; and deficiencies of iron, folate, and vitamin B_{12}. Biopsy is nondiagnostic. Deeper ulcerative lesions that heal with scarring are part of the spectrum of aphthous stomatitis (Sutton's disease; periadenitis mucosa necrotica recurrens). Antimetabolite therapy for neoplasia or psoriasis produces similar lesions. Behçet's syndrome is multiple aphthalike lesions with ocular ulcers, uveitis, genital ulcers, neurologic disease, and thrombophlebitis as components of a multisystemic chronic disease.

▪ **Treatment**
Identification and treatment of underlying causes. Oral tetracycline swishes are frequently helpful. Potent topical steroids; low-dose oral corticosteroids.

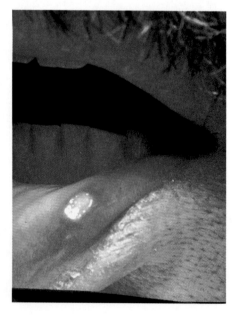

Chancre

▪ Morphology
A clean-based, indurated ulcer (1 to 3 cm in diameter).

▪ Distribution
Lips and tongue most common sites but can be anywhere.

▪ Patient Profile
Adults of both sexes.

▪ Diagnosis
Treponema pallidum can be demonstrated by dark-field examination. The presence of normal oral spirochetes complicates this test. A history of exposure to another person with syphilis will increase the suspicion of the diagnosis. Routine serologic tests may be negative early in the course of a chancre. Biopsy shows perivascular plasma-cell infiltrates, and silver stains demonstrate spirochetes.

▪ Treatment
Systemic antibiotics per STD protocol (see p. 588).

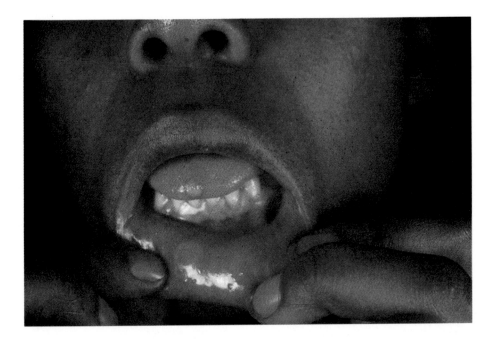

Vincent's Stomatitis
(Necrotizing Gingivitis)

▪ **Morphology**
Necrosis, sloughing, and ulceration of the interdental gingivae. The area is covered with a crust forming a pseudomembrane.

▪ **Distribution**
Gingivae.

▪ **Patient Profile**
Adults of both sexes. Disease characterized by pain, fever, malaise, and a fetid odor.

▪ **Diagnosis**
The rapid onset of necrotic disease limited to the gingivae is suggestive. Underlying systemic diseases should be ruled out. *Treponema vincentii* and *Fusobacterium nucleatum* can be demonstrated in the infected areas.

▪ **Treatment**
Metronidazole systemically.

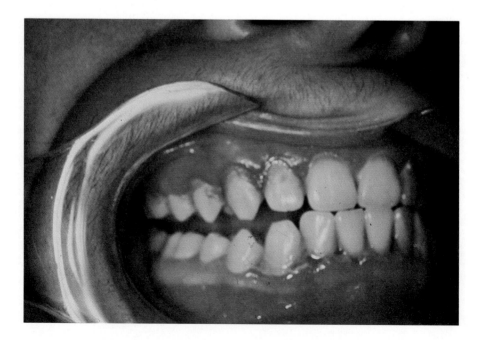

Herpes Simplex

▪ Morphology
Multiple erosions, oozing, and crusts. Discrete, grouped, umbilicated vesicles may be seen.

▪ Distribution
Entire oral mucosa including lips, general epidermis, and genitals may be involved.

▪ Patient Profile
Usually occurs in childhood; adults can be affected. Both sexes. Headache, fever, malaise, and clinical adenopathy common. Painful lesions. Acute course. Lesions are preceded by a burning sensation. Chronic herpes simplex lesions are seen in HIV-positive and other immunosuppressed patients.

▪ Diagnosis
Tzanck smear (see p. 16) showing multinucleated giant cells is diagnostic. Recurrent herpes simplex commonly involves the lips but only rarely the oral mucosa.

▪ Treatment
Systemic acyclovir 400 mg five times a day for 10 days.

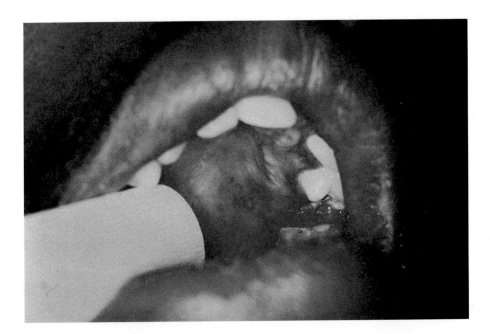

Herpes Zoster

■ **Morphology**
Closely grouped vesicles.

■ **Distribution**
Groups stop at midline and are in the distribution of a sensory nerve.

■ **Patient Profile**
This disease is most common in patients older than 40 years and in HIV-positive and other immunosuppressed patients. Frequently begins with pain and burning in a dermatomal distribution. After 3 to 4 days, groups of erythematous papules erupt that develop into characteristic umbilicated vesicles. Lesions and surrounding skin frequently are hyperalgesic.

■ **Diagnosis**
Multinucleated giant cells (see p. 16) can be demonstrated in the floor of the vesicle with the Tzanck smear.

■ **Treatment**
Systemic acyclovir 800 mg five times a day or famciclovir 500 mg three times a day in an immunosuppressed patient.

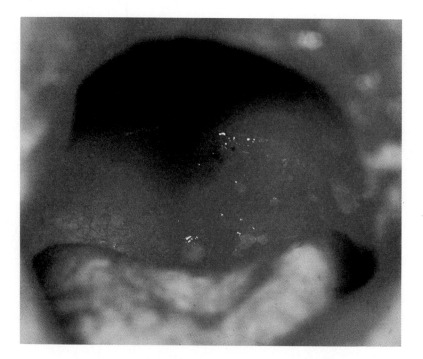

Other Viral Diseases

Chickenpox (see p. 312) may have intra-oral, umbilicated vesicles. In chickenpox, the multinucleated giant cell preparation (see p. 16) is positive.

Hand-foot-and-mouth disease (see p. 323) is characterized by oral lesions anywhere and painful palm and sole blisters.

Herpangina is a virally induced childhood disease with blisters limited to the back of the oral cavity (soft palate, tonsils, uvula, and pharynx).

Smallpox (see p. 310).

Vaccinia (see p. 311).

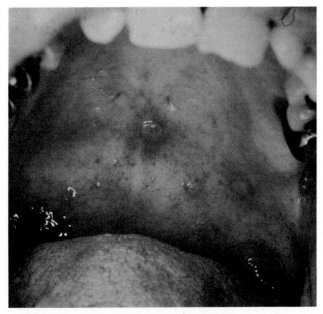

Hand-foot-and-mouth disease

Blistered or Ulcerated Mouth Lesions: Neoplastic

Eosinophilic Granuloma
(Histiocytosis X)

▪ **Morphology**
Loose teeth, swollen gingivae, and a non-healing ulceration may be present.

▪ **Distribution**
Gingivae.

▪ **Patient Profile**
Usually young adult.

▪ **Diagnosis**
X-rays show radiolucency in involved mandible or maxilla; biopsy shows sheets of histiocytes.

▪ **Treatment**
Systemic chemotherapy.

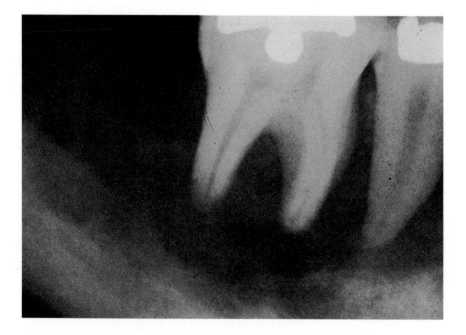

Blistered or Ulcerated Mouth Lesions: Other Etiologies

Reiter's Disease

■ **Morphology**
Polycyclic red erosions that may have intact vesicles.

■ **Distribution**
Anywhere.

■ **Patient Profile**
Most frequent in adult men. Circinate, red, eroded, and scaling lesions on the glans penis. Urethritis, conjunctivitis, and sacroiliitis often present.

■ **Diagnosis**
Patient very often HLA-B27 positive. Biopsy shows epithelial hyperplasia and intraepithelial microabscesses. Ordinary psoriasis very rarely has intraoral lesions.

■ **Treatment**
Systemic retinoids as used for pustular psoriasis (see p. 590).

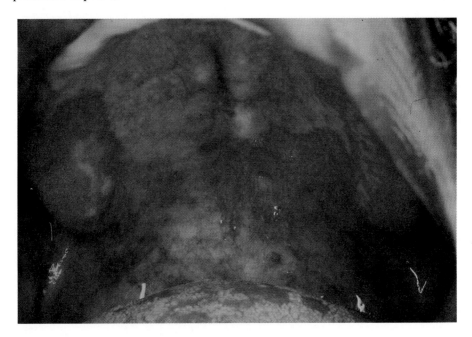

FLAT OR WHITE MOUTH LESIONS

DIAGNOSTIC OBSERVATIONS

A careful history and physical examination will establish the mechanical, chemical, and burn etiologies. Cultures for gonorrhea and diphtheria, smear for *Candida*, and a serologic test for syphilis are part of the evaluation for infectious causes. Acute white lesions of the oral mucosa are often painful and represent the inflammatory response to infection or trauma. Rather than true whiteness, many of the acute lesions have gray opacity.

MAJOR CATEGORIES

Acute
Chronic
Pigmented

Flat or White Mouth Lesions: Acute

CAUSES

Blistering Diseases
See pages 540–551.

Burn
Hot food or utensil
Electricity
Radiation: therapeutic to mouth, skin, and
  deeper structures

Chemical Trauma
Acid, alkali
Antimetabolite therapy
Camphor or phenol
Gold hypersensitivity

Infectious Disease
Aphthous stomatitis (see p. 544)
Candidiasis
Fusospirochetal infection
Gonorrhea (see p. 466)
Hand-foot-and-mouth disease: palmar and
  plantar blisters (see p. 323)
Measles: Koplik's spots (see pp. 70–71)
Secondary syphilis: mucous patches (see
  p. 262)

Mechanical Trauma
Lacerations, abrasions
Poorly fitting dentures: palate and gingi-
  vae

Candidiasis
(Moniliasis)

▪ Morphology
Thick, cheeselike white areas that can be rubbed off, leaving a raw, red base. Skin lesions (see p. 342) and perlèche (see p. 334) may be present.

▪ Distribution
Buccal mucosa and tongue most commonly. Fissures at corners of the mouth.

▪ Patient Profile
All ages, including infancy. Both sexes. Sometimes painful lesion. Often history of immunodeficiency, including HIV-positive patients, immunosuppressive drugs, diabetes, debilitating diseases, or broad-spectrum antibiotic treatment.

▪ Diagnosis
Identification of underlying cause in cases after infancy is mandatory. Candidiasis in infancy is often called thrush. Potassium hydroxide preparations of removed exudate show pseudomycelia and budding yeast. Culture reveals *Candida albicans.*

▪ Treatment
Oral nystatin suspension, amphotericin troches, and systemic imidazoles for 7 to 10 days. Identification of underlying causes.

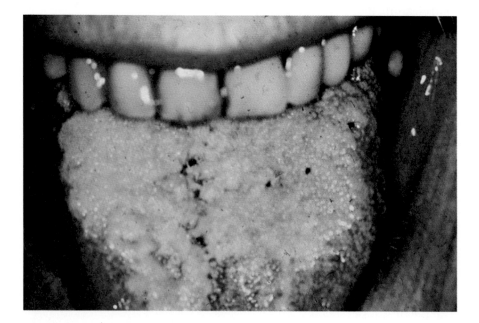

Flat or White Mouth Lesions: Chronic

DIAGNOSTIC OBSERVATIONS

Subacute or chronic white lesions of the mouth are usually not painful. Many individuals, especially African-Americans, have multiple white ridges or folds on the buccal mucosa. Stretching the mucosa with a finger or tongue blade removes these.

Many small, white lesions are in the bite line from trauma or the chewing of the buccal mucosa. Persistent white lesions require a definitive diagnosis because of the frequency of oral malignancy.

Major Categories

Candidiasis (see p. 342).
Discoid lupus erythematosus (see p. 384).
Fordyce's disease.
Genetic diseases: Five genetic diseases involving the mucosa and other organs present with persistent white oral plaque (Table 13–1). All these diseases begin in childhood, and their diagnosis is suggested by the family history and associated genetic features.
Geographic tongue.
HIV infection.
Leukoplakia.
Lichen planus.
Smoker's palate.
Squamous cell carcinoma.

TABLE 13–1. **Hereditary Diseases with White Oral Lesions**

Disease	Genetics	Associated Features
Benign intraepithelial dyskeratosis	Autosomal dominant	Raised, shiny, persistent conjunctival plaques
Darier's disease	Autosomal dominant	Scalp, face, upper back, and chest papules; palms and soles involved
Dyskeratosis congenita	X-linked or autosomal dominant	Absent lacrimal glands, reticular hyperpigmentation, atrophic nails, associated oral and epithelial malignancies, and aplastic anemia
Pachyonychia congenita	Autosomal dominant	Natal teeth, epidermal cysts, plantar hyperkeratosis, markedly hyperkeratotic nail beds
White sponge nevus	Autosomal dominant	Very swollen mucosa

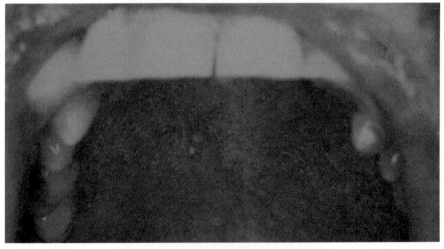

Darier's disease

Fordyce's Disease

▪ **Morphology**
White to yellow slightly raised lesions, 2 to 4 mm in diameter, that may be grouped together.

▪ **Distribution**
Buccal mucosa, lips, retromolar areas most common.

▪ **Patient Profile**
Adults of both sexes. Incidence increases with age.

▪ **Diagnosis**
The slightly yellow grains are diagnostic. Biopsy, which is rarely necessary, shows increased numbers of sebaceous glands.

In infancy, similar lesions are common. They are keratin-containing cysts called Epstein's pearls.

▪ **Treatment**
No treatment is necessary.

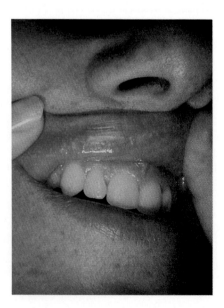

Geographic Tongue

■ **Morphology**
Multiple arcuate or annular white areas surrounding red areas in which filiform papillae are absent. The shape of the lesions changes over hours to days.

■ **Distribution**
Tongue.

■ **Patient Profile**
Adults; slightly more common in women. Increased association of lesions with congenitally fissured (scrotal) tongue and with psoriasis and Reiter's disease. Lesions usually asymptomatic; sometimes painful. Can be infected with *Candida albicans*.

■ **Diagnosis**
The changing morphology of the lesions over short periods of time is diagnostic.

■ **Treatment**
Topical corticosteroids (class I or II) or retinoic acid may be effective.

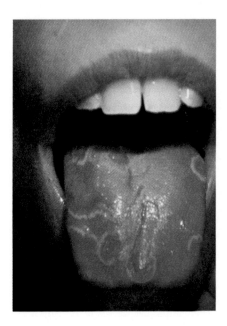

Leukoplakia

▪ **Morphology**
White, elevated papules that are often grooved or fissured. Varying degrees of underlying redness may be present.

▪ **Distribution**
Cheek, lips, mandibular mucosa most frequently involved sites. Palate in smokers. Can be anywhere.

▪ **Patient Profile**
Usually adults older than 40 years. More common in males. Chronic lesions.

▪ **Diagnosis**
Predisposing factors include smoking, snuff dipping, tobacco chewing, iron or vitamin deficiency, and chronic oral irritants. Biopsy may show hyperkeratosis, chronic inflammation, and definite dyskeratotic changes. Dyskeratotic cells on biopsy define the premalignant nature of this disease. Definitive diagnosis and therapy are required. Benign white hyperkeratotic lesions from trauma, for example, resolve within 3 to 4 weeks.

▪ **Treatment**
Surgical removal of suspicious lesions.

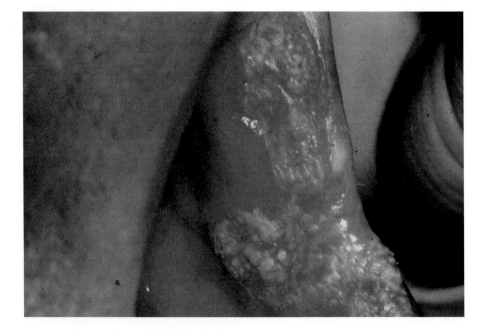

Lichen Planus

■ **Morphology**
Multiple white papules that are arranged in a netlike or lacelike pattern. Diffuse erythema and erosions of the gingivae may be present. White areas cannot be scraped off. May ulcerate.

■ **Distribution**
Cheek, lips, and tongue most common but can be anywhere.

■ **Patient Profile**
Adults of both sexes. Painful lesions when ulcerated. Lichen planus skin lesions elsewhere (see p. 251).

■ **Diagnosis**
Characteristic skin lesions (see p. 251) elsewhere confirm the diagnosis. Squamous cell carcinoma may develop within chronic lesions. Biopsy is diagnostic and shows hyperkeratosis, vacuolation of the basal layer, and a bandlike infiltrate of lymphocytes close to the epidermis.

■ **Treatment**
Topical (class I or II) or intralesional corticosteroids. Topical cyclosporine, cryosurgery, or Retin-A.

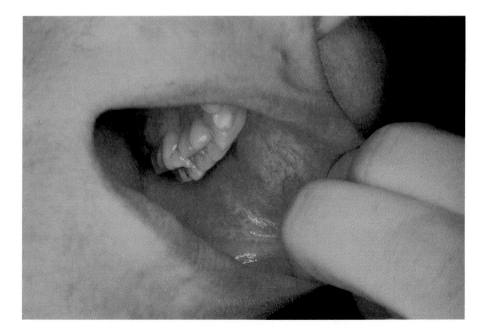

Smoker's Palate
(Stomatitis Nicotina)

▪ **Morphology**
White umbilicated papules on a red background.

▪ **Distribution**
Hard and soft palates.

▪ **Patient Profile**
Adults of both sexes. Smokers.

▪ **Diagnosis**
Distribution and rapid regression with the elimination of smoking distinguish this disease.

▪ **Treatment**
Stopping smoking.

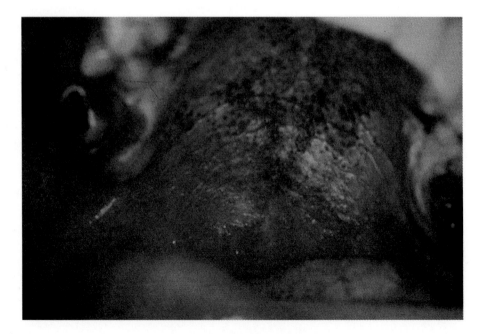

Squamous Cell Carcinoma

▪ Morphology
Disease presents as a white, raised area that may be ulcerated. Definite firmness can be felt around the borders of the lesions. On the lips, lesion appears as a scaling papule. Firm, enlarged regional lymph nodes may be present.

▪ Distribution
Tongue and floor of mouth most common intraoral locations. May be elsewhere. The lips are a common site.

▪ Patient Profile
Male adults older than 50 years most frequently affected. Smoking, tobacco chewing, snuff usage, and alcoholism are important predisposing factors. Chronic and persistent lesions.

▪ Diagnosis
Any persistent white lesion in the mouth must be biopsied. Biopsy is diagnostic and shows invasion of the underlying tissues by a neoplastic epithelium. Metastatic carcinoma may present in a similar fashion.

▪ Treatment
Surgical excision.

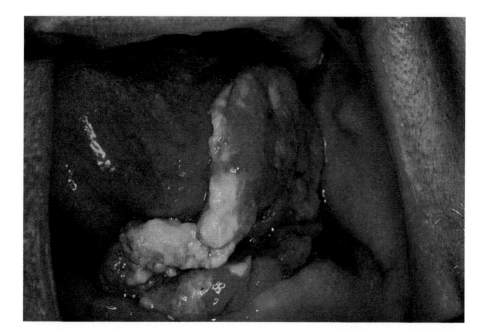

Pigmented Mouth Lesions

DIAGNOSTIC OBSERVATIONS
Many of the disorders causing generalized pigmentation of the skin (see p.
34) also cause hyperpigmentation of
the mucosa (Table 13–2). Patients of
color frequently have intraoral hyperpigmentation.

TABLE 13–2. **Conditions with Persistent Intraoral Hyperpigmentation**

Disease	Features and Diagnostic Clues
Acanthosis nigricans	Epidermal hyperplasia. Very high incidence of internal malignancy.
Addison's disease	Buccal, cutaneous, and systemic manifestations present.
Albright's syndrome and neurofibromatosis (see p. 39)	Other cutaneous and systemic manifestations present.
Amalgam tattoo	Discrete blue or black tattoo on gingivae or buccal mucosa.
Antimalarial drugs	Palate has bluish hue.
Black hairy tongue	Elongated and hyperpigmented papillae, sometimes related to tetracycline use.
Hemochromatosis (see p. 34)	Slate gray skin changes; increased serum iron and iron binding capacity.
Mercury, lead, or bismuth exposure	Most prominent on free gingivae, increased salivation.
Nevus, lentigo, or melanoma, blue nevus	Usually single.
Nevus of Ota	Diffuse blue on palate with associated skin lesions.
Phenothiazine tranquilizers	Palate has bluish hue.
Peutz-Jeghers syndrome (see p. 43)	Buccal mucosa and lips, gastrointestinal polyps.
Smoking	Palate.

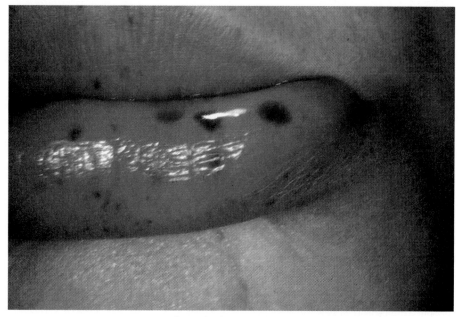

Peutz-Jeghers syndrome

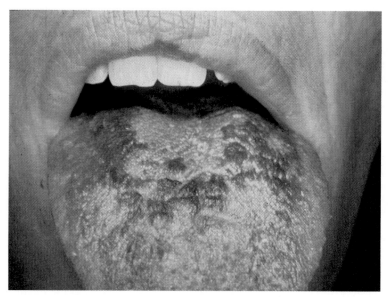

Black hairy tongue

RAISED MOUTH LESIONS

DIAGNOSTIC OBSERVATIONS

Various benign and malignant lesions can present as intraoral papules or cysts. Some discrete, definitely raised papular lesions seemingly grow out from the mucosa or infiltrate into the mucosa rather than represent diffuse thickening of the mucosa. Torus palatinus and torus mandibularis are hard, midline, exophytic, bony lesions, usually without clinical significance.

MAJOR CATEGORIES

Cysts
Mucocele
Rarer causes

Diffuse Thickening of Gingivae
Drug-induced: phenytoin (Dilantin), cyclosporine, calcium channel blockers
Hereditary fibromatosis and hypertrichosis syndrome
Inflammatory periodontal disease
Lymphoma, leukemia
Pregnancy
Scurvy

Papular Lesions
A persistent red or mucosal-colored plaque in the mouth should be biopsied. Possible diagnoses for such lesions include:
Acanthosis nigricans
Amyloidosis: associated with tongue enlargement
Benign tumors (see p. 408)
Foreign-body granulomas
Granular cell myoblastoma
Granuloma pyogenicum: friable and hemorrhagic (see p. 222)
Hairy leukoplakia
Histiocytosis X
Inflammatory periodontal disease: limited to gingivae
Irritation fibromas
Lipoid proteinosis: hoarseness and skin lesions (see pp. 174–175)
Lupus erythematosus
Lymphoma and leukemia
Median rhomboid glossitis: papules grouped posteriorly in midtongue with evidence of *Candida albicans*
Metastatic carcinoma (see p. 220)
Pregnancy tumor
Psoriasis
Sarcoidosis
Squamous cell carcinoma
Warts, condylomata
Other rarer causes (see pp. 598–601)

Vascular Lesions
Blue rubber bleb nevus syndrome: oral and cutaneous lesions associated with gastrointestinal bleeding (see p. 180)
Hemangiomas: especially with Sturge-Weber syndrome (see p. 96)
Kaposi's sarcoma (p. 138)
Telangiectasia: with Osler-Weber-Rendu disease and systemic sclerosis
Varicosities (vascular ectasia): especially under tongue and on lips; common in older adults, of no special significance

Raised Mouth Lesions: Cysts

Mucocele

■ **Morphology**
Single, compressible, bluish lesions, often with an intermittent mucoid discharge. Freely movable.

■ **Distribution**
Lip or tongue most common site.

■ **Patient Profile**
Any age, both sexes. Often secondary to trauma.

■ **Diagnosis**
Biopsy shows a mucous-containing cyst and chronic inflammation.

■ **Treatment**
Usually resolve spontaneously. If not, surgical excision required.

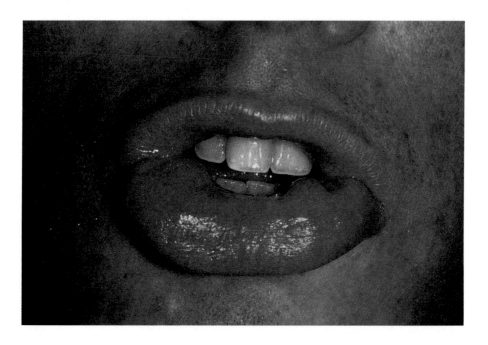

Rare Causes of Cystic Lesions

Cystic hygroma: A lymphangioma in the floor of the mouth and neck; appears in infancy.

Epidermal cyst: A keratin-containing cyst in the floor of the mouth.

Lymphangioma: Similar to lymphangioma circumscriptum (see p. 164). Appears on tongue or cheek at any age.

Ranula: A cyst associated with a sublingual gland or submaxillary gland in the floor of the mouth.

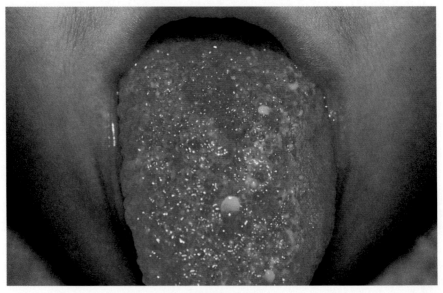

Lymphangioma

Raised Mouth Lesions: Diffuse Thickening of the Gingivae

Gingival thickening accompanies:
Drug-induced hyperplasia: phenytoin, cyclosporin A, calcium channel blockers
Hereditary fibromatosis and hypertrichosis syndromes
Inflammatory periodontal disease
Lymphomas, leukemia: hemorrhagic and friable
Pregnancy
Vitamin C deficiency (scurvy): hemorrhagic

A complete history and physical and laboratory examinations are indicated in these patients to exclude serious underlying diseases.

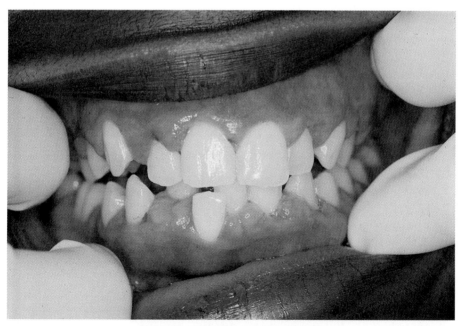

Phenytoin-induced gingival hyperplasia

Raised Papular Lesions of the Mouth

Foreign Body Granulomas

▪ **Morphology**
Single, raised, firm lesion that may drain.

▪ **Distribution**
Tongue, floor of mouth but may be anywhere.

▪ **Patient Profile**
Any age, both sexes.

▪ **Diagnosis**
History of preceding trauma. Biopsy may show foreign body reaction and evidence of foreign body, such as a bone spicula of fish or animal origin.

▪ **Treatment**
Surgical excision.

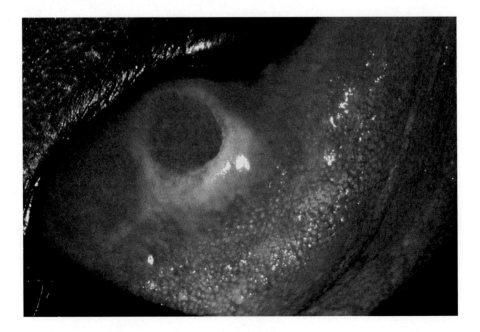

Granular Cell Myoblastoma

■ **Morphology**
Single, discrete, firm, white-topped papule
up to 4 cm in diameter.

■ **Distribution**
Tongue, especially dorsal and lateral surfaces.

■ **Patient Profile**
Adults of both sexes.

■ **Diagnosis**
Biopsy is diagnostic, showing hyperplastic
epithelium and cells with a very granular
cytoplasm.

■ **Treatment**
Surgical excision.

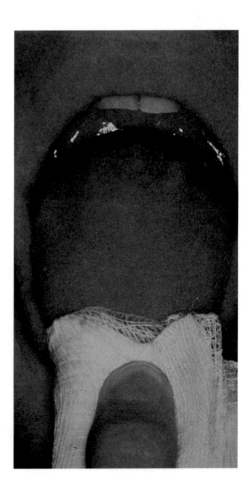

Hairy Leukoplakia

▪ **Morphology**
White to grayish-white verrucous plaques on the tongue that cannot be removed.

▪ **Distribution**
Single to multiple lesions that often involve the lateral margins of the tongue.

▪ **Patient Profile**
HIV-positive patient.

▪ **Diagnosis**
Usually a clinical diagnosis. Biopsy demonstrates acanthosis, parakeratosis, and ballooning degeneration of keratinocytes. Causative organism is Epstein-Barr virus.

▪ **Treatment**
May resolve spontaneously. Topical podophyllin.

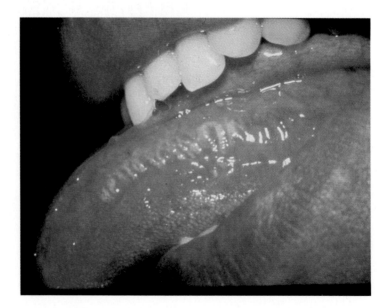

Irritation Fibroma

■ **Morphology**
Single pale papule, 2 mm to 2 cm in diameter.

■ **Distribution**
Anywhere.

■ **Patient Profile**
All ages, both sexes. Local irritation, as from dentures or infection.

■ **Diagnosis**
Most common tumorlike growth in oral cavity. Biopsy shows collagen proliferation. Similar lesions include peripheral fibromas, epulis granulomatosa (around extraction sites), and peripheral cell granuloma (broad-based lesions on edentulous ridges in older people).

■ **Treatment**
Intralesional corticosteroids.

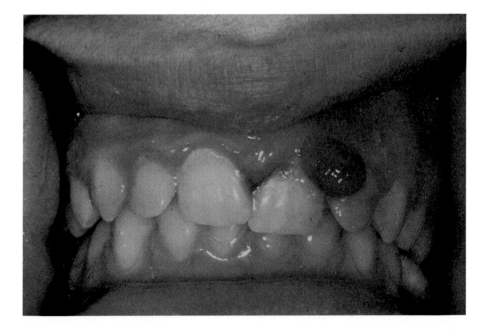

Squamous Cell Carcinoma

▪ **Morphology**

Lesion presents as a white, raised area that may be ulcerated. Definite firmness can be felt around the borders of the lesions. On the lips, lesion appears as a scaling papule. Firm, enlarged regional lymph nodes may be present.

▪ **Distribution**

Tongue and floor of mouth most common intraoral locations. May be anywhere. The lips are a common site.

▪ **Patient Profile**

Male adults older than 50 years most frequently affected. Smoking or chewing of tobacco, use of snuff, and alcoholism are important predisposing factors. Chronic and persistent lesions.

▪ **Diagnosis**

Any persistent white lesion in the mouth must be biopsied. Biopsy is diagnostic and shows invasion of the underlying tissues by a neoplastic epithelium. Metastatic carcinoma may present in a similar fashion.

▪ **Treatment**

Surgical excision.

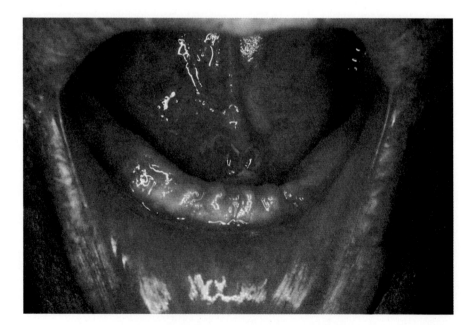

Warts
(Condylomata)

▪ Morphology
Multiple, stalklike folds are present in white to pink papillomatous lesions up to 2 cm in diameter.

▪ Distribution
Lips and palate but may be anywhere.

▪ Patient Profile
Warts: children of both sexes. Condylomata: adults of both sexes.

▪ Diagnosis
Warts may be present elsewhere. Biopsy shows papillomatous hyperkeratosis (see p. 241).

▪ Treatment
Cryotherapy or laser therapy.

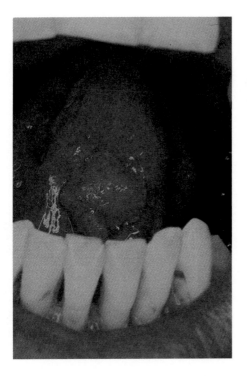

TONGUE LESIONS

MAJOR CATEGORIES

Atrophy
Geographic tongue (see p. 557)
Iron deficiency
Lichen planus (see p. 559)
Lichen sclerosus et atrophicus
Lupus erythematosus
Squamous cell carcinoma
Tertiary syphilis
Vitamin deficiency: pellagra, sprue, vita-
min B deficiency

Enlargement
Acromegaly
Amyloidosis
Angioneurotic edema
Down syndrome
Hemangioma or lymphangioma
Hypothyroidism
Neurofibroma
Squamous cell carcinoma
Superior vena cava syndrome
Thyroglossal duct cyst

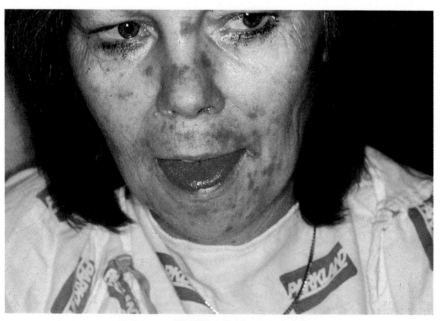

Vitamin deficiency

TOOTH DEFECTS ASSOCIATED WITH DISEASE

MAJOR CATEGORIES

Abnormal Color

Bluish Teeth
Ochronosis

Green Teeth
Biliary atresia or bile tract disease

Brown Teeth
Amelogenesis imperfecta (several forms)
Dentinogenesis imperfecta
Erythroblastosis fetalis
Junctional and dominant dystrophic epidermolysis bullosa
Tetracycline treatment

Purple Teeth
Hereditary opalescent dentin with osteogenesis imperfecta

Red-Brown Teeth That Fluoresce Red-Purple under Wood's Light
Erythropoietic porphyria

Peg-Shaped Teeth
Anhidrotic ectodermal dysplasia (see p. 494)
Chondroectodermal dysplasia
Incontinentia pigmenti (see p. 300)

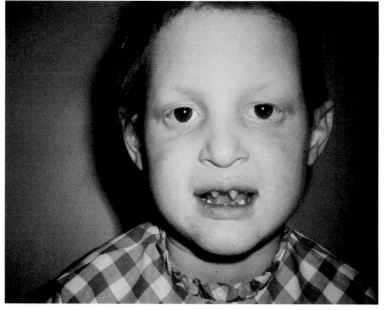

Anhidrotic ectodermal dysplasia

PART

3

Therapy

Chapter 14

■ ■

Principles of Therapy

PRINCIPLES OF THERAPY

Sound therapy is based on a definitive diagnosis. A diagnosis can be established by clinical criteria or clinical features, supplemented by biopsy or other laboratory tests. The therapeutic recommendations in this chapter assume that a definitive diagnosis has been established. Before prescribing any of the therapies outlined in this text, the prescriber should be fully familiar with the agents, their usage, and their side effects. This information can be obtained from pharmacology textbooks, the product insert, and sources such as the *Physicians' Desk Reference*. This chapter is not meant to substitute for such sources. The *Manual of Dermatologic Therapeutics* by K. A. Arndt, K. E. Bowers, and A. R. Chuttani and *Dermatology: Diagnosis and Therapy* by E. E. Bondi, B. J. Jegasothy, and G. S. Lazarus are excellent sources for details of various therapeutic regimens.

Amounts of Topical Agents

It takes approximately 30 g of cream or ointment to cover the entire body once; to cover the entire body twice daily for 2 weeks takes approximately 840 g (or 2 lb) of cream. Approximate amounts of topical agents needed to cover different body areas of a 70-kg person twice a day for 2 weeks are shown in Table 14–1.

Many failures of therapy using topical agents are related to the use of inadequate amounts. This is often directly related to the cost of an agent, especially in relation to the discretionary budget of the patient.

TABLE 14–1. Amounts of Topical Agents

	To Cover Once	bid for 2 Weeks
Entire body	30 g	840 g (30 oz)
Face, hands, feet	2 g	60 g
Arm	3 g	90 g
Trunk: anterior or posterior	3 g	90 g
Leg	4 g	120 g
Scalp	2 mL	60 mL

Types of Topical Agents

Topical medicines are available in four main forms: creams, ointments, gels, and solutions (or lotions). Creams are often in vanishing bases so that after application the skin will appear essentially normal. A thick, visible film on the skin suggests that too much medication has been applied. Creams are often used for mild to moderately scaly lesions.

Ointments are in a greasy base and are usually visible or perceptible on the skin after application. Ointments are more occlusive than creams, thereby enhancing penetration and moisturization when properly used. Getting ointments on clothes, papers, books, or other people often limits their use. Ointments are best suited for moderate to severe dry, scaling dermatoses. Ointments are not well tolerated by patients with atopic eczema and should be avoided in intertriginous areas.

Gels are clear, greaseless bases that sometimes contain alcohol. They may leave a sticky feeling and be irritating. Gels are

TABLE 14–2. **Antiseborrheic and Antipsoriatic Medications Used in Scalp**

Preparation	Active Ingredient
Baker's P&S	Salicylic acid 2%
Balnetar	Coal tar 2.5%
Capitrol	Chloroxine 2%
Denorex	Coal tar 1.8%
Derma-smoothe/FS topical oil*	Fluocinolone acetanide in oil 0.01%
Dovonex ointment†	Vitamin D
Dritho-Scalp	Anthralin 0.25% and 0.5%
Exsel	Selenium sulfide 2.5%
Head & Shoulders	Pyrithione zinc 1%
Ionil-T Plus	Coal tar 2%
Nizoral*	Ketoconazole 2%
Sebutone	Coal tar 0.5%
Selsun Blue	Selenium sulfide 1%
T/Gel	Coal tar 0.5%
T/Gel extra strength	Coal tar 1%
T Sal	Salicylic acid 2%
Tegrin	Coal tar 1.1%

*Prescription only.
†Can combine 1:1 with a conditioner and use overnight.

useful in hairy areas and for acute, exudative dermatoses.

Special Locations

Scalp
Solutions and gels are especially useful on the scalp and other hairy areas. To aid their penetration, some solutions are available as aerosols for locations like the scalp. Scales are best removed from the scalp by phenol and saline scalp solution applied overnight and then removed by shampooing in the morning. Antiseborrheic and antipsoriatic preparations are listed in Table 14–2.

Mouth
Many dermatologic conditions affect the oral mucosa. Topical corticosteroids can be useful for the treatment of lichen planus, aphthae, autoimmune blistering diseases, and lupus. Class I or II steroids may be used in either an ointment or gel, or as an aerosol. *Alcohol-based medications are flammable.* Topical Retin-A is used for lichen planus. Candidiasis is a potential complication of potent corticosteroids used in the mouth. Candidiasis of any cause can be treated with nystatin (Mycostatin) oral suspension swished around the mouth for 3 to 5 minutes three to five times a day. Troches containing imidazoles (Mycelex) are also available. Aphthous ulcers may benefit from a tetracycline swish (the contents of one 250-mg capsule tetracycline in 10 mL water) swished for 3 to 5 minutes and then expelled.

Occlusion
Occlusion increases the penetration of corticosteroids and other medications by increasing the moisture content of the stratum corneum and the ambient temperature of the skin. Occlusion can be obtained by applying cream under plastic wraps, a special dressing (e.g., Actiderm), or special nylonized suits (e.g., Sleep Sauna), or by using a tape impregnated with a medium-potency corticosteroid, which is effectively more potent under occlusion. Problems with occlusion include folliculitis, pruritus (often in patients with atopic dermatitis), and potentiation of all the side effects of topical corticosteroids. Side effects such as striae, telangiectasia, and atrophy may have permanent sequelae, so occlusion must be used in a rational therapeutic regimen. Occlusion is rarely indicated in children.

Drug Use in Pediatric Patients
The pediatric dosages of oral medicines are indicated in Table 14–3 and are based on milligrams per kilogram of body weight. In using topical agents, it is important to remember that the ratio of body surface to volume is higher in young children, especially neonates. Premature infants may have incomplete barrier functions of the stratum corneum, allowing higher absorption of topical agents. Many topical agents have not been tested or approved for use in children, and this information should be carefully checked before use.

As a general rule of thumb, it must be taken into consideration that all of the

TABLE 14–3. **Commonly Used Pediatric Preparations**

Brand	Generic	Concentration	Dosing
Amoxil	Amoxicillin	250 mg/5 mL	20 mg/kg, divided tid
Atarax	Hydroxyzine	10 mg/5 mL	2 mg/kg, divided qid
Augmentin	Amoxicillin with clavulanic acid	125 mg/5 mL	20 mg/kg, divided tid
Eryped	Erythromycin	200 mg/5 mL	40–50 mg/kg, divided qid
Fulvicin	Griseofulvin	125 mg/5 mL	15–20 mg/kg, divided bid with food
Keflex	Cephalexin	125 mg/5 mL	30–40 mg/kg, divided qid
Zovirax	Acyclovir	20 mg/5 mL	20 mg/kg, divided qid (herpes simplex)
Zovirax	Acyclovir	20 mg/5 mL	100 mg/kg, divided qid (herpes zoster)

ingredients in a topical agent may be absorbed, and the systemic effect must be calculated. This is especially important in infants with generalized epidermal disorders.

Topicals with Retin-A, salicylic acid, or lactic acid are not recommended in very young children, except over small areas not exceeding 1% of the body surface, such as when these agents are used to treat warts. As mentioned, occlusion is almost never used in treating young children because of the danger of hyperthermia and excess absorption.

Drug Use during Pregnancy

During pregnancy, pruritus, systemic skin diseases, intercurrent conditions such as severe contact dermatitis, the treatment of warts, and exacerbations of acne are all conditions challenging the therapeutic resourcefulness of a physician. Drugs have been rated as to possible adverse effects in the following standard system established by the Food and Drug Administration (FDA):

A – Controlled studies show no risk.
B – No evidence of risk in humans.
C – Risk cannot be ruled out.
D – Positive evidence of risk.
X – Contraindicated in pregnancy.

Drugs that can be used systemically during pregnancy, such as erythromycin, should be safe for topical use. Podophyllin is contraindicated during pregnancy, as is oral isotretinoin (Accutane). Although many articles suggest that topical retinoic acid can be safely used during pregnancy, we try to avoid doing so.

GENERAL THERAPIES

Antipruritics: Systemic and Topical

Cool baths and showers provide relief from itching. The addition of colloidal oatmeal preparations is often soothing as well. For those with chronic itching, keeping their surroundings cool, especially the bedroom, is recommended. Dry skin is often pruritic and its treatment includes attention to hydration, as described later.

A variety of antihistamines are available for oral use (Table 14–4). Hydroxyzine is preferred by many dermatologists because it has significant flexibility of dosage and low anticholinergic side effects. Side effects of all antihistamines include the anticholinergic effects of constipation, xerostomia, and precipitation of glaucoma. As indicated in Table 14–4, important cardiac arrhythmias occur with two of the newer antihistamines (astemizole and terfenadine), along with noteworthy drug interactions.

Topical antipruritics include lotions with 0.25% menthol, 1% phenol, or both; Sarna lotion; and topical anesthetics such as (pramoxine) Pramosone.

Topical antihistamines and benzocaine are not recommended because of their potential for allergic sensitization. Topical doxepin (Zonalon) is now available and is effective, but use over extensive areas can lead to drowsiness and anticholinergic side effects.

Corticosteroids: Systemic and Topical

Although a variety of systemic corticosteroids are available, prednisone is the oral

TABLE 14–4. **Antihistamines**

Class	Generic Name	Brand Name	Available Sizes	Frequency	Side Effects
		H₁ Blockers			
Alkylamines	Chlorpheniramine	Chlor-Trimeton	4, 8, 12 mg	q 4–12 h	Sedating
Ethanolamines	Diphenhydramine	Benadryl	25, 50 mg	q 6–8 h	Sedating
	Clemastine	Tavist	1.34, 2.68 mg	q 8–12 h	Sedating
Ethylenediamine	Tripelennamine	PBZ	25, 50 mg	q 4–6 h	Sedating
Phenothiazines	Promethazine	Phenergan	12.5, 25, 50 mg	q 6 h	Sedating
Piperidines	Cyproheptadine	Periactin	4 mg	q 6–8 h	Sedating
Piperazines	Hydroxyzine	Atarax	10, 25, 50, 100 mg	q 6–8 h	Sedating
Other	Astemizole*	Hismanal	10 mg	q d	Low sedating†
	Loratadine*	Claritin	10 mg	q d	Low sedating
	Terfenadine*	Seldane	60 mg	q 12 h	Low sedating†
	Cetirizine	Zyrtec	5, 10 mg	q d	Low sedating
		H₂ Blockers			
	Cimetidine	Tagamet	200, 300, 400, 800 mg	q d—bid	
	Famotidine*	Pepcid	20, 40 mg & 40 mg/5 mL	q d—bid	
	Nizatidine*	Axid	150, 300 mg	q d—bid	
	Ranitidine*	Zantac	150, 300 mg & 15 mg/mL	q d—bid	
		Topical Antihistamines			
	Diphenhydramine				
	1% cream	Benadryl	15 g		Nonsedating‡
	2% cream	Benadryl	15, 30 g		Nonsedating‡
	Doxepin 5% cream	Zonalon	30 g		Sedating‡

*High cost per unit.
†Not to be taken concurrently with erythromycin or ketoconazole due to potential cardiac arrhythmia.
‡Possible cutaneous sensitizer.

medicine of choice, and it is rare to use other steroids. Using systemic steroids for treating severe contact dermatitis initially requires 60 mg daily as a single dose. A single morning dose is usually therapeutic, increases compliance, and decreases steroid side effects. When high-dose corticosteroids are necessary for more than a month, one should attempt to use them on an every-other-day schedule, which decreases steroid side effects. When oral corticosteroids are being used for chronic conditions, they should be tapered slowly to prevent flare-up, usually at a rate of 2.5 to 5 mg per week.

In rare instances of chronic disease, intermittent injections of 40 mg of triamcinolone acetonide or its equivalent may be necessary; this decision is best made in consultation with a dermatologist.

Topical steroids come in several strengths and forms, as shown in Table 14–5. Side effects include atrophy, striae, folliculitis, hypopigmentation and hyperpigmentation, telangiectasia, perioral dermatitis, and even contact dermatitis. Most of these side effects are more likely with more potent agents; striae are especially common in adolescents. Use of steroids in unrecognized scabies or fungal infection can lead to partial resolution of symptoms but overgrowth of organisms. Extensive use of topical class I agents or class II and III corticosteroids under occlusion can lead to adrenal suppression. Repeated administration of topical corticosteroids often leads

TABLE 14–5. **Topical Steroids**

Class	Generic Name	Brand Name	Sizes (g Unless Noted)
I	Betamethasone dipropionate	Diprolene ointment 0.05%*	15, 45
	Clobetasol propionate	Temovate cream 0.05%*	15, 30, 45
		Temovate ointment 0.05%*	15, 30, 45
	Diflorasone diacetate	Psorcon cream	15, 30, 60
		Psorcon ointment 0.05%*	15, 30, 60
	Flurandrenolide	Cordran Tape*	
	Halobetasol propionate	Ultravate cream 0.05%*	15, 45
		Ultravate ointment 0.05%*	15, 45
II	Amcinonide	Cyclocort ointment 0.1%	15, 30, 60
	Betamethasone dipropionate	Diprolene AF cream 0.05%	15, 45
	Betamethasone dipropionate	Diprosone ointment 0.05%	15, 45
	Betamethasone dipropionate	Maxivate cream 0.05%	15, 45
		Maxivate ointment 0.05%	15, 45
	Desoximetasone	Topicort cream 0.25%	15, 60, 120
		Topicort gel 0.05%	15, 60
		Topicort ointment 0.25%	15, 60
	Diflorasone diacetate	Florone ointment 0.05%	15, 30, 60
	Diflorasone diacetate	Maxiflor ointment 0.05%	15, 30, 60
	Fluocinonide	Lidex cream 0.05%	15, 30, 60, 120
		Lidex gel 0.05%	15, 30, 60, 120
		Lidex ointment 0.05%	15, 30, 60, 120
		Lidex solution 0.05%	20, 60 mL
	Halcinonide	Halog cream 0.1%	15, 30, 60, 240
	Mometasone furoate	Elocon ointment 0.1%	15, 45
III	Amcinonide	Cyclocort cream 0.1%	15, 30, 60
	Betamethasone dipropionate	Diprosone cream 0.05%	15, 45
	Betamethasone dipropionate	Maxivate lotion 0.05%	60 mL
	Betamethasone valerate	Valisone ointment 0.1%	15, 45
	Desoximetasone	Topicort LP cream 0.05%	15, 60
	Diflorasone diacetate	Florone cream 0.05%	15, 30, 60
	Diflorasone diacetate	Maxiflor cream 0.05%	15, 30, 60
	Fluocinonide	Lidex E cream 0.05%	15, 30, 60, 120
	Fluticasone propionate	Cutivate ointment 0.0005%	15, 30, 60
	Halcinonide	Halog ointment 0.1%	15, 30, 60, 240
		Halog solution 0.1%	20, 60 mL
	Triamcinolone acetonide	Aristocort A ointment 0.1%	15, 60

(Continued)

to tachyphylaxis. Lower-potency agents should be used on the face, neck, and intertriginous areas such as axillae, submammary folds, groin, and pendulous abdominal folds.

Wet Dressings
Wet dressings are useful for cooling inflamed skin, decreasing pruritus, and removing crusts and adherent eschars. The main and most important ingredient in soaks is water. Additional ingredients are saline (1 teaspoon [5 g] table salt per pint) or aluminum sulfate (Domeboro, one tablet or packet per pint). The soak can be applied to old linen, loose mesh bandage, or soft gauze fluffs, which should be kept

TABLE 14–5. **Topical Steroids** (Continued)

Class	Generic Name	Brand Name	Sizes (g Unless Noted)
IV	Fluocinolone acetonide	Synalar ointment 0.025%	15, 30, 60, 120, 425
	Flurandrenolide	Cordran ointment 0.05%	15, 30, 60, 225
	Triamcinolone acetonide	Aristocort cream 0.1%	15, 60, 240
	Triamcinolone acetonide	Kenalog cream 0.1%	15, 60, 80, 240
		Kenalog ointment 0.025%	15, 60, 80, 240
	Mometasone furoate	Elocon cream 0.1%	15, 45
		Elocon lotion 0.1%	30, 60 mL
V	Betamethasone valerate	Valisone cream 0.1%	15, 45, 110, 430
	Desonide	Tridesilon ointment 0.05%	15, 60
	Fluocinolone acetonide	Synalar cream 0.025%	15, 30, 60, 425
	Flurandrenolide	Cordran cream 0.05%	15, 30, 60, 225
	Fluticasone propionate	Cutivate cream 0.05%	15, 30, 60
	Hydrocortisone butyrate	Locoid cream 0.1%	15, 45
		Locoid ointment 0.1%	15, 45
		Locoid solution 0.1%	20, 60 mL
	Hydrocortisone valerate	Westcort cream 0.2%	15, 45, 60, 120
		Westcort ointment 0.2%	15, 45, 60
	Triamcinolone acetonide	Kenalog lotion 0.1%	15, 60 mL
		Kenalog ointment 0.025%	15, 60, 80, 240
VI	Alclometasone dipropionate	Aclovate cream 0.05%	15, 45
		Aclovate ointment 0.05%	15, 45
	Betamethasone valerate	Valisone lotion 0.1%	20, 60 mL
	Desonide	Tridesilon cream 0.05%	15, 60
	Fluocinolone acetonide	Synalar cream 0.01%	15, 45, 60, 425
		Synalar lotion 0.01%	20, 60 mL
	Triamcinolone acetonide	Aristocort cream 0.025%	15, 60, 240
	Tramcinolone acetonide	Kenalog cream 0.025%	15, 60, 240
		Kenalog lotion 0.025%	60 mL
VII	Hydrocortisone	Hytone cream 1.0%	30, 120
		Hytone cream 2.5%	30, 60
		Hytone lotion 1.0%	120
		Hytone lotion 2.5%	60
		Hytone ointment 1.0%	30
		Hytone ointment 2.5%	30
	Hydrocortisone acetate and pramoxine HCl 1%	Pramosone cream 1.0%	1, 2, 4 oz; 1 lb
		Pramosone cream 2.5%	1, 2, 4 oz; 1 lb
		Pramosone lotion 1.0%	2, 4, 8 oz
		Pramosone lotion 2.5%	2, 4, 8 oz
		Pramosone ointment 1.0%	1, 4 oz; 1 lb
		Pramosone ointment 2.5%	1, 4 oz; 1 lb

*High cost per unit dose.

TABLE 14–6. Emollients

Aquaphor
Aveeno lotion
Cetaphil lotion
Curel Moisturizing lotion
Dermasil lotion
Eucerin lotion
Keri lotion
Lac-Hydrin lotion 5%
Lac-Hydrin lotion 12% (225, 400 g)*
Lubriderm lotion
Moisturel lotion
Neutrogena emulsion
Penecare lotion
White petrolatum

*Prescription only.

moist for 20 minutes and then gently removed. Soaks can be used two to three times a day.

Lubrication, Hydration, and Emollients
The basis of therapy for dry skin from any cause is that only water can make the skin more flexible and pliable. Soaps, chemicals, and diseases alter the water-retaining characteristics of the epidermis. Epidermal water loss increases in a low-humidity environment. Humidification of the room or the house is useful for increasing the ambient humidity. Lubricating lotions, creams, and especially ointments (Table 14–6) help retain epidermal moisture. The agents are best applied after hydration of the epidermis such as occurs during bathing. Water-free products such as petrolatum do not require preservatives and therefore have the lowest potential for a secondary sensitization dermatitis.

Preparations containing 5% to 12% lactic acid or alpha-hydroxy acids such as glycolic acid can cause superficial desquamation, which relieves the scaling that often accompanies dry skin. These agents, however, can be irritating to inflamed skin.

Physical Therapies

Lights
UVB (290 to 320 nm) and UVA (320 to 400 nm) light is useful for the therapy of skin disease. Eye protection is mandatory dur-

ing the use of lights for phototherapy. Experience with this therapy is critical to avoid serious harm to the patient. Medications taken for other conditions may act as photosensitizers and complicate phototherapy.

UVB therapy is commonly used to treat psoriasis, severe eczema, cutaneous T-cell lymphoma, pruritus of chronic renal disease, other forms of refractory pruritus, and pityriasis rosea. UVA therapy, in conjunction with oral psoralens (PUVA therapy), is helpful in treatment of psoriasis, cutaneous T-cell lymphoma, and vitiligo.

Cryotherapy
Liquid nitrogen is the usual mode of cryotherapy. Necrosis or subepidermal blistering leads to the diminution or removal of the lesion. Overtreatment can lead to atrophy, scarring, hypopigmentation, or hyperpigmentation. Cryotherapy is used to treat actinic keratoses, warts, seborrheic keratoses, keloids, and prurigo nodularis. Malignancies require special modes of therapy when using cryotherapy, and nevi should not be treated by this modality. Because there is no histologic confirmation of the diagnosis when cryotherapy is used, the physician must be certain of the diagnosis before initiating treatment.

Sun Protection
In addition to avoiding sun exposure and using physical protection, a variety of sunscreens are available that give both UVB and UVA protection. Some of these are listed in Table 14–7.

Surgical Approaches
The details of surgical approaches are beyond this basic text. Surgical skills should be learned under appropriate supervision before being performed.

TREATMENT OF SPECIFIC DISEASES

Infectious Diseases

Fungal Infections
Many topical agents are available to treat topical fungal infections (Table 14–8). Topi-

TABLE 14–7. **Sunscreens**

Brand Name	SPF	Active Ingredients
Coppertone Broad Spectrum Lotion	25	Avobenzone, benzophenones, cinnamates
DuraScreen	15	Benzophenones, cinnamates
Johnson's Baby Sunblock Lotion	30	Benzophenones, cinnamates, salicylates
Neutrogena Chemical-Free	17	Titanium dioxide
Neutrogena Sunblock	30	Cinnamates, menthyl anthranilate, octocrylene
PreSun	15, 25, 46	Benzophenones, cinnamates, PABA
Shade UVAGUARD	15	Avobenzone, benzophenones, cinnamates
Shade UVA/UVB	15, 25, 30, 45	Avobenzone, benzophenones, cinnamates
SolBar PF Cream	15	Benzophenones, PABA
Sundown Sport	15	Titanium dioxide, zinc oxide
Total Eclipse Lotion	15	Benzophenones, salicylates, PABA
Water Babies UVA/UVB	12, 25, 30, 45	Benzophenones, cinnamates, octocrylene

cal nystatin is effective against *Candida* but ineffective against dermatophytes.

Systemic fungal agents include griseofulvin, which is effective on dermatophytes but not on *Candida*; oral nystatin, which is not absorbed and is effective only in the gastrointestinal tract; and the new imidazoles, fluconazole and itraconazole, and the allylamine terbinafine (Table 14–9). Oral *Candida* may be treated with clotrimazole 10-mg oral troches or nystatin oral suspension.

Topical tinea versicolor infections may be treated with selenium sulfide suspension (e.g., Selsun Blue 2.5%), topical antifungal preparations, a short course of ketoconazole (200 mg daily), or a single dose of 400 mg ketoconazole.

Bacterial Infections

Tiny areas of folliculitis or pyoderma may be treated with topical 2% mupirocin (Bactroban) or neomycin. More extensive impe-

TABLE 14–8. **Topical Antifungals**

Generic Name/Form	Brand Name	Available Sizes
Sulconazole 1% cream	Exelderm	15, 30, 60 g
Sulconazole 1% solution	Exelderm	30 mL
Terbinafine 1% cream*	Lamisil	15, 30 g
Ciclopirox 1% cream	Loprox	15, 30, 90 g
Ciclopirox 1% lotion	Loprox	30, 60 mL
Clotrimazole 1% cream	Lotrimin	15, 30, 45, 90 g
Clotrimazole 1% lotion	Lotrimin	30 mL
Clotrimazole 1% solution	Lotrimin	10, 30 mL
Miconazole 2% cream	Monistat	15 g, 1, 3 oz
Nystatin cream	Mycostatin	15, 30 g
Naftifine 1% cream	Naftin	15, 30, 60 g
Naftifine 1% gel	Naftin	20, 40, 60 g
Ketoconazole 2% cream	Nizoral	15, 30, 60 g
Oxiconazole 1% cream*	Oxistat	15, 30, 60 g
Oxiconazole 1% lotion*	Oxistat	30 mL
Econazole 1% cream	Spectazole	15, 30, 85 g

*High cost per unit dose.

TABLE 14–9. **Systemic Antifungals**

Generic Name	Brand Name	Available Sizes
Fluconazole*	Diflucan	50, 100, 200 mg
Griseofulvin (microsize)	Fulvicin	250, 500 mg
Griseofulvin (ultramicrosize)	Grispeg, Fulvicin	125, 165, 250, 330 mg
Itraconazole*	Sporanox	100, 200 mg
Ketoconazole*	Nizoral	200 mg
Terbinafine*	Lamisil	250 mg

*High cost per unit dose.

tigo, folliculitis, or paronychia needs treatment with the appropriate antibiotics, usually dicloxacillin or erythromycin. Topical cleansing of the lesions to remove the crusts is also helpful. Infected cysts and carbuncles should be incised and drained and may require oral antibiotic therapy. Cellulitis requires systemic antibiotics. Nasal carriage of *Staphylococcus aureus* can be effectively treated with mupirocin applied to the anterior nares. "Hot tub folliculitis," caused by *Pseudomonas*, responds to systemic ciprofloxacin.

Parasitic Infections
Pyrethrins have become the standard therapies for scabies and lice (Table 14–10). Crotamiton (Eurax) can be used in patients who may be ragweed sensitive. Concern about neurotoxicity of lindane has led to its decreased use. Recurrence of scabies is almost always related to reinfection or incomplete treatment of the patient rather than to resistance of the mite.

Viral Infections
Primary and recurrent herpes simplex is treated with oral acyclovir 200 mg five times a day for 5 days. Acyclovir 200 mg two or three times a day can prevent the recurrence of simplex infections.

TABLE 14–10. **Antiparasitic Agents**

Generic Name/Form	Brand Name	Available Sizes	Indications
Lindane 1% cream	Kwell	60 g	Scabies and lice
Lindane lotion	Kwell	2 oz	Scabies and lice
Lindane shampoo	Kwell	2 oz	Scabies and lice
Permethrin 5% cream	Elimite	60-g tube	Scabies
Crotamiton cream or lotion	Eurax	60 g	Scabies
Permethrin spray	Rid	5 oz	Lice
Permethrin shampoo	Rid	2, 4, 8 oz	Lice

TABLE 14–11. **Antiviral Agents**

Agents	Brand Name	Available Sizes	Indications	Dosing*
Acyclovir, oral	Zovirax	200-mg capsules	Initial herpes simplex	200 mg 5×/d × 10 d
		200-mg capsules	Intermittent herpes simplex	200 mg 5×/d × 5 d
		200-mg capsules	Suppressive dose for simplex	200 mg bid
Acyclovir 5% ointment	Zovirax	3-, 15-g tubes	Herpes simplex	6×/d × 7 d
Acyclovir	Zovirax	800-mg capsules	Herpes zoster	800 mg 5×/d × 10 d
Valacyclovir	Valtrex	500-mg capsules	Herpes zoster	1 g tid × 7 d
Famciclovir	Famvir	500 mg	Herpes zoster	500 mg tid × 7 d

*In patients with normal renal function.

TABLE 14–12. **Treatments for Sexually Transmitted Diseases**

Disease	Primary Treatment	Alternate Treatment
Chancroid	Azithromycin 1 g PO × 1 or ceftri-axone 250 mg IM × 1 or erythro-mycin base 500 mg PO qid × 7 d	Augmentin 500 mg tid × 7 d or ciprofloxacin 500 mg bid × 3 d
Lymphogranuloma venereum	Doxycycline 100 mg bid × 21 d	Erythromycin 500 mg qid × 21 d or sulfisoxazole 500 mg qid × 21 d
Syphilis (primary)	Benzathine penicillin 2.4 million units IM × 1	Doxycycline 100 mg bid × 2 wks
Syphilis (late latent)	Benzathine penicillin 2.4 million units IM weekly × 3 wks	Tetracycline 500 mg qid × 2 wks
Nongonococcal urethritis	Doxycycline 100 mg bid × 7 d	Azithromycin 1 g PO × 1 or erythro-mycin 800 mg qid × 7 d
Gonococcus	Ceftriaxone 125 mg IM × 1 or cefixime 400 mg PO × 1 or ciprofloxacin 500 mg PO × 1 or ofloxacin 400 mg PO × 1 (plus doxycycline 100 mg PO bid)	

Herpes zoster is treated with oral acyclovir 800 mg five times a day for 7 to 10 days, or famciclovir 500 mg three times a day for 7 days (Table 14–11). Protocols for treating other sexually transmitted diseases appear in Table 14–12.

Acne

A staged approach to the treatment of acne is indicated. For predominantly comedonal and inflammatory papules, initial therapy involves benzoyl peroxide preparations with 2.5% to 10% of the active ingredient; topical antibiotics are used initially as well (Table 14–13). Preparations combining erythromycin and benzoyl peroxide are available (Benzamycin). Tretinoin (vitamin A acid, Retin-A) is effective for comedonal and papular acne. Because these agents or their bases may be irritating to the skin, very mild soaps such as Neutrogena, Basis, Purpose, Dove, or Tone are recommended. Abrasive scrubs are not usually recommended. Therapy should not be altered for 6 to 8 weeks, because that much time is usually needed to observe therapeutic effects.

For inflammatory papules and cystic disease, patients benefit from systemic antibiotics, usually starting in the range of 1 g of tetracycline, erythromycin, or other broad-spectrum antibiotic (Table 14–14). With a good response, dosage can be gradually decreased. At least 6 or 8 weeks are required before considering changing antibiotics. Minocycline (Minocin) is often effective, but it may lead to skin pigmentation, which is not seen with other antibiot-

TABLE 14–13. **Topical Antibiotics**

Generic Name/Form	Brand Name	Available Sizes	Adult Dose for Skin Infection
Clindamycin solution or lotion	Cleocin	30, 60 mL	bid
Erythromycin			
2% solution	A/T/S	60 mL	bid
2% gel	A/T/S	30 g	bid
Mupirocin 2% ointment	Bactroban	1, 15, 30 g	bid
Silver sulfadiazine 1%	Silvadene	20, 50, 85, 400, 1000 g	bid
Meclocycline	Meclan	1% cream: 20, 45 g	bid
Metronidazole	MetroGel	1% gel: 1 oz, 45 g	bid

TABLE 14–14. **Systemic Antibiotics**

Generic Name	Brand Name	Available Sizes	Adult Dose for Skin Infection
Amoxicillin	Amoxil	125, 250, 500 mg	250 mg q 8 h × 7–10 d
Amoxicillin with clavulanic acid	Augmentin*	125, 250, 500 mg	250 mg q 8 h × 7–10 d
Azithromycin	Zithromax*	250 mg	250 mg q d × 5 d
Cephalexin	Keflex	250, 500 mg	250 mg q 6 h × 7–10 d
Ciprofloxacin	Cipro*	250, 500, 750 mg	500–750 mg q 12 h × 7–10 d
Clarithromycin	Biaxin*	250, 500 mg	250 mg q 12 h × 7 d
Clindamycin	Cleocin	75, 150, 300 mg	150 mg q 6 h
Dicloxacillin			250–500 mg q 6 h × 7–10 d
Doxycycline	Doryx	100 mg	100 mg q 12 h
Erythromycin	E-Mycin	250, 333 mg	250–333 mg q 6–8 h × 7–10 d
Minocycline	Minocin*	50, 100 mg	100 mg q 12 h
Tetracycline	Achromycin	250, 500 mg	500–1000 mg q 12 h
Trimethoprim/ sulfamethoxazole	Bactrim	Regular/double strength	1 tablet bid × 7–10 d

*High cost per unit dose.

ics. The colitis seen with systemic clinda-mycin has led to the infrequent use of that drug for acne.

For severe acne, patients may need isotretinoin (13-*cis*-retinoic acid, Accutane) and should be seen by someone very familiar with the use of that drug. It is essential that the patient not become pregnant during therapy. Before beginning this agent, studies for abnormal androgen production may be indicated in females. Estrogens in birth control pills may be effective in controlling acne, but this is usually not a prime therapeutic modality. Intralesional steroids may be used in individual cystic, inflammatory lesions. Atrophy may be seen with corticosteroid injections and it is advised that this therapy be used only by physicians familiar with this treatment.

Alopecia

Alopecia Areata
Class I to class III topical steroids (see Table 14–5) under occlusion or intralesional corticosteroids are often effective in growing hair in alopecia areata. When intralesional steroids are given, the total dose must be monitored to avoid systemic symptoms and signs of steroid excess. Topical anthralin (0.2% to 1%), starting with short-contact therapy (15 to 30 min-

utes) and advancing to overnight therapy, is often effective. Systemic steroids are rarely indicated. PUVA therapy or sensitization with potent contact sensitizers (not FDA-approved) may lead to hair growth.

Male Pattern Alopecia
A small percentage of patients, both men and women, with male pattern alopecia responds to twice daily application of 2% minoxidil. Usually those patients who respond have early disease. If therapy is discontinued, a rapid acceleration of hair loss ensues.

Eczematous Dermatitis

Atopic Dermatitis
Decreasing physical and psychic stimuli that aggravate itching is the mainstay of therapy for atopic dermatitis. This includes adequate hydration of the skin, decreasing exposure to wool and other physical agents that precipitate itching, use of systemic antihistamines, and judicious use of systemic antibiotics for the cutaneous infections to which these patients are prone. Rarely there is superinfection with herpes simplex, but should this occur, systemic treatment with acyclovir is needed. Very rarely does the patient with atopic dermatitis require systemic ste-

roids; the decision to start them should be made in conjunction with a dermatologist. Class II to IV topical steroids can be used on selected lesions. UVB, combined UVB and UVA, or PUVA therapy have been used in severely affected patients. Topical tars (e.g., liquor carbonis detergens [LCD]) are a useful adjuvant to therapy.

Acute Contact Dermatitis

Patients with acute contact dermatitis frequently need systemic corticosteroids for relief of their pruritus and edematous lesions, which frequently involve the face or genitals. Cool soaks as described previously are also useful. A tapering course of oral steroids over 10 to 14 days beginning at 60 mg of prednisone is often necessary to resolution. Shorter courses of therapy may be associated with flaring up of lesions. For limited disease, class I topical corticosteroids may be used.

Chronic Dermatitis (Lichen Simplex Chronicus)

Localized sites of dermatitis may be resistant to topical corticosteroid therapy even with class I agents. Intralesional steroids, Cordran tape, tars, or ultraviolet light may be necessary in such refractory cases.

Diaper Rash

Diaper rash is usually an irritant dermatitis, an eczematous dermatitis, or seborrheic dermatitis with or without superimposed candidal infection. It can be treated with class IV or V corticosteroid creams with the addition of an anticandidal agent. Stronger steroids with or without antifungal agents are not indicated for diaper dermatitis.

Life-Threatening Reactions

Toxic Epidermal Necrolysis

Toxic epidermal necrolysis is best treated by supportive therapy; patients with extensive disease benefit from hospitalization on a burn unit. Topical antibiotics and systemic steroids are of little proven benefit. Scrupulous attention should be given to fluid and electrolyte balance and treatment of systemic infection.

Drug Eruptions

Anaphylactic reactions may require epinephrine to maintain adequate respiration and should be treated as a medical emergency.

Urticaria can be treated with antihistamines (see Table 14–4). Topical antipruritics are of some benefit. Systemic steroids may be necessary to control symptoms in some patients.

Psoriasis

Treatment is with class I to class III topical corticosteroids; classes IV and V are used for intertriginous lesions, which are common. Topical tars and anthralin are effective, as are Cordran tape or intralesional steroids for resistant plaques. The scalp often requires keratolytic agents before steroids and occlusion can be effective. Topical vitamin D analogues (Dovonex) and vitamin A analogues (tazarotene) are also effective.

Systemic antistreptococcal antibiotics can be effective when given for 2 to 4 weeks for pharyngitis-associated flare-ups and early episodes of guttate psoriasis. Systemic antihistamines may help relieve pruritus.

UVB or PUVA therapies are helpful for more extensive disease. Systemic retinoids (acitretin), antimetabolites (e.g., methotrexate), or immunosuppressives (cyclosporine) should be reserved for more advanced and refractory disease (Table 14–15).

Rosacea

Mild rosacea may respond to topical antibiotics, topical metronidazole (MetroGel), or 10% sodium sulfacetamide 5% sulfur (Sulfacet-R). More severe cases require abstaining from alcoholic beverages, very hot beverages, caffeine, and spicy foods, in conjunction with the use of systemic broadspectrum antibiotics such as tetracycline (1 g qd) or minocycline (100 to 200 mg qd).

Seborrheic Dermatitis

Topical corticosteroids (class III or IV) combined with topical antifungal agents are effective in controlling this disorder, which often needs life-long intermittent therapy. Very refractory disease should raise the possibility of HIV infection.

TABLE 14–15. **Immunosuppressive Agents and Antimetabolites**

Generic Name	Brand Name	Available Sizes	Adult Doses	Laboratory Follow-up
Azathioprine	Imuran	50 mg tablets	50–100 mg/d	CBC, LFTs
Cyclophos-phamide	Cytoxan	25, 50 mg tablets	1–5 mg/kg per day	CBC, UA
Cyclosporine	Sandimmune	25, 100 mg capsules	3–6 mg/kg per day	Electrolytes, creatinine
Methotrexate	Rheumatrex	2.5 mg tablets	5–25 mg/wk	CBC, LFTs
Prednisone	Deltasone	2.5, 5, 10, 20, 50 mg	5–60 mg/d	Glucose
Tacrolimus	Prograf	1, 5 mg	0.15–0.30 mg/kg per day	Electrolytes, creatinine

CBC = complete blood count; LFTs = liver function tests; UA = urinalysis.

Ulcers

Appropriate antibiotic therapy, usually systemic, is required for lesions that are truly infected. Elevation of the legs and elimination of edema is an important therapeutic modality. A variety of dressings are available to aid the healing of lesions (Table 14–16).

Urticaria

Urticaria may require one or more of the antihistamines listed in Table 14–4. The search for inciting agents is often unsuccessful. Avoidance of food additives and over-the-counter medications should be tried. Long-term systemic steroids should be avoided but short-term treatment may be necessary in symptomatic patients with very refractory disease.

Warts

This common dermatologic disease can be treated by occlusion with lactic or salicylic acid preparations (e.g., DuoFilm or Occlusal), electrodessication, curettage, or cryotherapy with liquid nitrogen. Flat warts on the face frequently respond to tretinoin cream. Condylomata respond to cryotherapy, topical podophyllin, or both. The podophyllin may be applied by the physician as podophyllum resin or by the patient as an alcoholic extract (Condylox). Podophyllin is contraindicated during pregnancy. Refractory lesions have been treated with laser or intralesional bleomycin. Interferon alfa-2 and imiquimod 5% cream have been used for refractory condylomata.

TABLE 14–16. **Wound Dressings**

Dressing	Transmits O₂	Transmits H₂O Vapor	Excludes Bacteria	Absorbs Fluids	Transparent	Adhesive
Biooclusive	+	+	–	–	+	+
Duoderm	–	–	+	+	–	+
Geliperm	+	+	+	+	+	+
Intrasite	–	–	+	+	–	+
Opsite	+	+	+	–	+	+
Replicare	–	–	+	–	–	+
Tegasorb	–	–	+	+	–	+
Tegoderm	+	+	?	–	+	+
Vigilon	+	–	–	+	+	–
Zenoderm	+	+	+	+	+	+

PART

4

Index

Chapter 15

■ ■

Index of Differential Diagnosis

MACULES (Chapter 3, pp. 23–124)

Blue Macules
Congenital
Mongolian spot (congenital dermal melanocytosis)
Nevus of Ota or Ito

Acquired
Blue nevus
Drug-induced blue macule
Erythema dyschromicum perstans
Maculae ceruleae
Malignant melanoma
Ochronosis
Tattoo

Brown Macules

Generalized Hyperpigmentation

Common Causes
Addison's disease (Nelson's syndrome)
Arsenic ingestion
Biliary cirrhosis
Cushing's syndrome, exogenous adrenocorticotropic hormone (ACTH) (melanocyte-stimulating hormone), or ACTH-secreting tumor
Drug-induced hyperpigmentation
Hemochromatosis
Hyperthyroidism
Malignant melanoma with generalized melanomatosis
POEMS syndrome (adult onset)
Porphyria cutanea tarda (and variegate porphyria)

Scleroderma
Sprue malabsorption
Whipple's disease
Wilson's disease

Rare Causes
Acromegaly
Central nervous system disease:
 Schilder's disease, catatonic
 schizophrenia
Chronic disease: infection, lymphoma,
 neoplasia
Felty's syndrome
Gaucher's disease, Niemann-Pick disease
Pheochromocytoma
POEMS syndrome
Pregnancy
Preasthmatic attack melanoderma
Vitamin B$_{12}$ deficiency

Localized Hyperpigmentation

**Brown Macules in Sun-Exposed Areas or
 Non–Sun-Exposed Areas**
Acanthosis nigricans
Becker's nevus
Café au lait spot: Albright's syndrome,
 neurofibromatosis
Erythrasma
Fungal infection (dermatophyte)
Lentigo syndromes
Mastocytosis (telangiectasia macularis
 eruptiva perstans, urticaria
 pigmentosa)
Nevi
Postinflammatory hyperpigmentation:
 dermatitis, dyskeratosis congenita,
 fixed drug eruption, incontinentia
 pigmenti, lichen planus, macular
 amyloid, pinta
Progressive pigmentary purpura
Stasis dermatitis
Tinea versicolor

Brown Macules on Palms or Soles
Acral lentiginous melanoma
Cronkhite-Canada syndrome
Secondary syphilis
Talon noir
Tinea nigra palmaris

Brown Macules in Sun-Exposed Areas
Actinic lentigo
Berlock dermatitis
Drug-induced hyperpigmentation
Freckle (ephelis)

Lentigo maligna
Melasma
Pellagra
Xeroderma pigmentosum

Purple Macules and Purpura
Caput succedaneum
Dysproteinemia
Ecchymoses: trauma, senile purpura,
 venous stasis, clotting abnormalities,
 Cushing's syndrome, corticosteroid
 usage, chronic renal disease, primary
 amyloidosis, psychogenic purpura
Kaposi's sarcoma
Platelet abnormalities
Progressive pigmentary purpura
Scurvy
Severe physical exertion
Viral infection and immune disorders:
 Wiskott-Aldrich syndrome,
 histiocytosis X

Red Macules
Red Exanthems

Red Exanthems with Adenopathy
Brucellosis
Echovirus 16, Boston exanthem
Collagen vascular disease, systemic lupus
 erythematosus, rheumatoid arthritis
Cytomegalovirus
Gianotti-Crosti syndrome
HIV infection, primary
Infectious mononucleosis
Mucocutaneous lymph node syndrome,
 Kawasaki's disease
Rubella, German measles
Syphilis, congenital
Syphilis, secondary
Toxoplasmosis

Red Exanthems without Adenopathy
*Common Exanthems Not Associated with
 Systemic Lymphadenopathy*
Collagen vascular disease, systemic lupus
 erythematosus, rheumatoid arthritis,
 rheumatic fever
Drug-induced eruption
Enterovirus echo or coxsackievirus
Erythema infectiosum, parvovirus B19
Infectious hepatitis
Measles
Rocky Mountain spotted fever
Roseola infantum (echovirus 16 may be
 very similar)
Scarlet fever

*Uncommon Exanthems Not Associated with
  Systemic Lymphadenopathy*
Acrodynia
Infectious hepatitis
Rat-bite fever (*Spirillum minus*)
Typhoid fever
Typhus

Reticulated Red Macules
Erythema ab igne
Erythema infectiosum
Larva migrans
Livedo reticularis

Scattered Red Macules
Atopic dermatitis
Burns
Cellulitis
Dermatomyositis
Erysipelas
Fixed drug eruption
Herpes zoster
Intertrigo
Leprosy
Lupus erythematosus
Seborrheic dermatitis

Telangiectasia

**Telangiectatic Lesions without Other
  Skin Lesions**
Ataxia-telangiectasia
Essential telangiectasia
Hereditary hemorrhagic telangiectasia
  (Osler-Weber-Rendu disease)
Lupus erythematosus
Nevus flammeus
Posterior nail fold telangiectasia
Scleroderma
Telangiectasia macularis eruptiva
  perstans (mastocytosis)

Telangiectasia with Other Skin Changes
Actinically damaged skin
Atrophy from systemic or topical
  administration of corticosteroids
Dermatomyositis
Goltz's syndrome (focal dermal
  hypoplasia)
Lupus erythematosus
Necrobiosis lipoidica diabeticorum
Poikiloderma atrophicans vasculare
Radiodermatitis
Rare childhood diseases with atrophy
Rosacea
Scleroderma

Telangiectasia and prominent
  hyperpigmentation

Transient Red Macules
Cholinergic urticaria
Erythromelalgia
Flushing syndromes: carcinoid syndrome,
  pheochromocytoma, mastocytosis,
  nervous system diseases, Riley-Day
  syndrome
Juvenile rheumatoid arthritis (Still's
  disease)
Raynaud's phenomenon
Rheumatic fever (erythema marginatum)
Transient erythemas of the newborn
Urticaria (hives)

White Macules
Congenital or Genetic White Macules

Generalized Depigmentation
Albinism: Chédiak-Higashi syndrome,
  phenylketonuria, vitiligo

Localized Hyperpigmented Lesions
Nevus anemicus
Piebaldism: Waardenburg's syndrome,
  deafness, and piebaldism syndromes
Tuberous sclerosis
Other causes of hypopigmentation:
  dyskeratosis congenita, incontinentia
  pigmenti achromians, nevus
  depigmentosus

Acquired White Macules

Nonatrophic Lesions
Halo nevus
Pityriasis alba
Postinflammatory hypopigmentation:
  arsenical hypopigmentation, chemical
  depigmentation, idiopathic guttate
  hypomelanosis, kwashiorkor, leprosy,
  pinta, sarcoidosis
Tinea versicolor
Vitiligo

Atrophic Lesions
Discoid lupus erythematosus
Lichen sclerosus et atrophicus
Malignant atrophic papulosis (Degos'
  disease)
Poikiloderma vasculare atrophicans
Potent topical steroid use (atrophy)
Scleroderma, morphea
Sclerosis, scar, morphea
X-ray dermatitis

DIFFUSE SCALING (Chapter 4, pp. 125–132)

Scaling of Palms and Soles
Arsenical keratoses
Hereditary keratodermas
Postdermatoses
Scaling without discrete papules
Tyrosinemia II

Generalized Scaling
Epidermolytic hyperkeratosis
Erythema craquele
Exfoliative dermatitis: AIDS, drug reaction, eczematous dermatitis, idiopathic dermatitis, lymphoma, mycosis fungoides, pityriasis rubra pilaris, psoriasis, seborrheic dermatitis
Ichthyosis vulgaris
Lamellar ichthyosis
X-linked ichthyosis
Xerosis

PAPULES (Chapter 5, pp. 133–280)

Blue-Black Papules

Single
Atypical nevi
Blue nevus
Ecthyma gangrenosum
Malignant melanoma

Multiple (Including Vascular Lesions)
Angioma
Fabry's disease
Hemangioma
Kaposi's sarcoma
Lichen planus
Malignancy: lymphoma, leukemia, mycosis fungoides, metastatic melanoma
Open acne comedones
Venous lakes and blue rubber bleb nevus syndrome

Brown Papules

Single
Basal cell carcinoma
Dermatofibroma
Malignant melanoma
Mastocytoma

Multiple
Acanthosis nigricans
Atypical nevi
Cat scratch disease
Deep fungal disease
Foreign body disease
Histiocytosis X
Lichen amyloidosis
Leishmaniasis
Mastocytoma (urticaria pigmentosa)
Mycobacterial disease: tuberculosis, atypical mycobacterial disease, swimming pool granuloma
Nevi (moles)
Porokeratosis
Sarcoidosis
Seborrheic keratoses
Syphilis and yaws
Tinea versicolor

Flesh-Colored Papules, Including Linear and Painful Papular Lesions
Acne comedone
Actinic elastosis
Basal cell carcinoma
Condyloma acuminatum
Dermatofibroma
Fox-Fordyce disease
Granuloma annulare
Keloids
Lichen nitidus
Lichen planus
Lymphangioma circumscriptum
Metastatic tumors
Milia
Molluscum contagiosum
Neurofibromata
Nevi (moles)
Pretibial myxedema
Prurigo
Sarcoidosis
Skin tags (acrochordons)
Warts (flat)
Rare, single flesh-colored papules: amelanocytic melanoma, apocrine hidrocystoma, Malherbe's calcifying epithelioma, connective tissue nevus, hidradenoma papilliferum, mastocytoma, Merkel cell tumor, metastatic tumors, pilonodal sinus
Rare, small, persistent flesh-colored papules on the face: acne, adenoma sebaceum (tuberous sclerosis), amyloidosis, basal cell nevus syndrome, colloid milium, Cowden

disease, eccrine hidrocystomas, lipoid proteinosis, sarcoid, syringomas, trichoepitheliomas

Rare, small, persistent flesh-colored papules (anywhere): adnexal tumors (cylindroma, syringoma), amyloidosis, connective tissue nevus, colloid milium, Degos' disease, generalized eruptive histiocytosis, Hunter's syndrome, knuckle pads, lichen amyloidosis, multicentric reticulohistiocytosis, multiple cysts (hair cysts, steatocystoma multiplex), papular mucinosis (lichen myxedematosus), xanthogranuloma (juvenile nevoxanthoendothelioma), xanthoma disseminatum

Linear Papular Lesions
Darier's disease
Focal dermal hypoplasia
Herpes zoster
Incontinentia pigmenti
Lichen nidus
Lichen planus
Lichen striatus
Molluscum contagiosum
Papular mucinosis
Psoriasis
Sarcoid
Warts

Painful Papules
Angiolipoma
Blue rubber bleb nevus
Chondrodermatitis nodularis chronica helicis
Chordoma cutis
Dercum's disease
Eccrine spiradenoma
Endometrioma
Glomus tumor
Leiomyomas
Neurilemoma
Neuroma

Purpuric Papules
Atheroembolism
Consumption coagulopathy
Coumadin necrosis
Leukocytoclastic vasculitis: allergic vasculitis, collagen vascular disease, drug-induced cutaneous vasculitis, dysproteinemia, idiopathic, rheumatoid arthritis, Schönlein-Henoch purpura, thrombotic thrombocytopenic purpura
Rocky Mountain spotted fever
Septicemia
Subacute bacterial endocarditis

Smooth, Red Papules with Abrupt Onset

Grouped
Contact dermatitis
Eccrine neutrophilic hidradenitis
Folliculitis
Insect bites
Herpes infection: herpes zoster, herpes simplex
Miliaria

Multiple
Autoeczematization
Bacillary angiomatosis
Drug-induced eruption
Erythema multiforme
Graft-versus-host disease (GVHD)
Pityriasis rosea
Polymorphous light eruption
Psoriasis
Secondary syphilis
Systemic lupus erythematosus
Vasculitis

Single
Coma induced
Erysipelas
Fixed drug reaction
Leishmaniasis

Transient (Appear and Disappear within Hours to Days)
Burns: chemicals, heat, sunlight, ultraviolet irradiation
Cholinergic urticaria
Goose bumps (cutis anserina)
Grover's disease
Jellyfish sting
Juvenile rheumatoid arthritis
Urticaria

Smooth, Red Papules with Gradual Onset

Any Location
Angiokeratoma and cherry angiomas
Configurate erythema and Lyme disease
Erythema elevatum diutinum
Fabry's disease
Granuloma annulare
Granulomatous diseases: cat scratch

disease, deep fungal disease, foreign body disease, leishmaniasis, mycobacterial disease, sarcoidosis, syphilis, yaws
Hemangioma
Kaposi's sarcoma, bacterial angiomatosa, and malignant angioendothelioma
Kawasaki's disease
Leprosy
Leishmaniasis
Lichen planus
Lymphomatoid papulosis
Malignancy: adnexal tumors, leukemia, lymphoma, metastatic carcinoma, mycosis fungoides
Molluscum contagiosum
Pityriasis lichenoides et varioliformis acuta (PLEVA)
Pyogenic granuloma
Sarcoidosis
Scabies
Syphilis

Smooth, Red Papules in Specific Locations (Gradual Onset)

Digits
Glomus tumor

Genitals
Erythroplasia of Queyrat

Head and neck
Acne vulgaris and rosacea
Follicular mucinosis
Granuloma faciale
Lupus erythematosus
Lymphocytic infiltrate
Lymphocytoma cutis
Perioral dermatitis
Polymorphous light eruption
Relapsing polychondritis

Scaly Papules

Limited Lesions (<10)
Actinic keratoses (can be multiple)
Bowen's disease
Keratoacanthoma
Lichen simplex chronicus
Paget's disease
Squamous cell carcinoma
Warts, including condylomata

Multiple Lesions
Atopic dermatitis (eczema)
Darier's disease

Dermatophyte infection
Drug eruptions
Exfoliative dermatitis: drug reaction, eczematous dermatitis, idiopathic cause, lymphoma, mycosis fungoides, pityriasis rubra pilaris, psoriasis, seborrheic dermatitis
Kawasaki's disease
Keratosis pilaris
Lichen amyloidosis and lichen myxedematosus
Lichen planus
Lupus erythematosus
Mycosis fungoides and parapsoriasis
Neurodermatitis
Nummular eczema
Pityriasis rosea
Pityriasis rubra pilaris
Prurigo nodularis
Psoriasis
Seborrheic dermatitis
Seborrheic keratoses
Secondary syphilis
Tinea versicolor
Warts and condyloma acuminatum
Rare causes: acquired perforating dermatoses, elastosis perforans serpiginosa, epidermal nevus, epidermodysplasia verruciformis, Kyrle's disease, lichen amyloidosis, multiple keratoacanthoma, pemphigus foliaceus, perforating collagenosis, perforating folliculitis, perforating granuloma annulare

Yellow Papules
Actinic elastosis
Eruptive xanthomas
Necrobiosis lipoidica diabeticorum
Noneruptive xanthomas
Pseudoxanthoma elasticum
Sebaceous hyperplasia
Other yellow lesions: Goltz's syndrome, lupus vulgaris, nevus lipomatosus, nevus sebaceous, xanthogranuloma

Palm and Sole Papules with Scaling
Arsenical keratoses
Diffuse palm and sole scaling: acanthosis nigricans, arsenic ingestion , chronic eczematous dermatitis, dermatophyte infection, drug-related eruption,

hidrotic ectodermal dysplasia,
ichthyosis secondary to other diseases
(HIV, carcinoma, lymphoma),
ichthyosis vulgaris, lamellar ichthyosis,
lupus erythematosus, psoriasis
Digital fibromas
Hereditary keratodermas
Hyperhidrosis
Tyrosinemia II

BLISTERS, EROSIONS, AND EXCORIATIONS (Chapter 6, pp. 281–336)
Blisters with Red Papules
Multiple, Symmetric Lesions
Autoeczematization
Bullous pemphigoid
Contact dermatitis
Dermatitis herpetiformis
Erythema multiforme
Vasculitis

Asymmetric Lesions
Bullous pemphigoid
Contact dermatitis
Dermatophyte infection
Insect bites
Nummular eczema
Scabies

Rare Causes of Blisters with Red Papules
Congenital syphilis
Erysipelas
Fixed drug reaction
Gas gangrene
Herpes gestationis
Lichen planus
Lupus erythematosus
Pemphigus vegetans
Pityriasis lichenoides et varioliformis acuta
Rickettsialpox
Tumor

Blisters with Nonred Papules
Dystrophic epidermolysis bullosa
Incontinentia pigmenti
Linear IgA disease
Lymphangioma circumscriptum
Porphyria cutanea tarda
Urticaria pigmentosa (infants)

Rare diseases with blistering and nonred papules: Darier's disease, lichen sclerosus et atrophicus, urticaria pigmentosa (diffuse, cutaneous, severe mastocytosis)

Umbilicated Blisters
Herpes simplex
Herpes zoster (shingles)
Kaposi's varicelliform eruption
Orf and milker's nodule
Smallpox
Vaccinia
Varicella (chickenpox)

Blisters without Other Lesions
Pinpoint, Tiny Vesicles
Dyshidrosis (hands, feet)
Miliaria

Vesicles and Bullae
Bites
Bullous impetigo
Burns
Cicatricial pemphigoid
Coma, drug-related, and neuropathic bullae
Dystrophic epidermolysis bullosa
Epidermolysis bullosa acquisita
Epidermolysis bullosa letalis
Epidermolysis bullosa simplex
Familial benign pemphigus
Hand-foot-and-mouth disease
IgA bullous dermatoses
Pemphigoid, bullous lupus erythematosus
Pemphigus foliaceus
Pemphigus vulgaris
Toxic epidermal necrolysis (staphylococcal or drug related)

Erosions and Crusting
Candidiasis
Dermatophyte infection
Fragile skin: actinically damaged skin, Ehlers-Danlos syndrome, epidermolysis bullosa; epidermolytic hyperkeratosis, porphyria cutanea tarda, corticosteroid ingestion, or topical application
Impetigo
Intertrigo
Pemphigus: foliaceus, vulgaris, and

Hailey-Hailey disease
Perlèche
Toxic epidermal necrolysis

Excoriations

Skin Diseases That May Be Extremely Pruritic and Result in Excoriations
Atopic dermatitis
Drug eruptions
Insect bites and infestations
Lichen planus
Mycosis fungoides
Neurodermatitis
Prurigo nodularis
Scabies
Stasis dermatitis
Swimmers' itch

Pruritus and Excoriations without Skin Disease
Central nervous system disease
Delusions of parasitism
Diabetes
Drug reactions: codeine, amphetamines
Hyperparathyroidism
Hyperthyroidism
Infestations: pubic or body lice, worms
Leukemia
Liver disease
Lymphoma
Neuropathy
Polycythemia rubra vera
Pregnancy
Psychosis
Renal disease: often with uremia
Sarcoidosis
Secondary hyperparathyroidism

PUSTULES, ABSCESSES, AND SINUSES (Chapter 7, pp. 337–371)

Pustules in Generalized or Nonspecific Locations
Acrodermatitis enteropathica
Acute generalized exanthematous pustulosis
Blastomycosis
Candidiasis (moniliasis)
Dermatophyte infection
Drug-related eruptions
Folliculitis
Impetigo

Pustular psoriasis
Septic vasculitis
Subcorneal pustular dermatoses
Rare pustular eruptions: impetigo herpetiformis, myiasis, pyoderma gangrenosum, secondary syphilis, swimmers' itch

Pustules or Abscesses on the Face
Acne
Rosacea
Sycosis barbae (folliculitis)
Tinea barbae

Pustules or Abscesses on the Scalp
Dermatophyte infection
Dissecting cellulitis
Folliculitis decalvans

Pustules or Abscesses on the Palms and Soles
Acropustulosis
Dermatophyte infection
Dyshidrosis
Epidermolysis bullosa simplex
Pustular psoriasis
Septic vasculitis

Abscesses
Anthrax
Furuncle-carbuncle
Hidradenitis suppurativa

Sinuses
Actinomycosis and nocardiosis
Dental sinus
Hidradenitis suppurativa
Mycetoma
Scrofuloderma

INDURATION, SCLEROSIS, AND ATROPHY (Chapter 8, pp. 373–393)

Induration and Sclerosis
Edema
Lymphedema
Mastocytosis
Pachydermoperiostosis
Scleredema
Scleroderma
Rare scleroderma-like diseases:

acromegaly, amyloidosis, ataxia-telangiectasia, carcinoid syndrome, congenital generalized fibromatosis, diffuse infiltrating carcinoma *(peau d'orange)*, erythropoietic protoporphyria, graft-versus-host reactions, leprosy, lipoid proteinosis, mucopolysaccharide storage disorders (Hurler's syndrome, Hunter's syndrome), myxedema, phenylketonuria, porphyria cutanea tarda, progeria, scleromyxedema

Atrophy

Lichen sclerosus et atrophicus
Lupus erythematosus
Lupus vulgaris
Morphea
Necrobiosis lipoidica diabeticorum
Poikiloderma
Porphyria cutanea tarda
Striae
Trauma or injection
Varioliform or chickenpox-like scarring: postinflammatory causes, lymphomatoid papulosis, malignant atrophic papulosis (Degos' disease), pityriasis lichenoides et varioliformis acuta
Rare causes of subcutaneous atrophy: acrodermatitis chronica atrophicans, acrogeria, anetoderma, facial hemiatrophy (Parry-Romberg syndrome), focal dermal hypoplasia (Goltz's syndrome), Gower's panatrophy, partial lipodystrophy, progeria, total lipoatrophy (Lawrence-Seip syndrome), Weber-Christian disease, Werner's syndrome

NODULES AND CYSTS
(Chapter 9, pp. 395–434)

Cysts

Epidermal cyst
Pilar cyst
Dermoid cyst
Steatocystoma multiplex
Parasitic cyst

Flesh-Colored to Red Nodules

Deep nodules peculiar to newborns
Dermatofibrosarcoma protuberans
Eccrine poroma
Eccrine spiradenoma
Fibromatosis
Foreign body
Gummatous syphilis
Hemangioma: blanching with pressure
Juxta-articular nodules: rheumatoid arthritis, rheumatic fever, gout, calcinosis cutis, granuloma annulare, synovial cysts or ganglia, chondroma, osteoarthritis (Heberden's node), billonodular synovitis, multicentric reticulohistiocytosis, xanthoma
Lipoma: common
Lupus profundus
Malignancies and metastatic carcinoma
Phlebolith
Prurigo nodularis
Sarcoidosis
Systemic mycosis or mycobacterial disease
Vasculitis: often tender lesions

Purple Nodules

Hemangiomas (on unusual occasions, may present as deep blue nodules)
Kaposi's sarcoma
Lymphoma, leukemia, mycosis fungoides
Melanoma

Tender Red Nodules

Calcinosis cutis
Carbuncle (boil)
Erythema induratum (nodular vasculitis)
Erythema nodosum
Hidradenitis suppurativa
Leishmaniasis
Lymphogranuloma venereum
Nodules peculiar to tropical or subtropical areas: Buruli ulcer (atypical mycobacteria), deep fungi (especially South American blastomycosis), leishmaniasis (protozoa), leprosy, myiasis (insect larvae), nematodes (round worms, flat worms), rhinoscleroma, yaws
Panniculitis with pancreatic disease
Polyarteritis nodosa
Subacute migratory panniculitis
Suppurative adenitis
Systemic mycosis or mycobacterial disease
Temporal arteritis (cranial arteritis)

Thrombophlebitis
Trauma or cold
Weber-Christian disease

ULCERS (Chapter 10, pp. 435–467)
Anesthetic Ulcers
Neuropathic ulcers, mal perforans
Diabetes mellitus
Leprosy
Polyneuropathy

Painful and Ischemic Ulcers
Arteriosclerosis
Atrophie blanche
Bacterial emboli
Cholesterol emboli
Consumption coagulopathy
Cryoglobulinemia
Cutaneous polyarteritis nodosa
Diabetes mellitus
Dysproteinemia
Ergotism
Giant cell arteritis
Hemoglobinopathy
Hyperparathyroidism
Hypertensive cardiovascular disease
Insect bites (especially of the brown
  recluse spider)
Lupus erythematosus
Lethal midline granuloma
Polyarteritis nodosa
Polycythemia rubra vera
Raynaud's disease
Rheumatoid vasculitis
Scleroderma
Thromboangiitis obliterans (Buerger's
  disease)
Thrombotic thrombocytopenic purpura
Wegener's granulomatosis

Ulcers in Areas of Primary Dermatologic Disease
Bites
Calcinosis cutis
Decubitus ulcer
Erythema induratum
Factitial ulceration
Gout
Leishmaniasis
Milker's nodule
Necrobiosis lipoidica diabeticorum

Nodular liquefying panniculitis
  (panniculitis with pancreatitis)
Orf
Pyoderma gangrenosum
Radiodermatitis
Stasis dermatitis
Trauma
Tumor nodules

Purulent Ulcers
Purulent Ulcers without Marked Adenopathy
Anthrax
Atypical mycobacterial infection
Blastomycosis
Botryomycosis
Coccidioidomycosis
Cryptococcosis
Diphtheria
Herpes simplex
Lupus vulgaris
Pasteurella multocida
Progressive bacterial synergistic gangrene
Pseudomonas
Tuberculosis orificialis

Purulent Ulcers with Marked, Often Painful Adenopathy
Atypical mycobacteria
Cat scratch fever
Glanders
Plaque
Sporotrichosis
Tularemia

Purulent Ulcers in Patients Who Have Been in Tropical and Subtropical Areas
Amebiasis
Blastomycosis (South American)
Buruli ulcer
Chromomycosis
Leishmaniasis
Leprosy
Yaws

Ulcers in Specific Locations
Nasal Septum
Collagen vascular disease
Infection
Trauma
Tumor

Genital Ulcers
Syphilis (chancre)
Chancroid

HAIR AND SCALP DISEASES
(Chapter 11, pp. 469–510)

Acquired Hair Loss

Normal Scalp
Alopecia areata
Androgenetic alopecia
Dermatophyte infection
Follicular mucinosis
Traumatic alopecia
Trichotillomania

Hair Loss with Systemic Disorders
Telogen effluvium

Scarred Scalp
Congenital scalp defect (cutis aplasia)
Discoid lupus erythematosus
Folliculitis decalvans
Hot comb alopecia (follicular
   degeneration syndrome)
Infections: bacterial, fungal, and viral
Kerion (dermatophyte infection)
Lichen planopilaris
Linear morphea (coup de sabre)
Necrobiosis lipoidica diabeticorum
Neoplasia
Nevus sebaceous
Radiodermatitis
Trauma and rarer causes

Congenital or Genetic Disorders of Hair

Alopecia with Normal Hair Shaft
Anhidrotic ectodermal dysplasia
Hidrotic ectodermal dysplasia

Alopecia with Abnormal Hair Shaft
Monilethrix
Pili torti: Menkes' syndrome and
   uncombable hair syndrome
Trichothiodystrophy
Trichorrhexis nodosa

Other Alopecias

Generalized
Cartilage—hair hypoplasia
Dyskeratosis congenita
Hallermann-Streiff syndrome
Myotonic dystrophy
Netherton's syndrome
Pachyonychia congenita
Rothmund-Thomson syndrome
Trichorhinophalangeal syndrome

Turner's syndrome
Unna's hair dystrophy
Werner's syndrome

Localized
Congenital skin defects
Poland's syndrome
Testicular feminization syndrome

Abnormal Hair without Alopecia
Pseudofolliculitis barbae
Ringed hair
Wooly hair nevus

Abnormal Color of Hair
Use of hair preparations

Focal Areas of White or Gray Hair
Alopecia areata
Piebaldism
Tuberous sclerosis
Vitiligo
Vogt-Koyanagi syndrome
White forelock

Diffuse Diminution in Pigment
Albinism
Chédiak-Higashi syndrome

Gray Hair (Poliosis)
Aging

Green Hair
Copper exposure
Pernicious anemia
Phenylketonuria

White Hair
Chloroquine

Increased Hair Growth

Acquired
Anorexia nervosa and malnutrition
Dermatomyositis
Drug-related hypertrichosis:
   diphenylhydantoin, streptomycin,
   diazoxide, and corticosteroids (systemic
   or topical), cyclosporine, minoxidil
Epidermolysis bullosa dystrophica
Hypothyroidism, especially in children
Porphyrias: hexachlorobenzene
   intoxication, erythropoietic porphyria,
   porphyria cutanea tarda
Pretibial myxedema
Central nervous system disease or injury
Surrounding wounds

Congenital or Genetic

Generalized
Congenital macrogingivae syndrome
Cornelia de Lange's syndrome
Hurler's syndrome
Hypertrichosis lanuginosa (congenital
and acquired)
Increased mucopolysaccharide in skin
and urine
Leprechaunism
Lipodystrophic diabetes

Localized
Becker's nevus
Fauntail nevus
Fetal alcohol syndrome
Giant hairy nevus
Waardenburg's syndrome

Scalp and Hair Scaling

Scaling of the Scalp
Atopic dermatitis
Dandruff
Dermatophyte infection
Cutaneous lupus erythematosus
Neurodermatitis
Psoriasis
Seborrheic dermatitis
Tinea amiantacea

Firmly Adherent Material on the Hair
Pediculosis capitis
Piedra
Trichomycosis axillaris

NAIL DISEASES (Chapter 12, pp. 511–538)

Disorders of the Nail Plate

Loss of the Nail Plate (Acquired)

Permanent Nail Plate Loss (Complete or Partial)
Inflammatory, infiltrative blistering or
vascular diseases of the nail matrix, nail
folds, or nail beds may cause
permanent loss of portions of the nail
plate. These diseases include:
Amyloidosis
Arterial occlusion: especially scleroderma,
Raynaud's phenomenon, and diabetes
mellitus
Darier's disease (associated with thin and
brittle nail plates)
Dyskeratosis congenita: childhood and
adolescence

Epidermolysis bullosa and other
blistering diseases (especially junctional
and dystrophic forms)
Lichen planus
Lupus erythematosus
Radiodermatitis
Severe trauma

Temporary Nail Plate Loss
Candida infections including
mucocutaneous candidiasis
Dermatophyte infection
Exfoliative erythroderma of any cause
Psoriasis, pityriasis rubra pilaris, and
acropustulosis
Radiation therapy
Reiter's disease
Scabies

Nail Plate Loss Due to Separation of the Nail Plate from the Nail Bed (Onycholysis)
Dermatophyte infection
Dermatitis
Drug-related separation
Hidrotic ectodermal dysplasia
Hyperthyroidism and hypothyroidism
Nail cosmetic treatments
Paronychia
Porphyria cutanea tarda
Psoriasis (Reiter's)
Trauma: physical or chemical
Weed killers: paraquat and diquat

Absence of Nail Plate: Congenital

Color Change in the Nail Plate
Addison's disease (black-brown)
Antineoplastic drugs (black-brown)
Arsenic (Mees' lines) (white)
Arsenic or gold exposures (black-brown)
Chronic malaria (black-brown)
Film-developing chemicals (black-brown)
Fungi (*Scopulariopsis brevicaulis*) (white)
Fungi (*Trichophyton mentagrophytes*)
(white)
Hair dyes (black-brown, yellow)
Hereditary (leukonychia totalis) (white)
Infection with *Pseudomonas aeruginosa*
(green) or *Candida albicans* (green,
yellow)
Melanoma (black-brown)
Melanoma with diffuse melanosis
(black-brown)
Metallic dyes (Grecian Formula) (black-
brown)
Nevus (black-brown)

Nicotine (yellow)
Psoriasis (black-brown, yellow)
Thallium poisoning, associated with
 systemic illness (white)
Trauma (white)
Yellow nail syndrome (yellow)
Zidovudine (AZT) (black-brown)

Increase in Size of Nail Plate
Intestinal diseases
Pulmonary and cardiac diseases
 (including lung carcinoma)
Thyroid acropachy with pretibial
 myxedema

Pits and Grooves

Systemic Causes
Bacterial and viral infections
Coronary occlusions
Hypocalcemia

Dermatologic Causes
Generalized diseases: psoriasis, alopecia
 areata, dermatitis of posterior nail fold
Localized diseases: median nail
 dystrophy, paronychia, trauma

Increased Thickness of the Nail Plate
Dermatophyte infection
Impaired circulation
Pachyonychia congenita
Psoriasis and pityriasis rubra pilaris
Yellow nail syndrome

Thinning of the Nail Plate
Darier's disease
Dyskeratosis congenita
Epidermolysis bullosa
Familial tendency
Iron deficiency
Lichen planus
Raynaud's disease

Disorders Involving the Nail Folds
Acute paronychia
Chronic paronychia
Ingrown nails
Mucous cysts
Papules and cysts: tuberous sclerosis
 (fibroma), glomus tumor, melanoma,
 multicentric reticulohistiocytosis, nevi,
 pyogenic granuloma, subungual
 exostoses, warts
Telangiectasia

Disorders Involving the Nail Bed

Color Changes
Addison's disease (brown)
Anemia (white)
Antineoplastic drugs (brown)
Argyria (blue)
Chronic renal disease (white)
Chronic renal disease (half-and-half nails)
 (brown)
Cyanosis (blue)
Fixed drug reaction (blue)
Glomus tumor (red to brown)
Hypoalbuminemia (Muehrcke's lines)
 (white)
Low plasma albumin (white)
Melanoma (brown)
Nevus and melanoma (brown)
Ochronosis (blue)
Phenothiazine reaction (blue)
Splinter hemorrhages: psoriasis, subacute
 bacterial endocarditis, trauma,
 trichinosis, vasculitis (red to brown)
Trauma (red to brown)
Wilson's disease (blue)

Subungual Hyperkeratosis
Bowen's disease
Dermatitis
Dermatophyte infection
Epidermal nevi
Exfoliative erythroderma
Incontinentia pigmenti
Lichen planus
Mycosis fungoides
Pachyonychia congenita
Parakeratosis pustulosa (children)
Psoriasis, pityriasis rubra pilaris
Squamous cell carcinoma
Tyrosinemia II

Tumors
See Table 12–6 (pp. 537)

MOUTH LESIONS (Chapter 13, pp. 539–575)

Blistered or Ulcerated

Hypersensitivity-Related Diseases
Benign mucous membrane pemphigoid
 and other blistering diseases
Contact dermatitis

Dermatitis herpetiformis
Epidermolysis bullosa
Erythema multiforme and toxic
  epidermal necrolysis
Lupus erythematosus
Lethal midline granuloma
Pemphigoid
Pemphigus
Wegener's granulomatosis

Infectious Diseases
Aspergillosis
Aphthous stomatitis
Cryptococcus candidiasis
Histoplasmosis
Mucormycosis (in diabetics)
Mycobacterial infection: tuberculosis,
  leprosy
Spirochetal etiology: chancre, tertiary
  syphilis (gumma), yaws
Vincent's stomatitis (necrotizing
  gingivitis)
Viral etiology: herpes simplex, herpes
  zoster, chickenpox, hand-foot-and-
  mouth disease, herpangina, smallpox,
  vaccinia

Neoplastic Diseases
Eosinophilic granuloma (histiocytosis X)
Lymphoma, leukemia
Squamous cell carcinoma
Metastatic carcinoma

Other Etiologies
Agranulocytosis
Antimetabolite therapy
Lichen planus
Parulis (ruptured periodontal abscess)
Pemphigus
Reiter's syndrome
Trauma

Flat or White Mouth Lesions

Acute

Blistering Diseases
Behçet's syndrome
Benign mucous membrane pemphigoid
Contact dermatitis
Dermatitis herpetiformis
Epidermolysis bullosa
Erythema multiforme
Pemphigoid
Pemphigus
Toxic epidermal necrolysis

Burn
Hot food or utensil
Electricity
Radiation: therapeutic to mouth, skin,
  and deeper structures

Chemical Trauma
Acid, alkali
Camphor or phenol
Gold hypersensitivity
Antimetabolite therapy

Infectious Disease
Aphthous stomatitis
Candidiasis
Fusospirochetal infection
Gonorrhea
Hand-foot-and-mouth disease
Measles (Koplik's spots)
Secondary syphilis

Mechanical Trauma
Lacerations, abrasions
Poorly fitting dentures

Chronic Flat or White Mouth Lesions
Candidiasis
Discoid lupus erythematosus
Fordyce's disease
Genetic disease: Darier's disease,
  dyskeratosis congenita, benign
  epithelial dyskeratosis, pachyonychia
  congenita, white sponge nevus
Geographic tongue
HIV infection
Leukoplakia
Lichen planus
Smoker's palate (stomatitis nicotina)
Squamous cell carcinoma

Pigmented Mouth Lesions
Acanthosis nigricans
Addison's disease
Albright's syndrome and
  neurofibromatosis
Amalgam tattoo
Antimalarial drugs
Black hairy tongue
Hemochromatosis
Mercury, lead, or bismuth exposure
Nevus, lentigo, or melanoma, blue nevus
Nevus of Ota
Phenothiazines
Peutz-Jeghers syndrome
Smoking

Raised Mouth Lesions

Cysts
Mucocele
Rare causes: cystic hygroma, epidermal
cyst, lymphangioma, ranula

Diffuse Thickening of Gingivae
Drug-induced: phenytoin, cyclosporin A,
calcium channel blockers
Hereditary fibromatosis and
hypertrichosis syndrome
Inflammatory periodontal disease
Lymphoma, leukemia
Pregnancy
Scurvy

Papular Lesions
Benign tumors
Foreign-body granulomas
Granular cell myoblastoma
Granuloma pyogenicum
Hairy leukoplakia
Irritation fibromas
Lymphoma and leukemia
Metastatic carcinoma
Pregnancy tumor
Squamous cell carcinoma
Warts, condylomata
Rare causes: acanthosis nigricans,
amyloidosis, histiocytosis X, lipoid
proteinosis, lupus erythematosus,
median rhomboid glossitis, periodontal
disease, plasma cell infiltration,
psoriasis, sarcoidosis

Vascular Lesions
Blue rubber bleb nevus syndrome
Hemangiomas: especially with Sturge-
Weber syndrome
Kaposi's sarcoma
Telangiectasia: with Osler-Weber-Rendu
disease and systemic sclerosis
Varicosities (vascular ectasia)

Tongue Lesions

Atrophy
Geographic tongue
Iron deficiency
Lichen planus
Lichen sclerosus et atrophicus
Lupus erythematosus
Squamous cell carcinoma
Tertiary syphilis
Vitamin deficiency: pellagra, sprue,
vitamin B deficiency

Enlargement
Acromegaly
Amyloidosis
Angioneurotic edema
Down syndrome
Hemangioma, lymphangioma
Hypothyroidism
Neurofibroma
Squamous cell carcinoma
Superior vena cava syndrome
Thyroglossal duct cyst

Tooth Defects

Abnormal Color
Amelogenesis imperfecta
Biliary atresia
Dentinogenesis imperfecta
Epidermolysis bullosa
Erythroblastosis fetalis
Erythropoietic porphyria
Ochronosis
Osteogenesis imperfecta
Tetracycline therapy

Peg-Shaped Teeth
Anhidrotic ectodermal dysplasia
Chondroectodermal dysplasia
Incontinentia pigmenti

Bibliography

Cutaneous Medicine and Surgery. Arndt KA, LeBoit PE, Robinson JK, et al (eds). WB Saunders, Philadelphia, 1996.

Dermatological Signs of Internal Disease. Callen JP, Jorizzo JL, Greer KE, et al (eds). WB Saunders, Philadelphia, 1995.

Dermatology: Diagnosis and Therapy. Bondi EE, Jegasothy BV, and Lazarus GS (eds). Appleton and Lange, Norwalk, CT, 1991.

Dermatology in General Medicine. Fitzpatrick TB, Eisen AZ, Wolff K, et al (eds). McGraw-Hill, New York, 1993.

Diagnosis of Skin Disease. Lazarus GS and Goldsmith LA. FA Davis, Philadelphia, 1980.

Fisher's Contact Dermatitis, 4th ed. Reitschel RL and Fowler JR Jr (eds). Williams & Wilkins, Baltimore, 1995.

Manual of Dermatologic Therapeutics, 5th ed. Arndt KA, Bowers KE, and Chuttani AR. Little, Brown and Company, Boston, 1995.

Pathology of the Skin. Farmer ER and Hood AF (eds). Appleton and Lange. Norwalk, CT, 1990.

Pediatric Dermatology, 2nd ed. Schachner LA and Hansen RC (eds). Churchill Livingstone, New York, 1995.

Index

Page numbers followed by an 'f' indicate figures; page numbers followed by a 't' indicate tables.

COMMON GYNECOLOGIC DERMATOSES

HYPERPIGMENTED MACULES
Acanthosis nigricans
Addison's disease
Cushing's syndrome
Junctional nevus
Lentigines
Melanoma
Postinflammatory
Pregnancy

HYPOPIGMENTED MACULES
Corticosteroids (topical)
Lichen sclerosus et atrophicus
Morphea
Postinflammatory
Vitiligo

BLUE-BLACK PAPULES
Blue nevus
Kaposi's sarcoma
Melanoma
Varicosity

FLESH-COLORED/BROWN PAPULES
Acrochordons
Basal cell carcinoma
Dermatofibroma
Fordyce spots
Keloid
Melanoma
Milia
Molluscum
Neurofibroma
Nevus
Sarcoid
Seborrheic keratosis
Syringoma
Tinea versicolor
Wart

RED PAPULES
Atopic dermatitis
Candidiasis
Contact dermatitis
Dermatophyte
Fixed drug eruption
Folliculitis
Hemangioma
Intertrigo
Lichen planus
Lichen simplex chronicus
Lupus erythematosus
Lymphangioma
Molluscum contagiosum
Paget's disease
Psoriasis
Pyogenic granuloma
Scabies
Seborrheic dermatitis
Squamous cell carcinoma
Trauma

BLISTERS
Autoimmune blistering diseases
Contact dermatitis
Dermatophyte
Epidermolysis bullosa
Erysipelas
Erythema multiforme
Herpes simplex/zoster
Impetigo
Insect bites
Lichen sclerosus et atrophicus
Lymphangioma circumscriptum
Toxic epidermal necrolysis
Trauma

PUSTULES/ABCESSES
Candidiasis
Folliculitis

Infected Bartholin's cyst
Herpes simplex/zoster
Hidradenitis suppurativa

INDURATION/SCLEROSIS
Keloid
Lichen sclerosus et atrophicus
Lymphedema
Lymphogranuloma venereum
Morphea
Scar
Squamous cell carcinoma

ATROPHY
Corticosteroids (topical)
Lichen sclerosus et atrophicus
Morphea
Trauma

NODULE/CYST
Bartholin's cyst
Epidermoid cyst
Granular cell tumor
Hemangioma
Hidradenitis suppurativa
Hidradenoma papilliferum
Leiomyoma
Pilar cyst

ULCER
Aphthous ulcer
Beçet's syndrome
Candidiasis
Chancroid
Granuloma inguinale
Herpes simplex/zoster
Squamous cell carcinoma
Syphilis
Trauma